Ibn Edriss. A. M
Abd Elmoneim. M. A

Histological Techniques

Ibn Edriss. A. M
Abd Elmoneim. M. A

Histological Techniques

Quick Review

Noor Publishing

Publisher:
Noor Publishing
is a trademark of
Dodo Books Indian Ocean Ltd., member of the OmniScriptum S.R.L Publishing group
str. A.Russo 15, of. 61, Chisinau-2068, Republic of Moldova Europe
Printed at: see last page
ISBN: 978-620-4-72022-7

HISTOLOGICAL TECHNIQUES

QUICK REVIEW

First Edition

IBN EDRISS. A. M
Assistant professor
Department of histopathology
University of El-Imam El-Mahdi

ABD ELMONEIM. M. A
BSc (Honours). MSc
Department of histopathology
University of Omdurman Islamic

To the memory of who that said: There is no histochemistry without chemistry and no understanding of the methods without knowledge of their chemical background.

A. G . E. Pearse.

Preface

Many years' experience of teaching undergraduates and postgraduates, and daily consultations with colleagues both in hospitals, privates and universities have brought home very clearly the problems experienced by most students (and practitioners) in histopathology laboratories. Histopathological techniques are very difficult to teach at the undergraduate level because the curriculum is necessarily fragmented across different years of study, and often separated considerably in time. However, it requires insight into several distinct aspects such as anatomy, biochemistry, molecular biology and immunology. Although many excellent texts and references were available covering various aspects and methods of Histopathological techniques, the lack of a concise comprehensive guide to using these methods was a major motivation for writing this book. Our intention was to create an easy-to-read and focused resource based on state-of-the-art information for a broad readers ranging from students and technical assistants to experienced researchers. This book has a concise format, with protocols and instructions for methods immediately following the short introductory theoretical material in each chapter. It is suitable for those with limited time and immediate information needs. This guide provides practical advice on best-practice techniques and simple ways to avoid common errors. Each aspect of the histology process is covered: specimen collection, processing, embedding, sectioning and staining (routine, special, immunohistochemistry and in situ hybridization). Ultimately, we hope that we have produced a modern and relevant histotechnology text which will be of use to those in training as well as established practitioners worldwide. We hope each step provides a valuable reminder of good histology practice and also helps with troubleshooting when unacceptable results do occur. Thanks are due to many people who have given advice and criticism over the years. Among present and former colleagues, we thank **Abbashar. M & Omnia. K** for sharing their wisdom and expertise. Finally, we thank those special people, too numerous to mention, on whom we relied for support, encouragement, and patience.

Abd elmoneim. M. A   *Ibn edriss. A. M*

Contents

Histopathology is the microscopic examination of tissue to study disease manifestations. It is the central to biological and medical science, it stands at the cross–road between molecular biology biochemistry, and physiology on the one side and diseases and their effects on the other side.

The study of histology began with the development of simple light microscopes and techniques for preparing thin slices of biological materials to make them suitable for examination. Despite their simple histologists equipment and somewhat in adequately prepared material, early learned a surprising amount about the structure of biological materials. Such studies led Virchow to propound his cellular theory of the structure of living organism that established the cell as the basic building block of most biological material.

Medical picture now offers the opportunity to view histological samples of gastro intestinal tract, female genital tract and many more. Histological examination of such samples is an increasing important and direct way of diagnosing disease. Until recently the only way to look at the fine intracellular details was by using electron microscopy which greatly increases resolution allowing the sub-cellular composition of cell to be defined. This technique is now complemented by the increasing use of immunohistochemical methods. Antibodies are applied to specific cell constituents to visualize details within cells at the light microscopic level that are not visible by other techniques. It is also now possible to demonstrate specific deoxyribonucleic acid (DNA) and ribonucleic acid (RNA) sequence in tissues by the techniques of *In Situ Hybridization*, there by gaining of fundamental insight into the molecular mechanism of the cells. Histology has never been such an important part of the medical and biological curriculum as it is today (I.G. Ilegbedion, *et al.* 2013).

WORK FLOW:

There are many reasons to examine human cells and tissues under the microscope. Medical and biological research is under-pinned by knowledge of the normal structure and function of cells and tissues and the organs and structures that they make up. In the normal healthy state, the cells and other tissue elements are arranged in regular recognizable patterns. Changes induced by a wide range of chemical and physical influences are reflected by alterations in structure at a microscopic level and many diseases are characterized by typical structural and chemical abnormalities that differ from the normal state. Identifying these changes and linking them to particular diseases is the basis of histopathology and cytopathology.

Microscopy:

There are many different forms of microscopy but the one most commonly employed is light (bright field) microscopy, where the specimen is illuminated with a beam of light that passes through it (as opposed to a beam of electrons as in electron microscopy). The general requirements for a specimen to be successfully examined using brightfield microscopy are that:

· The cells and other elements in the specimen are preserved in a "life-like" state (this process is called "fixation")
· The specimen is transparent rather than opaque, so that light can pass through it.
· The specimen is thin and flat so that only a single layer of cells is present. Some components have been differentially coloured (stained) so that they can be clearly distinguished.

Preparation options:

For microscopy requirements, options for preparing specimens are limited to:

· Whole-mounts, where an entire organism or structure is small enough or thin enough to be placed directly onto a microscope slide (e.g. a small unicellular or multicellular organism or a membrane that can be stretched thinly on to a slide).

· Squash preparations, where cells are intentionally squashed or crushed onto a slide to reveal their contents (e.g. botanical specimens where cells are disrupted to reveal chromosomes).

· Smears, where the specimen consists of cells suspended in a fluid (e.g. blood, semen, cerebro-spinal fluid, or a culture of microorganisms), or where individual cells have been scraped (brushed) or aspirated (sucked) from a surface or from within an organ (exfoliative cytology). Smears are the basis of the well-known "Pap test" that is used to screen for cervical cancer in women.

· Sections, where specimens are supported in some way so that very thin slices can be cut from them, mounted on slides, and stained. Sections are prepared using an instrument called a "microtome". Of these options only whole-mounts and sections preserve the structural relationships between individual cells and extracellular components. Smears and squash preparations provide detail about individual cells and relative cell numbers, but structural relationships are lost.

SECTION PREPARATION

Most fresh tissue is very delicate, easily distorted and damaged and it is thus impossible to prepare thin sections (slices) from it unless it is supported in some way whilst it is being cut. Usually the specimen also needs to be preserved or "fixed" before sections are prepared. Broadly there are two strategies that can be employed to provide this support.

■ The tissue can be rapidly frozen and kept frozen while sections are cut using a cryostat microtome (a microtome in a freezing chamber). These are called "frozen sections". Frozen sections can be prepared very quickly and are therefore used when an intra-operative diagnosis is required to guide a surgical procedure or where any type of interference with the chemical makeup of the cells is to be avoided (as in some histochemical investigations).

■ Alternatively, specimens can be infiltrated with a liquid agent that can subsequently be converted into a solid that has appropriate physical properties that will allow thin sections to be cut from it. Various agents can be used for infiltrating and supporting specimens including epoxy and methacrylate resinsbut paraffin wax-based histological waxes are the most popular for routine light microscopy. This produces so-called "paraffin sections". These sections are usually prepared with a "rotary" microtome. "Rotary" describes the cutting action of the instrument. In all histopathology laboratories paraffin sections are routinely prepared from almost every specimen and used in diagnosis.

The following paragraphs describe the major steps in preparing paraffin sections. These steps generally dictate the layout and workflow in large, specialist histopathology laboratories where hundreds of specimens are handled every day.

Specimen reception:

Specimens received for histological examination may come from a number of different sources. They range from very large specimens or whole organs to tiny fragments of tissue. For example, the following are some of the specimen-types commonly received in a histopathology lab.

· Excisional specimens (surgical biopsies), where whole organs or affected areas are removed at operation.
· Incisional biopsy specimens, where tissue is removed for diagnosis from within an affected area.
· Punch biopsies, where punches are used to remove a small piece of suspicious tissue for examination (often from the skin).
· Shave biopsies, where small fragments of tissue are "shaved" from a surface (usually skin).
· Curettings, where tissue is removed in small pieces from the lining of the uterus or cervix.
· Core biopsies, where a small tissue sample is removed using a special needle sometimes through the skin (percutaneously).

Specimens are usually received in fixative (preservative) but sometimes arrive fresh and must be immediately fixed. Before specimens are accepted by a laboratory the identification (labelling) and accompanying documentation will be carefully checked, all details recorded and "specimen tracking" commenced. It is vital that patient or research specimens are properly identified and the risk of inaccuracies minimized.

*Note:*Specimens to which the following conditions apply will be rejected (Rejection Criteria), returned to the originating site or specimen processing delayed. The physician office will be notified.

- Specimen is received without a requisition.
- Requisition is received without a specimen.
- Requisition or specimen label lacks two patient identifiers.
- Requisition or specimen label information is illegible.
- Requisition and specimen label information is not identical.
- Requisition and/or specimen mislabeled (Patient identifiers inaccurate).
- Incorrect specimen container/tube is used.
- Date of collection is not recorded.
- Time of collection is not recorded.
- Specimen is clotted.
- Specimen is sent without fixation.
- Specimen container is leaking.
- Specimen quantity is insufficient.
- Specimen contamination, dilution or other interfering substances affect specimen integrity.

Fixation:

Fixation is a foundation step in preparing specimens for microscopic examination. Its objective is to prevent decay and preserve cells and tissues in a "life-like" state. It does this by stopping enzyme activity, killing microorganisms and hardening the specimen while maintaining sufficient of the molecular structure to enable appropriate staining methods to be applied (including those involving antigen-antibody reactions and those depending on preserving DNA and RNA). Immediate fixation is necessary following separation of a specimen from its blood supply to obtain accurate result. The most popular fixing agent is formaldehyde, usually in the form of a phosphate-buffered solution (often referred to as "formalin"). Ideally specimens should be fixed by immersion in formalin for six to twelve hours before they are processed.

Grossing:

Grossing, often referred to as "cut-up", involves a careful examination and description of the specimen that will include the appearance, the number of pieces and their dimensions. Larger specimens may require further dissection to produce representative pieces from appropriate areas. For example, multiple samples may be taken from the excision margins of a tumor to ensure that the tumor has been completely removed. In the case of small specimens, the entire specimen may be processed. The tissues selected for processing will be placed in cassettes (small perforated baskets) and batches will be loaded onto a tissue processor for processing through to wax.

Processing:

Where large batches of specimens are processed for paraffin section preparation automated instruments called "tissue processors" are used. These instruments allow the specimens to be infiltrated with a sequence of different solvents finishing in molten paraffin wax. The specimens are in an aqueous environment to start with (water-based) and must be passed through multiple changes of dehydrating and clearing solvents (typically ethanol and xylene) before they can be placed in molten wax (which is hydrophobic and immiscible with water). The duration and step details of the "processing schedule" chosen for a particular batch of specimens will depend on the nature and size of the specimens. Schedules can be as short as one hour for small specimens or as long as twelve hours or more for large specimens. In many labs the bulk of processing is carried out overnight. At present there is considerable pressure on laboratories to use processors capable of rapid processing in an effort to improve workflow and reduce turnaround times.

Embedding:

After processing the specimens are placed in an embedding Centre where they are removed from their cassettes and placed in wax-filled molds. At these stage specimens are carefully orientated because this will determine the plane through which the section will be cut and ultimately may decide whether an abnormal area will be visible under the microscope. The cassette in which the tissue has been processed carries the specimen identification details and it is

now placed on top of the mold and is attached by adding further wax. The specimen "block" is now allowed to solidify on a cold surface and when set the mold is removed. The cassette, now filled with wax and forming part of the block, provides a stable base for clamping in the microtome. The block containing the specimen is now ready for section cutting.

Sectioning:

Sections are cut on a precision instrument called a "microtome" using extremely fine steel blades. Paraffin sections are usually cut at a thickness of 3 - 5μm ensuring that only a single layer of cells makes up the section (a red blood cell has a diameter of about 7μm). One of the advantages of paraffin wax as an embedding agent is that as sections are cut they will stick together edge-to-edge, forming a "ribbon" of sections. This makes handling easier. Sections are now "floated out" on the surface of warm water in a flotation bath to flatten them and then picked up onto microscope slides. After thorough drying they are ready for staining.

The micrometer (μM) is standard unit for measurement of the section thickness in histopathology, (μM) = 1/1000 mm = (10^{-3}). Most histological sections are 3–5 μM.

Staining:

Apart from a few natural pigments such as melanin on the cells and other elements making up most specimens are ***colorless***. In order to reveal structural detail using bright field microscopy (light microscope) some form of *staining is required*. The routine stain used universally as a starting point in providing essential structural information, is the hematoxylin and eosin (H&E) stain. With these method cell nuclei are stained blue and cytoplasm and many extra-cellular components in shades of pink. In histopathology many conditions can be diagnosed by examining an H&E alone. However sometimes additional information is required to provide a full differential diagnosis and this requires further, more specialized staining techniques. These may be "special stains" using dyes or metallic impregnations to define particular structures or microorganisms, or immunohistochemical methods (IHC) involving the location of diagnostically useful proteins using labelled antibodies. Molecular methods such as *in situ* hybridization (ISH) may also be required to detect specific DNA or RNA sequences. These methods can all be applied to paraffin sections and in most cases the slides produced are completely stable and can be kept for many years.

After staining, the sections are covered with a glass cover slip and are then sent to a pathologist who will view them under a microscope to make an appropriate diagnosis and prepare a report.

Further reading:

- Allan stevens and James S. Human histology, second edition, Oxoford University, London 1998; 1: pp 1.
- Drury R B and Wallington E A. Carleton Histological Techniques, fifth edition, Oxoford University press, London 1980; pp 36-44.
- http://www.leicabiosystems.com/pathologyleaders/an-introduction-to-specimen-preparation/30-May-2011.
- John Crocker & David Burnett. The Sciences of Laboratory Diagnosis, second edition, John Wiley & Sons Ltd, The Atrium, Southern Gate, Chichester, West Sussex PO19 8SQ, England 2005, pp 3 – 12.
- Identifying and Evaluating Hazards in Research Laboratories (2013) Guidelines developed by the Hazards Identification and Evaluation Task Force of the American Chemical Society's Committee on Chemical Safety: American Chemical Society.
- Banks I, Gamble M. (2002) Managing the Laboratory, Chapter 1. In: Bancroft J.D. and Gamble M, eds. Theory and Practice of Histological Techniques, 2nd ed. London: Churchill Livingstone, IL.

OPTICAL MICROSCOPE:

The optical microscope, often referred to as the "light microscope", is a type of microscope which uses visible light and a system of lenses to magnify images of small samples. There are two basic configurations of the optical microscope, the simple (one lens) and compound (many lenses).

Simple microscope:

A simple microscope is a microscope that uses only one lens for magnification, and is the original design of light microscope. Van Leeuwenhoek's microscopes consisted of a small, single converging lens mounted on a brass plate, with a screw mechanism to hold the sample or specimen to be examined.

Principle

A simple microscope works on the principle that when a tiny object is placed within its focus, a virtual, erect and magnified image of the object is formed at the least distance of distinct vision from the eye held close to the lens.

The parts of simple microscope

Eyepiece: It is the lens that is used to study the samples and is placed at the top. It has a magnification of 10X to 15X.

Base: This provides support to the microscope.

Tube: This is used to connect the eyepiece to the objective lenses.

Objective lenses: These are found with the magnification of 10X, 40X and 100X and are colour coded. The lower power lenses are the shortest lens and the highest power lenses are the longest lens.

Revolving nose-piece: This is also known as the turret. It is used for holding of other objective lens and can be rotated while viewing the samples.

Diaphragm: It is used to control the amount of light that passes through the stage.

Stage: It is the platform used for placing the slides with samples.

Stage clip: These are used to hold the slides in the proper place.

Coarse adjustment knob: It is used to focus on scanning.

Fine adjustment knob: It is used to focus on oil.

Arm: It is used to support the tube and connects to the base of the microscope.

Power switch: The main power switch used to turn on or off the microscope.

Condenser: It is used to focus the light on the sample and 400X power lenses are used.

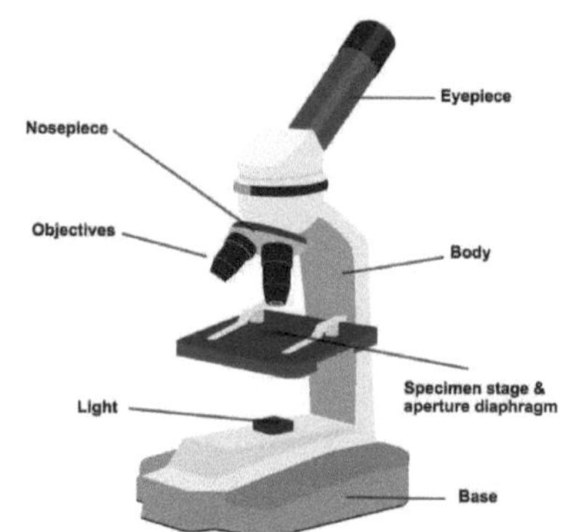

Compound microscope:

A compound microscope is a microscope which uses multiple lenses to collect light from the sample and then a separate set of lenses to focus the light into the eye or camera. Compound microscopes are heavier, larger and more expensive than simple microscopes due to the increased number of lenses used in construction.

Working principle

When light from the light source is passed through a thin transparent object, condensation of rays is brought about by the substage condenser through the numerical aperture. There is a substage condenser located between the stage and light source that helps in condensing the light rays. This type of light condensing and gathering capacity of the condenser is called the numerical aperture of the condenser. The first lens, called objective lens, collects the light passing through the object from the light source and then focuses it on forming a real image of an object inside the microscope. Then, the formed image is magnified by a second lens called as eyepiece lens and is perceived as "virtual image" by the observer.

Component parts of a compound microscope

Eyepiece (ocular):
The eyepiece, or ocular, is a cylinder containing two or more lenses; its function is to bring the image into focus for the eye. The eyepiece is inserted into the top end of the body tube. Eyepieces are interchangeable and many different eyepieces can be inserted with different degrees of magnification. Typical magnification values for eyepieces include 2×, 5× and 10×.

Objective turret or Revolver:
Objective turret or Revolver is the part that holds the set of objective lenses, it allows changing them.

Objective:
At the lower end of a typical compound optical microscope there are one or more objective lenses that collect light from the sample. The objective is usually in a cylinder housing containing a glass single or multi-element compound lens. Typically, there will be around three objective lenses screwed into a circular nose piece which may be rotated to select the required objective lens. These arrangements are designed to be parfocal, which means that when one changes from one lens to another on a microscope, the sample stays in focus. Microscope objectives are characterized by two parameters, namely, magnification and numerical aperture. The former typically ranges from 5× to 100× while the latter ranges from 0.14 to 0.7, corresponding to focal lengths of about 40 to 2 mm, respectively. Objective lenses with higher magnifications normally have a higher numerical aperture and a shorter depth of field in the resulting image.

Oil-immersion objectives:
Some microscopes make use of oil-immersion objectives or water-immersion objectives for greater resolution at high magnification. These are used with index-matching material such as immersion oil or water and a matched cover slip between the objective lens and the sample.

The refractive index of the index-matching material is higher than air allowing the objective lens to have a larger numerical aperture (greater than 1) so that the light is transmitted from the specimen to the outer face of the objective lens with minimal refraction.

Numerical apertures as high as 1.6 can be achieved. The larger numerical aperture allows collection of more light making detailed observation of smaller details possible. An oil immersion lens usually has a magnification of 40 to 100×.

Focus wheels:
Adjustment wheels move the stage up and down with separate adjustment for coarse and fine focussing. The same controls enable the microscope to adjust to specimens of different thickness.

Frame:
The whole of the optical assembly is traditionally attached to a rigid arm which in turn is attached to a robust U shaped foot to provide the necessary rigidity. The arm angle may be adjustable to allow the viewing angle to be adjusted.

The frame provides a mounting point for various microscope controls. Normally this will include controls for focusing, typically a large knurled wheel to adjust coarse focus, together with a smaller knurled wheel to control fine focus.

Light source:

Many sources of light can be used. At its simplest, daylight is directed via a mirror. Most microscopes, however, have their own adjustable and controllable light source – often a halogen lamp, although illumination using LEDs and lasers are becoming a more common provision.

Condenser:

The condenser is a lens designed to focus light from the illumination source onto the sample. The condenser may also include other features, such as a diaphragm and/or filters, to manage the quality and intensity of the illumination.

Stage:

The stage is a platform below the objective which supports the specimen being viewed. In the center of the stage is a hole through which light passes to illuminate the specimen. The stage usually has arms to holdslides (rectangular glass plates with typical dimensions of 25×75 mm, on which the specimen is mounted). At magnifications higher than 100x moving a slide by hand is not practical. A mechanical stage, typical of medium and higher priced microscopes, allows tiny movements of the slide via control knobs that reposition the sample/slide as desired. If a microscope did not originally have a mechanical stage it may be possible to add one.

All stages move up and down for focus. With a mechanical stage slides move on two horizontal axes for positioning the specimen to examine specimen details. Focusing starts at lower magnification in order to center the specimen by the user on the stage. Moving to a higher magnification requires the stage to be moved higher vertically for re-focus at the higher magnification and may also require slight horizontal specimen position adjustment. Horizontal specimen position adjustments are the reason for having a mechanical stage.

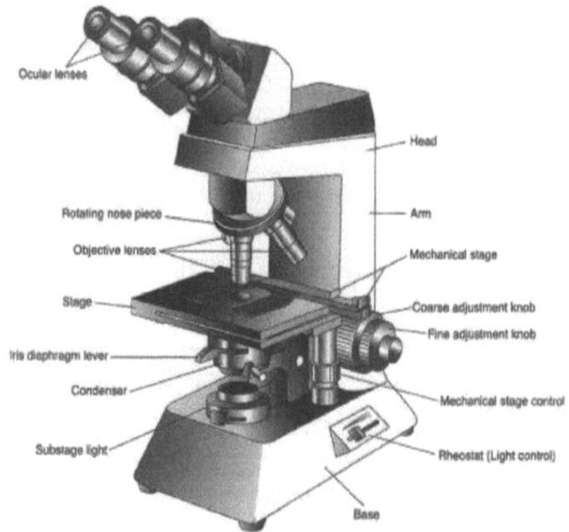

PHASE CONTRAST MICROSCOPE

Phase contrast microscopy is an optical microscopy illumination technique in which small phase shifts in the light passing through a transparent specimen are converted into amplitude or contrast changes in the image. As light travels through a medium other than vacuum, interaction with this medium causes its amplitude and phase to change in a way which depends on properties of the medium. Changes in amplitude give rise to familiar absorption of light, which is wavelength dependent and gives rise to colours. The human eye measures only the energy of light arriving on the retina, so changes in phase are not easily observed, yet often these changes in phase carry a large amount of information.

Principle

In this microscope, the objects having different refractive indices are identified as they produce different contrasts. The object with scattered light is identified from the illuminating background light. If the light passes through a transparent object, then due to the change of refractive index of the object, the pathway of light will be deviated slightly, and the light wave is retarded. In case of denser particle (higher refractive index) in the object, the deviation of light will be more, and the light wave is more retarded. This is known as phase difference. Usually these phase differences are invisible to us; however, the phase contrast microscope makes these changes significantly visible.

Components and work flow

Phase-contrast microscopy consists of a phase ring (located in a conjugated aperture plane somewhere behind the front lens element of the objective) and a matching annular ring, which is located in the primary aperture plane (location of the condenser's aperture).

Two selected light rays, which are emitted from one point inside the lamp's filament, get focused by the field lens exactly inside the opening of the condenser annular ring. Since this location is precisely in the front focal plane of the condenser, the two light rays are then refracted in such way that they exit the condenser as parallel rays. Assuming that the two rays in question are neither refracted nor diffracted in the specimen plane (location of microscope slide), they enter the objective as parallel rays. Since all parallel rays are focused in the back focal plane of the objective, the back focal plane is a conjugated aperture plane to the condenser's front focal plane (also location of the condenser annulus). To complete the phase setup, a phase plate is positioned inside the back focal plane in such a way that it lines up nicely with the condenser annulus. Only through correctly centering the two elements can phase contrast illumination be established. A phase centering telescope that temporarily replaces one of the oculars is used, first to focus the phase element plane and then center the annular illumination ring with the corresponding ring of the phase plate.

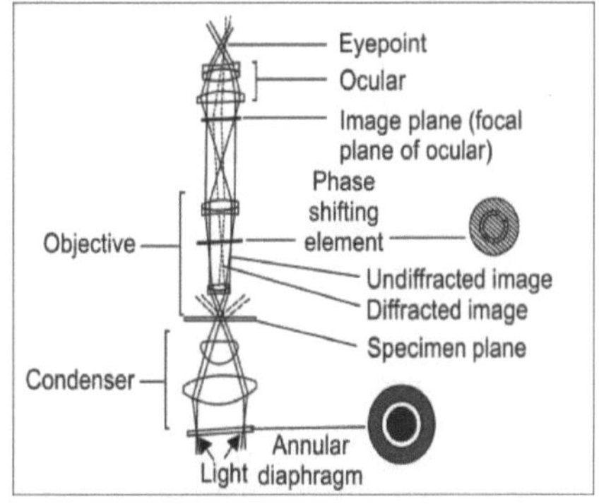

Polarized light microscopy can mean any of a number of optical microscopy techniques involving polarized light. Simple techniques include illumination of the sample with polarized light. These illumination techniques are most commonly used on birefringent samples where the polarized light interacts strongly with the sample and so generating contrast with the background. Polarized light can distinguish between isotropic and anisotropic substances. Furthermore, the contrast-enhancing technique exploits the optical properties specific to anisotropy and reveals detailed information concerning the structure and composition of materials that are invaluable for identification and diagnostic purposes.

The principle

In a polarized light microscope, a polarizer intervenes between the light source and the sample. Thus, the polarized light source is converted into plane-polarized light before it hits the sample. This polarized light falls on a doubly refracting specimen which generates two wave components that are at right angles to each other. These two waves are called ordinary and extraordinary light rays. The waves pass through the specimen in different phases.

They are then combined using constructive and destructive interference, by an analyzer. This leads to the final generation of a high-contrast image.

Microscope components:

Polarizers
Polarizing filters are the most critical part of the polarized light microscope. There are usually two polarizing filters: the polarizer and the analyzer. The polarizer is located below the specimen stage and can be rotated through 360°. It helps to polarize the light which falls on the specimen. The analyzer is placed above the objective and may be rotatable in some cases. It combines the different rays emerging from the specimen to generate the final image.

Specialized Stage
This is the specimen stage and it can rotate 360° to facilitate the correct orientation of the specimen with the objective plane. In several stages, a Vernier scale is also provided to provide an accuracy of 0.1° in the rotational angle of the stage.

Strain-Free Objectives
Any stress on the objective during installation can lead to a change in the optical properties of the lens which can reduce the performance. Strain can also be introduced if the lens is mounted too tightly on the frame. Also, anti-reflection coatings and refractive properties must be accurately assessed in order to ensure polarization and increased contrast.

Revolving Nosepiece
As the stage and objectives can revolve in many polarizing microscopes, a revolving nosepiece is also often fitted such that the specimen can be visualized in the center of the view field even if the stage is rotated.

Compensator and Retardation Plates
Several polarization microscopes have compensators and/or retardation plates. This is placed between the crossed polarizers to increase the difference in the optical path in the specimen. This would further increase the contrast of the image quality. Thus, polarizing microscopes are being used to increase the image contrast to visualize many anisotropic sub-cellular structures.

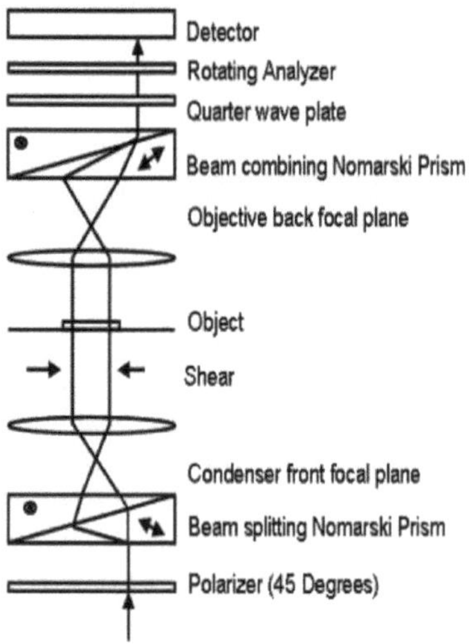

FLUORESCENCE MICROSCOPE

A fluorescence microscope is an optical microscope used to study properties of organic or inorganic substances using the phenomena of fluorescence and phosphorescence instead of, or in addition to, reflection and absorption.

Principle:

All fluorescence microscopy methods share the same principle. A sample is illuminated with light of a wavelength which causes fluorescence in the sample. The light emitted by fluorescence, which is at a different, longer, wavelength than the illumination, is then detected through a microscope objective.

<u>**Main components of a fluorescence microscope:**</u>

Fluorecent dyes (Fluorophore): A fluorophore is a fluorescent chemical compound that can re-emit light upon light excitation.They typically contain several combined aromatic groups, or plane or cyclic molecules with several π bonds. Many fluorescent dyes have been designed for a range of biological molecules. Some of these are small molecules which are intrinsically fluorescent and bind a biological molecule of interest. Major examples of these are nucleic acid stains like DAPI and Hoechst which bind the minor groove of DNA, thus labelling the nuclei of cells. Others are drugs or toxins which bind specific cellular structures and have been derivatised with a fluorescent reporter. A major example of this class of fluorescent stain is fluorescently labelled-phalloidin which is used to stain actin fibres in mammalian cells.

Light source: Four main types of light sources are used, including xenon arc lamps or mercury vapor lamps with an excitation filter, lasers, and high- power LEDs.

The excitation filter: The exciter is typically abandpass filter that passes only the wavelengths absorbed by the fluorophore, thus minimizing the excitation of other sources of fluorescence and blocking excitation light in the fluorescence emission band.

The emission filter: The emitter is typically a bandpass filter that passes only the wavelengths emitted by the fluorophore and blocks all undesired light outside this band – especially the excitation light.

The dichroic mirror: A dichroic filter is a very accurate color filter used to selectively pass light of a small range of colors while reflecting other colors.

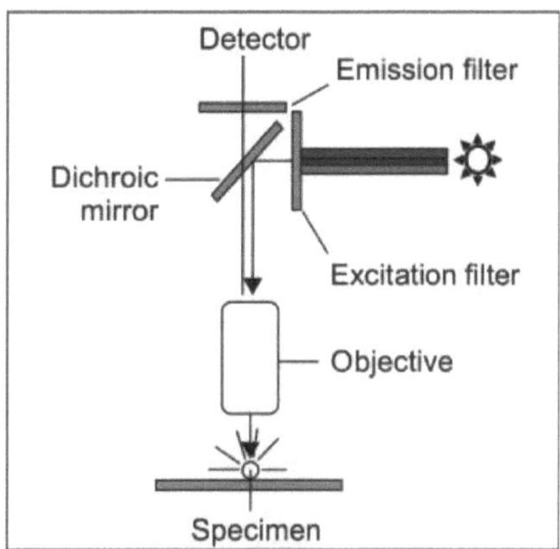

ELECTRON MICROSCOPY

An electron microscope is a type of microscope that uses a particle beam of electrons to illuminate the specimen and produce a magnified image. Electron microscopes (EM) have a greater resolving power than a light-powered Optical microscope, because electrons have wavelengths about 100,000 times shorter than visible light (photons), and can achieve better resolution and magnifications of up to about 10,000,000x, whereas ordinary, non-confocal light microscopes are limited by diffraction to about 200 nm resolution and useful magnifications below 2000x.

The electron microscope uses electrostatic and electromagnetic "lenses" to control the electron beam and focus it to form an image. These lenses are analogous to, but different from the glass lenses of an optical microscope that form a magnified image by focusing light on or through the specimen. The real image thus formed is magnified by a factor ranging from a few hundred to many hundred thousand times, and can be viewed on a detecting screen or recorded using photographic film or plates or with a digital camera. Electron microscopes are used to observe a wide range of biological and inorganic specimens including microorganisms, cells, large molecules, biopsy samples, metals, and crystals. Industrially, the electron microscope is primarily used for quality control and failure analysis in semiconductor device fabrication (Erni, Rolf *et al.*2009).

Principle

The electronic beam is obtained from a heated tungsten filament which generates electrons. A large voltage is applied between the cathode (the tungsten filament) and the anode, which excites the electrons and it travels with high velocity towards the condenser lens. The condenser lenses focus the electronic beams through the specimen and electrons are scattered depending upon the thickness or refractive index of different parts of the specimen.

The denser regions in the specimen scatter more electrons and therefore appear darker in the image since fewer electrons strike that area of the screen. In contrast, transparent regions are brighter. The electron beam coming out of the specimen passes to the objective lens, which has high power and forms the intermediate magnified image. The projector throws its image onto a fluorescent screen which may be substituted by a photographic plate to make a permanent record.

Components of an electron microscope

Source of light: The source of light is replaced by a beam of very fast-moving electrons. These electro beams are obtained when the tungsten filament in an electron microscope, is heated by applying a high voltage current, which is used as a light beam.

Electromagnetic fields (instead of lenses): The lenses that make the specimen seem bigger are replaced by a series of coil-shaped electromanets through which the electron beam travels also known as electromagnetic lenses. There are 3 sets of electromagnetic lenses in an electron microscope as compared to two in light microscopes. In addition to the condenser and objective lenses, a third projector lens is also present. The magnetic lens of an electron microscope can have different powers (focal lengths and magnification) depending on the amount of current flowing through the electrical coils. In an ordinary microscope, the glass lenses bend (or refract) the light beams passing through them to produce magnification. In an electron microscope, the coils bend the electron beams the same way.

Image viewing and recording system: The magnified image of the specimen is formed as a photograph (called an electron micrograph) or as an image on a TV screen.

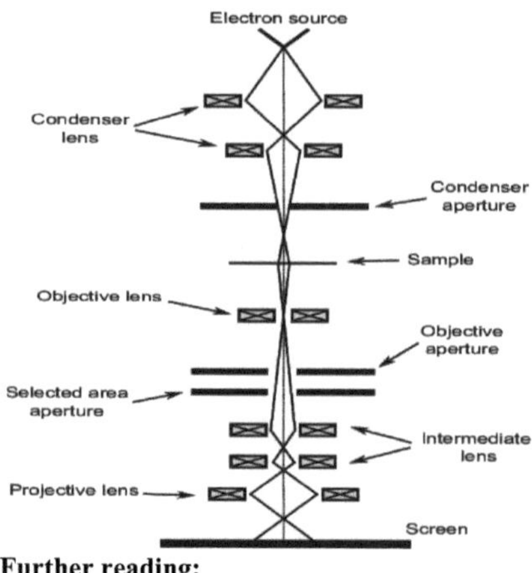

Further reading:

- Antonovsky, A. (1984). "The application of colour to sem imaging for increased definition". Micron and Micro scopica Acta **15** (2): 77–84. doi:10.1016/0739-6260(84)90005-4.

- Erni, Rolf; Rossell, MD; Kisielowski, C; Dahmen, U (2009). "Atomic-Resolution Imaging with a Sub-50-pm Electron Probe". Physical Review Letters **102** (9): 96101.Bibcode:2009PhRvL.102i6101E. doi:10.1103/PhysRevLett.102.096101. PMID 19392535.
- http://research.omicsgroup.org/index.php/Polarized_light_microscopy.
- http://www.microscopesmall.com/aboutmicroscopeshow.asp?id=19.
- http://www2.warwick.ac.uk/services/ris/business/analyticalguide/optical/.
- https://dmohankumar.files.wordpress.com.

Fixation is the most critical step in histotechnology, it is defined as the chemical (fixative solutions) or physical (heat, desiccation) process that allows tissue sections to be viewed in a close approximation to the living tissue (Eltoum I, *et al.* 2001). Histological fixation practices have been derived from many other fields, such as the leather tanning industry. Fixation is the single most important factor in achieving a well-prepared section for microscopic analysis (Sheehan, D. 1980). Fixation processes should be standardized so that subtle changes in microanatomy may be detected by comparing similarly fixed sections. When tissue is removed from the host, a good fixative will stop autolysis (the dissolution of cells by intracellular enzymatic digestion) and putrefaction (the breakdown of tissue by bacterial action) by inactivating the enzymes, bacteria, and molds that begin to form immediately after death. It will also protect the tissue from excessive shrinkage and swelling, and it will not dissolve or distort the tissue. Dehydrating agents and clearing agents can cause distortion of tissue, so the chosen fixing agent will also protect the cellular constituents from alterations (artifacts) caused by these chemicals. The fixative must also protect the tissue during the embedding process, which involves polymer impregnation at a high temperature. Finally, it must protect the tissue during sectioning, where the potential for mechanical damage is high (Sheehan, D. 1980).

In histopathology most tissues are fixed before they examined microscopically. It flows that fixation is a foundation step for the subsequent stages. The specimen must be fixed immediately after harvesting to avoid artifacts. Specimens should be rough-cut into small pieces. Large specimens may require perfusion fixation or vacuum-assisted infiltration of fixative solutions. Although each fixative has advantages, they all have many disadvantages. The fixative brings about cross linking of proteins which produces denaturation or coagulation of proteins, thus semifluid state is converted into semisolid state; so that it maintains everything in vivo in relation to each other. There may be several undesirable effects of fixation, including shrinkage and hardening of tissue. Ideally, the choice of a fixative should be governed by the tissue type and by enzyme or histochemical needs (Sanderson C. 1997). An easy way to remember is **PRISM; P**enetrate tissue easily, **R**apid in action, **I**sotonic, **S**afe to handle, **Mi**nimal loss or damage to tissue constituents.

AIM AND EFFECTS OF FIXATION:

If a fresh tissue is kept as such at room temperature it will become liquefied with a foul odour mainly due to action of bacteria (putrefaction) and autolysis, so the most aims of fixation are:

- The major objective of fixation in pathology is to maintain clear and consistent morphological features (Eltoum et al. 2001a, 2001b; Grizzle *et al.* 2001).
- Minimizing the loss of cellular components, including proteins, peptides, mRNA, DNA, and lipids, prevents the destruction of macromolecular structures such as cytoplasmic membranes, smooth endoplasmic reticulum, rough endoplasmic reticulum, nuclear membranes, lysosomes, and mitochondria.
- *Hardening*: Converts the normal semifluid consistency of cells (gel) to an irreversible semisolid consistency (solid). The hardening effect of fixatives allows easy manipulation of soft tissue like brain, also fixation fortify the tissue against the deleterious effects during tissue processing and allow good sectioning.
- *Optical differentiation:* It alters to varying degrees the refractive index of the various components of cells and tissues so that fixed unstained components are more easily visu-

alized than when unfixed (Drury and Wallington, 1980).

- *Effects on staining:* Certain fixatives like formaldehyde intensifies the staining character of tissue especially with hematoxylin (Eltoum I, Fredenburgh J, Myers RB,*et al.* 2001).

Hydrogen ion concentration (pH) and buffers:

The pH values of the different fixatives vary. In general, the hydrogen ion concentration is usually adjusted to the physiological range by use of suitable buffer. Satisfactory fixation occurs between pH 6 and 8. When acetic acid or other acids are added to a fixative solution, they will lower the pH. The normal tertiary and quaternary structures of proteins are stable over a fairly limited pH about neutrality.

Many buffer systems are available for use in fixation. The most common ones are phosphates-collidine, veronal acetate, bicarbonate, Tris and cacodylate. Care must be taken that the buffer chosen does not react with the fixative, as this will reduce both the buffering power and the fixation ability. The pH chosen for the histochemical reaction should be as near to the biochemical optimum as possible, although some compromise may be necessary.

Osmolality of fixatives and ionic composition:

The osmolality of the buffer and fixative is important; hypertonic and hypotonic solutions lead to shrinkage and swelling, respectively. The best morphological results are obtained with solutions that are slightly hypertonic (400–450 mOsm), though the osmolality for 10% NBF is about 1500 mOsm. Similarly, various ions (Na^+,

K^+, Ca^{2+}, Mg^{2+}) can affect cell shape and structure regardless of the osmotic effect.The ionic composition of fluids should be as isotonic as possible to the tissues.

Temperature:

The diffusion of molecules increases with rising temperature due to their more rapid movement and vibration; i.e. the rate of penetration of a tissue by formaldehyde is faster at higher temperatures. Microwaves therefore have been used to speed formaldehyde fixation by both increasing the temperature and molecular movements. Care is required to avoid cooking the specimen.

Concentration of fixative:

Effectiveness and solubility primarily determine the appropriate concentration of fixatives. Concentrations of formalin above 10% tend to cause increased hardening and shrinkage. In addition, higher concentrations result in formalin being present in its polymeric form, which can be deposited as white precipitate, as opposed to its monomeric form $HO(H2CO)$ H, which at 4% provides for greatest solubility. Ethanol concentrations below 70% do not remove free water from tissues efficiently.

Duration of fixation and size of specimens:

The factors that govern diffusion of a fixative into tissue were investigated by Medawar (1941). He found that the depth (d) reached by a fixative is directly proportional to the square root of duration of fixation (t) and expressed this relation as: $d = k \sqrt{t}$. The constant (k) is the coefficient of diffusability, which is specific to each fixative. Examples are 0.79 for 10% formaldehyde, 1.0 for 100% ethanol, and 1.33 for 3% potassium dichromate. Thus, for most fixatives, the time of fixation is approximately equal to the square of the distance which the fixative must penetrate. Most fixatives, such as NBF, will penetrate tissue to the depth of approximately 1 mm in one hour; hence for a 10 mm sphere, the fixative will not penetrate to the center until $(5)^2$ or 25 hours of fixation. It is important to note that the components of a compound fixative will penetrate the tissue at different rates, so that these aspects of the fixative will be best manifest in thin specimens.

Gross specimens should not rest on the bottom of a container of fixative, they should be separated from the bottom by wadded fixative-soaked paper or cloth, so allowing penetration of fixative or processing fluids from all directions. In addition, unfixed gross specimens which are to be cut and stored in fixative prior to processing should not be thicker than 0.5 cm. When surgical specimens are to be processed to paraffin blocks, the time of penetration by fixative is more critical. The fixative volume should be at least 10 times the volume of the tissue specimen for optimal, rapid fixation. Currently, in some laboratories, thin specimens may be fixed in NBF for only 5–6 hours including the short time of fixation in tissue processors (S. Kim Suvarna, *et al.* 2012).

METHODS OF FIXATION:

Fixation of tissues can be accomplished by physical and/or chemical methods. Physical methods such as heating, microwaving, and freeze-drying are independent processes and not used commonly in the routine practice of medical or veterinary pathology, anatomy, and histology, except for the use of dry heat fixation of microorganisms prior to Gram staining. Most methods of fixation used in processing of tissue for histopathological diagnosis rely on chemical fixation carried out by liquid fixatives (immersion and perfusion).

Heat fixation (physical fixation):

After a smear has dried at room temperature, the slide is gripped by tongs or a clothespin and passed through the flame of a Bunsen burner several times to kill and adhere the organism to the slide.

Effects of heat during fixation:

When the temperature of a fixative is raised or lowered (as is sometimes recommended for particular histochemical procedures), the rate of diffusion into the specimen is affected, as is the rate of the chemical fixation reactions occurring with the various tissue components. Increasing temperature accelerates the process of fixation. Excessive heat, however, particularly if it is prolonged, can damage cells and cause substantial shrinkage and hardening of the specimen.

In the days before the widespread use of the cryostat it was standard practice to rapidly fix small specimens in boiling formalin prior to preparing frozen sections using the freezing microtome. This process produced specimens which could be sectioned but showed indifferent and very variable microscopic results. Today, most laboratories carry out primary fixation of specimens at ambient temperature and only after specimens are loaded onto the processor, where staff have some protection from the vapours produced.

Temperatures between 37°C and 45°C are commonly employed. Another form of the problems of using hot fixative solutions to initially fix larger specimens (greater than 3 mm thick), is that the outside of the specimen fixes rapidly whilst it may take quite some time for the fixative to penetrate to the center of the specimen and this area may be poorly fixed or not fixed at all. Specimen then show an exaggerated "zonal" fixation effect with different morphological and staining characteristics on the outside as compared to the inside of the specimen. Thus, for these reasons microwave fixation is used in some laboratories (Geoffrey Rolls. 2012).

Microwave fixation:

Microwave heating as a means of tissue fixation was first reported in 1970. From this time there has been increasing use of microwave ovens in histopathology for fixation and other purposes such as antigen retrieval and to accelerate staining of sections (Mayers CP. 1970).

Broadly, there are two ways in which microwave technology is used for tissue fixation. Fresh tissue, placed in saline or other isotonic solution, can be irradiated to produce primary fixation referred to as "microwave fixation (Leong AS. 1991), or microwave stabilization (Kok LP & Boon ME, 1992). No chemical fixative is used at this stage. Alternatively, specimens can be placed in buffered formalin or some other fixative and, at a later stage, microwaved to assist the fixative action of the fixing agent (referred to as 'microwave-assisted fixation") (Ainley CD & Ironside JW, 1994). In this latter case, the microwaving may be carried out while the tissue is in fixative, in which case there may be some hazard from toxic fumes produced. Either way, fixative solution must be present within the tissue for microwave-assisted fixation to occur. Microwave-assisted fixation is much more commonly used than primary microwave fixation. Proprietary fixatives of relatively low toxicity, containing glyoxal, have been developed for use in microwave-assisted fixation (Ruijter ET, *et al.* 1997).

Microwaves are a form of non-ionizing radiation produced by the magnetron in domestic and scientific microwave ovens, at a frequency of 2.5 GHz, they have the capacity to generate instantaneous heat when dipolar molecules such as water or polar side chains of proteins are exposed to their alternating magnetic fields at 2.5 billion cycles per second. The rate at which the microwave energy will generate heat during tissue fixation depends on a number of factors including the power setting and power output of the oven, the volume and nature of the holding solution, the composition, shape and number of containers (including cassettes), the agitation or movement of the containers, also volume and dimensions of the specimens being fixed. According to Kok and Boon, 2.5 GHz microwaves have little effect on tissue beyond a depth of 4 cm and for primary microwave fixation tissue slices should not exceed 3 cm in thickness. After microwaving, they should immediately be sliced to 2 mm and placed in 70% ethanol (Kok LP & Boon ME, 1992).

For microwave assisted fixation, Leong suggests 2 mm thick slices should be prepared from tissues initially fixed in formalin prior to microwave treatment. Because of the many variables involved in microwave fixation, it is vital that every aspect of the technique is fully standardized (including consistent of specimen dimensions), the microwave oven is properly calibrated and that staff performing the fixation step is fully understanding the factors that will influence the outcome (Buesa RJ. 2002).

Heat is considered to be the major factor responsible for the effects of microwaves during tissue fixation. Apart from increasing diffusion rates, heat will increase molecular kinetics and speed up chemical reactions. There has been considerable discussion as to what other effects microwaves might have including the degradation of the oligomers in aldehyde fixatives to dimers and monomers, field-induced alterations in macromolecular hydrogen bonding, proton tunneling and disruption of bound water (Leong AS-Y. 1994). It appears to be necessary to achieve a temperature in excess of 60°C within the specimen for primary microwave fixation, whilst lower temperatures may be acceptable for microwave-assisted fixation (Lemire TD. 2000).

Freezing and Freeze Drying Fixation:

Frozen section techniques were developed in an attempt to eliminate artifacts in tissue specimens caused by exposure to normal processing procedures. Boyle, who sectioned frozen eyes, accomplished the first recorded frozen section in 1663. The initial freezing techniques were accomplished by outdoor freezing in cold weather or with volatile chemicals such as ether and rigolene. As the techniques advanced, freezing was accomplished by using carbon dioxide, Freon, isopentane, liquid nitrogen slush and other cryogens. Thermoelectric cooling is now also an accepted method for routine cryotomy for light microscopic evaluation.

If tissue is to be frozen, the histologic features are best preserved by very rapid freezing. This is best achieved by covering a small tissue sample with an appropriate commercial embedding medium, immersing the tissue in liquid nitrogen, and obtaining a frozen section with the use of a cryostat. Cryostat is formulated to freeze at a specific temperature and optimized to have sectioning characteristics similar to frozen tissue specimens. The compound can be used to either serve as a glue to attach the specimen to the holder, leaving the specimen exposed and reducing rolling during sectioning, or to surround the specimen and act as a support medium during the sectioning process. When the compound surrounds the specimen it becomes a thermal insulator, so care must be taken during the freezing process to prevent freezing artifacts (ice crystal damage). The compound can also be used to provide a protective covering to prevent desiccation (drying out) of the specimen during storage. Proper freezing techniques are extremely important and must be selected according to the requirements and resources available in individual laboratories. Techniques for suitable freezing include:

- Liquefied nitrogen (−190°C)
- Isopentane (2-methylbutane) cooled by liquid nitrogen (−150°C)
- Dry ice (−70°C)
- Carbon dioxide gas (−70°C)
- Aerosol sprays (−50°C)

Sectioning specimens at the proper temperature is critical. If the specimen is too warm, sections will compress and bunch up on the knife edge. If the specimen is too cold, it breaks and shatters under the pressure of the blade. Each type of biological specimen and industrial material will have its own optimum cutting temperature range. It is common for a specimen to have constituents that have very different characteristics for adequate sectioning and, when this occurs, it is preferable to freeze to the temperature of the constituent with the lowest optimum temperature. If the previously frozen specimen, knife or anti-roll plate becomes too warm, they can be cooled by spraying with an aerosol cryogen.

Although artifacts related to freezing and subsequent thawing are inevitable, the artifacts are not as severe as when a specimen is simply placed in a conventional freezer.

Under optimal conditions, frozen sections obtained as described here yield relatively good morphology. However, it should be recognized that red blood cells and the granules within neutrophils are lysed by freezing, so their presence must be determined by other clues at the time of slide interpretation (such as the distinctive shape of the nucleus in the case of neutrophils). Slow freezing produces ice crystals that can drastically distort the tissue, and slow thawing encourages autolysis.

The preparation of frozen sections is technically difficult and may lead to poor-quality sections, especially with relatively thick sections of more than 4-μm thickness. This in turn may lead to difficulties in the evaluation of tissue details, and the histochemical or immunohistochemical staining may give nonhomogenous distribution of the stain.

The interpretation of frozen sections can be helpful in determining the presence or absence of infection at the time of revision arthroplasty, and frozen sections play an important role in the diagnosis and staging of tumors. Finally, some proteins and other antigens are best identified with the use of immunohistochemical and other staining techniques that require the use of frozen tissue. Therefore, recognizing artifacts related to frozen tissue may be a necessary aspect of biomaterials research.

Conclusion: frozen sections used for:

- Rapid production of section for urgent diagnosis.
- Immunofluorescent method.
- Immunocytochemical method.
- Enzyme histochemistry.
- Some silver methods and research.

Perfusion Fixation (chemical):

The fixative is injected into the heart, with the injection volume matching cardiac output. The fixative spreads through the entire body, and the tissue doesn't die until it is fixed. This has the advantage of preserving perfect morphology, but the disadvantages that the subject dies, and the cost is high (Ryter, 1988).

Immersion (chemical):

It is the most routinely used method, performed by placing small pieces of tissue into a relatively large volume of fixative (minimum 10 times of tissue volume). This ratio is chosen to facilitate an interaction between the tissue and fixative. The rate of diffusion, which is dependent on the properties of both the fixative and tissue type, is obviously a limiting factor for optimal preservation.

PREPARATION OF SPECIMEN FOR FIXATION:

For achieving good fixation, it is important that the fixative penetrates the tissue well, hence the specimen should be > 4 mm thick, so that fixation fluid penetrates from the periphery to the centre of the tissue. For fixation of large organs perfusion method is used i.e. fixative is injected through the blood vessels into the organ. For hollow viscera, fixative is injected into the cavity e.g. urinary bladder, eyeball etc.

Ratio of fixative volume to the specimen volume should be 20:1.

Time necessary for fixation is important, routinely 10% aqueous formalin at room temperature takes 12 hours to fix the tissue. At higher temperature (60-65°C) the time for fixation is reduced to 2 hours (Chan, 2001).

CLASSIFICATION OF FIXATIVES:

The fixatives can be classified on the basis of the following criteria

- Action on tissue protein
- Component present
- Uses
- Nature of fixation

According to the action on tissue protein:

Traditionally, fixing agents were termed "coagulant" or "non-coagulant" based on their effect on soluble proteins in solution. Coagulant fixatives were said to result in a permeable meshwork of protein strands whereas non-coagulant fixatives, which are additive in nature, formed extensive cross-links producing a less permeable gel. These terms are still encountered in modern histological literature, but a more systematic approach has recently been taken to classification.

There are two major mechanisms which are important in fixation of proteins and protein complexes: coagulation and cross-linking.

Coagulation:

It subdivides into:

1. Dehydrant

Methanol (CH_3OH) and ethanol (C_2H_5OH) are the only alcohols which have a role as fixatives.

Methanol is closely related in structure to water thus it competes almost as effectively as ethanol for hydrogen bonds.

The action mechanism brought about by these fixative is primarily due to disruption of the protein tertiary structure. The tertiary structure of protein result from ionic bonding (Between positively and negatively charged side chains of amino acids) disulphide bonding (Between two cysteine amino acid units) hydrophobic bonding (Between hydrocarbon- like sick chains of leucine, isoleucine, valine, phenylalanine and tyrosine) hydrogen bonding (Between highly electro negative oxygen atom or nitrogen atom and hydrogen atom attached to another oxygen or nitrogen atom).

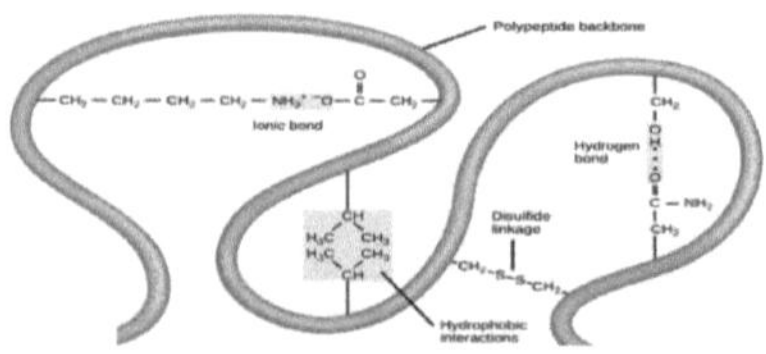

These reagents are capable of disrupting the side chain intra molecular hydrogen bonding beside interaction with hydrophobic residues.

The disrupting of hydrophobic bonding release the hydrophobic areas (found on the inside of protein) from the repulsion of water to become free and occupy greater area. On the other hand, disrupting of hydrogen bonding remove the free water bounded by hydrophilic areas (found on the outside of protein). These change reordered normal protein tertiary structure arrangement (hydrophilic out & hydrophobic in) to become partially reversed (hydrophilic in & hydrophobic out) and finally the protein become insoluble (Horobin 1982).

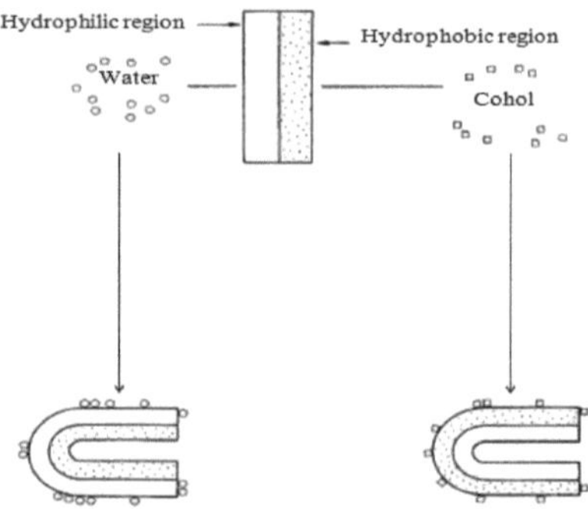

The protein solubility influence by many factors such as type of denaturing agent, temperature, pressure, pH, ion strength of the solute, the salting – in and the salting-out (Eltoum 2001).

2. Acidic

This group joined:

a) Picric Acid:

The amino acid picrates are important in fixation mechanism and the reaction may be due to dipole induction between nitro groups of picric acid and surface groups of fibrous proteins in addition to intermolecular salt links due to polarity in the amino acid side chains (pearse 1980).

b) Acetic Acid:

It is swelling proteins but not able to coagulates it and baker (1958) explained swelling by breaking both ionic and hydrogen bonds in proteins by undissociated part of acetic acid and hydronium ion in its solution that finally expose hydrophilic groups in proteins to attract water and swell it.

Also, precipitate nucleoprotein due to action of the acetate ion in splitting off DNA from histone (Baker, 1958).

c) Trichloroacetic Acid:

It coagulates proteins due to electrostatic interaction of trichloroacetate anion (-C-COO-)

with proteins positively charged groups of amino acids (Kiernan 2008).

The highly non-polar group (Cl3C-) enables the trichloroacetic acid molecule to penetrate into hydrophobic domains within proteins (Kiernan 2008).

Cross-linking:

These fixatives are chemically reacting with proteins and other cell and tissue components, becoming bound to them by forming inter-molecular and intra-molecular cross-links as the following examples:

a) Formaldehyde:

The simple addition of formaldehyde to an active hydrogen atom forming a hydroxyl methyl which finally condenses with other an active hydrogen atom to forming methylene bridge (-CH-).

Gustavson (1956) reported that one of the most important cross-links in over-fixation i.e. in tanning that between lysine and the amide group of the protein backbone (Kiernan 2008 & Eltoum 2001).

b) Glutaraldehyde:

Glutaraldehyde cross-links with several functional groups of proteins like amine, thiol, phenol and amidazole, but the termin-

al amino groups of lysine are the most important groups that forming cross-linking with glutaraldehde.

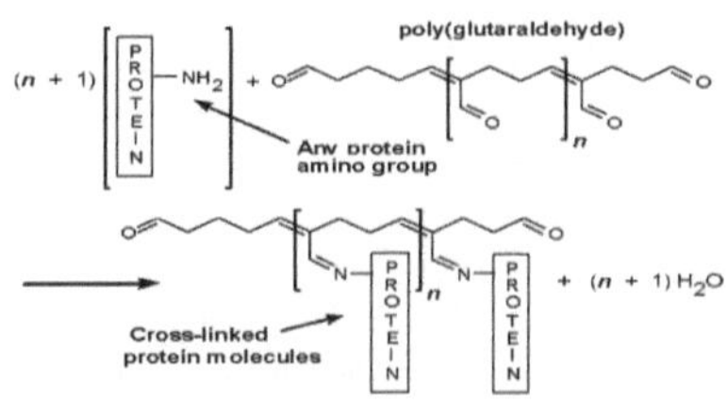

c) Osmium Tetroxide:

The most known cross-linking reaction of osmium tetroxide is that of the double bonds of unsaturated fatty acids.

d) Mercuric Chloride:

The main reaction of mercuric chloride is that by sulfhydryl group of cysteine.

$$Sulfydryl - 2\,(R-S-H) + HgCl_2 \rightleftharpoons (R-S)_2 - Hg + 2H^+ + 2Cl^-$$

Special Mechanisms

The fixation mechanism of chromium compounds (chromic acid and dichromate) in general depend on the reduction of hexavalent chromium to trivalent chromium which the later is cationic and able to form six coordinate bonds with water.

The anionic carboxylic groups (COO⁻) react with this cationic hydrated complex by displacement of coordinating bounded water (Kiernan 2008).

$$2\ \boxed{\text{PROTEIN}}-\underset{\underset{O}{\|}}{C}-O^- + [Cr(H_2O)_6]^{3+} \longrightarrow$$

$$\boxed{\text{PROTEIN}}-\underset{\underset{O}{\|}}{C}-O-\underset{\underset{H_2O\ \ OH_2}{\overset{H_2O\ \ OH_2}{\overset{+}{Cr}}}}-O-\underset{\underset{O}{\|}}{C}-\boxed{\text{PROTEIN}} + 2H_2O$$

According to their components

Fixatives are classified into:

- Simple fixative: Contains a single chemical, e.g. formaldehyde (10% formalin), glutaraldehyde, ethyl alcohol, etc.
- Compound fixative: Contains more than one chemical and used as mixtures.
  - *Formalin based:* 10% neutral buffered formalin, 10% neutral buffered formal saline and formal calcium.
  - *Mercurial fixatives:* Zenker's solution, Helly's solution and B5
  - *Dichromate fixatives:* Regaud's solution, Möller's solution and Orth's solution.
  - *Picric acid fixatives:* Bouin's solution and Gendre's fluid.
  - *Alcohol-containing fixatives:* Carnoy's and acetic alcohol formalin (AAF).

According to their uses:

Fixatives are classified in to:

- Fixatives used in histopathology which they are of two types:
  - *Microanatomical fixatives:* Preserves the microscopic structure of the tissue, e.g. formal saline, formal calcium, Zenker's fluid, etc.
  - *Histochemical fixatives:* To demonstrate enzymes, e.g. buffered neutral formalin absolute alcohol.

- Cytological fixatives: intended to preserve intracellular structures. They are divided into two types:
  - *Nuclear fixatives:* Carnoy's fluid, Clarke's fluid and Flemming's fluid.
  - *Cytoplasmic fixatives:* Champy's fluid and alcohol fixatives.

According to the nature of fixation

Fixatives are classified in to:

- Physical methods, e.g. heating, microwaving and freeze drying.
- Chemical methods, such as Formaldehyde, glutaraldehyde Osmium tetroxide and ethyl alcohol.

Formulas of fixatives

- **Fixatives used in histopathology:**

Over 600 formulations for fixatives are listed by Gray (1954), the following are the most commonly used formulas as presented in standard textbooks of histochemistry (Sheehan & Hrapchak, 1980; Carson, 1990; Kiernan, 1999). It is slightly varying from text to text.

Ferdinard Blum has been credited as the first person used formaldehyde as a tissue fixative (Puchtler and Meloan, 1996). It has been the routine fixative of choice for many years, but this has now been replaced by buffered formalin or by formol calcium acetate. Formaldehyde is a gas soluble in water up to 40%, commercially called formalin and contain about 14% added methanol as stabilizer.

It is a colour less clear solution become turbid on long storage through formation of paraformaldehyde $(CH_2O)_n$, this substance does not affect fixation process if it is removed by filtration. Also, formalin may become acid through formation of formic acid which effect on fixation, so neutralization is done by buffers. Acidic formalin favours the formation of formalin pigment which is brown to black deposits similar to malaria pigment, but it found extracellular (Drury and Wallington, 1980). Formalin fixes tissue by cross-linking the proteins, primarily the residues of the basic amino acid lysine. Its effects are reversible by excess water. Other benefits include: Long term storage and good tissue penetration. It is particularly good for immunohistochemistry techniques (Fox, et al.1985).

10% Neutral Buffered Formalin: (NBF).	
Formalin	10 ml
Acid sodium phosphate	0.4 gm
Anhydrous disodium phosphate	0.65 gm
Distilled water	90 ml
Note	
The pH should be 7.2–7.4.	

Formal calcium:	
Formalin	10 ml
Calcium acetate	2.0 gm
Distilled water	90 ml
Notes:	
It has a near neutral pH.	
Formalin pigment (acid formaldehyde hematin) is not formed.	

Buffered formal sucrose:	
Formalin	10 ml
Sucrose	7.5 gm
M/15 phosphate to 100 ml buffer (pH 7.4)	
Notes:	
This is an excellent fixative for the preservation of fine structure phospholipids and some enzymes.	
It is recommended for combined cytochemistry and electron microscopic studies. It should be used cold (4°C) on fresh tissue.	

Alcoholic formalin:	
Formalin	10 ml
70-95% alcohol	90 ml

Acetic alcoholic formalin:	
Formalin	5 ml
Glacial acetic acid	5 ml
Alcohol 70%	90 ml

Formalin ammonium bromide:	
Formalin	15 ml
Distilled water	85 ml
Ammonia bromide	2.0 gm
Preservation of neurological tissues especially when gold and silver impregnation is employed	

Mercuric fixatives

Mercury is a very toxic, affecting the central nervous system, and may cause acute nephritis. Systemic mercury poisoning by skin absorption is possible. Mercury is a hazardous substance; fixative containing this chemical should not be disposed off in the sanitary sewer system (e.g. sink).

Heidenhain's Susa:	
Mercuric chloride	4.5 gm
Sodium chloride	0.5 gm
Tricholoracetic acid	2.0 gm
Acetic acid	4.0 ml
Distilled water to 100 ml	

Zenker's fluid:	
Mercuric chloride	5gm
Potassium dichromate	2.5 gm
Sodium sulphate	1.0 gm
Distilled water to 100 ml	
Add immediately before use glacial acetic acid 5 ml	

Notes:
It is not stable after the addition of acetic acid hence acetic acid (or formalin) should be added just before use.
Washing of tissue in running water is necessary to remove excess dichromate.

Zenker formal (Helly's fluid) :	
Mercuric chloride	5 gm
Potassium dichromate	2.5 gm
Sodium sulphate	1.0 gm
Distilled water to 100 ml	
Add 5 ml of formalin immediately before use.	

Notes:
Excellent fixative for bone marrow, spleen and blood containing organs. As with Zenker's fluid it is necessary to remove excess dichromate and mercuric pigment.

B5 stock solution:	
Mercuric chloride	12 gm
Sodium acetate	2.5 gm
Distilled water	200 ml
B5 Working solution	
B5 stock solution	20 ml
Formalin (40% w/v)	2 ml

Notes:
B5 is widely advocated for fixation of lympho-nodes biopsies both to improve the cytological details and to enhance immunoreactivity with immunoglobulin antiserum used in phenotyping of B cell neoplasm.
Note: Prepare working solution just before use. Fix small pieces of tissue (7x7x2.5mm) for 1-6 hours at room temperature then process routinely to paraffin.

Picric acid fixatives:

Bouin's fluid:	
Saturated aqueous picric acid	75ml
Formalin	25ml
Glacial acetic acid	5 ml

Notes:
Penetrates rapidly and evenly and causes little shrinkage.
Excellent fixative for testicular and intestinal biopsies because it gives very good nuclear details, in testes is used for oligospermia and infertility studies. Good fixative for glycogen.
It is necessary to remove excess picric acid by alcohol treatment.

Gender's fluid (for glycogen):	
Saturated picric acid in 95% v/v/ alcohol 180 ml.	
Formalin	15 ml.
Glacial acetic acid	5 ml.

- **CYTOLOGICAL FIXATIES:**

Subdivided into Nuclear fixatives and Cytoplasmic fixatives.

(I) Nuclear fixatives:

As the name suggests it gives good nuclear fixation. This group includes.

Carnoy's fluid:	
Absolute alcohol	60 ml
Chloroform	30 ml
Glacial acetic acid	10 ml

Notes:
It penetrates very rapidly and gives excellent nuclear fixation.
Good fixative for carbohydrates. Nissil substance and glycogen are preserved.
Causes considerable shrinkage and dissolves most of the cytoplasmic elements.
Fixation is usually complete in 1-2 hours. For small pieces 2-3 mm thick only 15 minutes is needed for fixation.

Clarke's fluid:	
Absolute alcohol	75 ml
Glacial acetic acid	25 ml.

Notes:
Rapid, good nuclear fixation and good preservation of cytoplasmic elements.
It is excellent for smear or cover slip preparation of cell cultures or chromosomal analysis.

New Comer's fluid:	
Isopropranolol	60 ml.
Propionic acid	40 ml.
Petroleum ether	10 ml.
Acetone	10 ml.
Dioxane	10 ml.

Notes:
Recommended for fixation of chromosomes. It fixes and preserves mucopolysaccharides. Fixation is complete in 12-18 hours (Drury and Wallington, 1980).

(II) Cytoplasmic Fixatives:

Champy's fluid:	
3g/dl Potassium dichromate	7 ml.
1% (V/V) chromic acid	7 ml.
2gm/dl osmium tetraoxide	4 ml.

Notes:
This fixative cannot be kept hence prepared fresh.
It preserves the mitochondrial fat and lipids.
Penetration is poor and uneven.
Tissue must be washed overnight after fixation (Geoffrey Rolls. 2012).

- **Coating Fixative**

Coating fixatives substitutes wet cytological fixatives. They are aerosols in nature, applied through spraying the smear immediately after spreading.

Coating fixatives composed of alcohol base, which fixes the cells and a wax-like substance, that forms a thin protective coating layer over the cells, such as Carbowax (polyethylene glycol) fixative. Diaphine fixative (hairspray) with a high alcohol content and a minimum of lanolin or oil is also an effective fixative.

Most of these agents have a dual action in that they fix the cells and on drying forms a thin protective coating over the smear. These fixatives have practical value, specially in situations where smears have to be mailed to another laboratory for evaluation.

The distance from which the slides are sprayed with an aerosol fixative affects on the cytological details. A 10–12 inches (25–30 cm) is the distance recommended for aerosol fixation. Aerosol sprays are not recommended for bloody smears, because they cause clumping of erythrocytes. Waxes and oils from fixatives can be removed by 95% alcohol. Smears are kept overnight in 95% alcohol for removal of the coating fixative.

Some basic guidelines to optimize fixation:

- Use at least 10–20 volumes of fixative for every volume of tissue.
- No fixative will penetrate more than 2–3 mm of solid tissue or 0.5 cm of porous tissue in a 24-hour period.
- Thickness will depend on the type of tissue, but no specimen should be thicker than 4 mm, for good fixation; 3 mm is preferable.
- Anatomical barriers to fixation will be removed (e.g. fascia, bone, feces, thick tissue) and large specimens must be sectioned (e.g. lung) or opened and cleaned (gastrointestinal tract) to allow penetration.
- Bodily fluids (e.g. bile, blood, feces) that contaminate the fixative solution may be affecting concentration thus fixative must be replaced to ensure effectiveness.
- Pinning specimens to corkboard or inserting a paper or gauze "wick" into tubular structures can improve fixation and reduce tissue distortion.
- Fix at room temperature unless otherwise specified. Heat will increase the rate of fixation, but it also increases the rate of autolysis. Raising the temperature from 25°C to 37°C can double the fixation rate. Vacuum can increase fixation rate at room temperature by about 2.5×.
- Sufficient time must be allowed.

EVIDENCE FOR COMPLEATE FIXATION:

The formation of cross-linkages between proteins by fixative can be measured by change in the following:
- Viscosity.
- Mechanical strength.
- Molecular weight.

If two protein molecules are cross-linked, then their molecular weight is doubled and, as the polymerization proceeds, so the molecular weight increases. This may be shown using gel filtration, gel electrophoresis or viscometry to give quantitative results.

Secondary fixation:

Following fixation in formalin, it is sometimes useful to submit the tissue to a second fixative e.g. mercuric chloride for 4 hours. It provided firmer texture to the tissues and gives brilliance to the staining.

Post chromation:

It is the treatment of tissues with 3% potassium dichromate following normal fixation. Post chromation is carried out either before processing, when tissue is left for 6-8 days in dichromate solution or after processing when the sections are immersed in dichromate solution for 12-24 hours, in both states washing well in running water is essential. This technique is used a mordant to tissues.

Washing out:

After the use of certain fixative, it is urgent that the tissues be thoroughly washed in running water to remove the fixative entirely (see table 3.2).

Washing should be carried out ideally for 24 hours. Tissues treated with potassium dichromate, osmium tetroxide and picric acid particularly need to be washed thoroughly with water prior to treatment with alcohol (for dehydration) (www.rmsc.nic, no date).

FIXATION OF INDIVIDUAL TISSUES

Brain: Adequate preautopsy intra-arterial embalming is done. Formal saline is perfused for a minimum of 2 weeks via the middle cerebral arteries. Distortion is prevented by suspending the brain in the fluid by a thread. The brain can then be sliced at a 1–2 cm interval after fixation.

Eyes: Fixed in the lower compartment of the refrigerator (2–8°C) for 48 hours after the optic nerve is removed. To speed up the fixation, one or two windows are made into the globe after 24 hours.

Renal biopsies: Immunofluorescence biopsies are snap frozen in liquid nitrogen for cryostat sections and then embedded in epoxy resin. Alternatively, most laboratories fix the biopsy in an OCT medium in the cryostat itself before sectioning:
For electron microscopy, fixation is done in 2–3% glutaraldehyde.
For paraffin section, neutral buffered formalin.

Gastrointestinal tract specimen: Flexible fiberoptic endoscopies and small biopsies (2–3 mm) in neutral buffered formalin.

Liver biopsies: Core biopsies (2 × 10 mm) fixed in neutral buffered formalin or in alcohol fixative.
Lungs: Infusion with 4% buffered formaldehyde through main bronchi for 1 week, then fixed in neutral buffered formalin.

Lymphoid tissue: Fixed in neutral buffered formal saline or B5.

Muscle: Open small biopsies are fixed in neutral buffered formal saline, while deep-frozen for histochemistry.

Testis: Neutral buffered formal saline, Helly's solution and Bouin's fluid gives clear nuclear details, i.e. azoospermia and oligospermia.

Uterus and cervix: Neutral buffered saline.
Bone: Neutral buffered saline

Fixation Artifact

Formalin pigment:

Produced by fixation of tissue in acid formaldehyde (hematein). It is dark brown, birefringant maximal in or around the blood vessels and congested tissues.
It prevented by using buffered formalin or neutral, and can be removed by 1% alcoholic solution of sodium hydroxide (NaOH) or by saturated alcoholic picric acid.

Mercury deposit:

Dark brown to black granular deposit, distributed uniformaly throughout the tissue, soluble in alcoholic iodine and not affecting stain after removal. The pigment is converted by iodine to mercuric iodide, which is alcohol soluble.

Chrome deposition:

Occur as fine brown or black granules after dichromate fixation (zinker). It can be removed from the tissue by washing in running tap water from section by acid alcohol.

Crush artifact

may be found in surgical specimens particularly in   liver biopsies, associated with an intense eosinophilic staining at the center of
the tissue in H&E stained sections.   This may
be due to partial coagulation of partially fixed
protein by ethanol or by incomplete   wax   impregnation   during   subsequent   histological
processing.

Streaming artifact

frequently occurs in formalin fixed tissues intended for glycogen demonstration. It is displacement and precipitation of glycogen. It can
be avoided by immediate freeze drying. If immediate fixation is not possible, the tissue
should be refrigerated until adequate fixation is
possible.

Conclusion:

Fixation is the single most influential factor in
the long sequence of steps between procurement
of the specimen and coverslipping the stained
slide; nearly any other step can be reversed to
ameliorate a problem. Tissues can be reverse-
processed and then reprocessed if a mistake or
breakdown occurs in tissue processing. Most
stains can be removed and reapplied to correct
problems with intensity or specificity. Bubbles
under the coverslip can be removed simply by
removing and resetting the coverslip. In sharp
contrast to these examples, ***errors infixation
are permanent***. On the positive side, properly
fixed tissue is nearly impervious to abuse during tissue processing and slide preparation. Understanding the role and mechanism of fixation
is crucial to producing quality slides and inter-
preting artifacts. Important aspects can be
grouped under four rules.

Rule (1): is that fixatives denature macromolecules; i.e., fixation changes the shape of large
molecules. This rule is the basis for the varied
functions of fixation and why fixed specimens
look the way they do under the microscope.
Thus:
a) Fixation kills cells because denatured mole-
    cules can no longer engage in life-
    supporting chemical reactions.
b) Fixation prevents autolysis because biologi-
    cal activity of the specimen's enzymes is
    destroyed as their shape is altered.
c) Fixation prevents microbial attack because
    substrates are no longer recognizable in
    their new conformation.
d) Fixation firms the tissue (making it easier to
    gross and to section) because denatured mo-
    lecules form new intermolecular bonds.
e) Fixation changes the tissue's receptivity to
    stains and histochemical procedures. In
    most cases the influence is positive because
    procedures have been optimized to work
    with fixed tissue, but prominent negative
    examples exist (e.g. masking of antigenic
    sites necessary for immunohistochemical
    staining).

Rule (2): is that different fixatives produce their
own morphological patterns. That is an objective fact that does not imply good or bad.
Whether we like what we see is a subjective
matter, predominantly based on our individual
training. Many chemicals act as fixatives in that
they denature macromolecules, but little produce "acceptable" results because each creates
its own unique pattern of changes visible at the
level of the light microscope.

Speak about "formaldehyde patterns" ("good")
versus "alcohol patterns" ("bad") in describing
how a specimen appears under the microscope.
Some observers give high preference to mercuric fixatives over neutral buffered formalin
(NBF) for lymphoid tissues, and picric acid for
gastric biopsies, because of the extra sharp images they produce. Defining "good" fixation,

then, is difficult because of varying personal preferences. However, there are well-documented and accepted minimum staining criteria that specify well-defined nuclear patterns, epithelial cell membranes, and cytoplasmic staining exhibited by well-fixed tissues.

Rule (3): is that fixation is a chemical reaction that is not instantaneous. Its rate is dependent upon the chemical nature of the fixative solution and its temperature. Closely correlated with this is **Rule (4):**, which says that a fixative must be present for any reaction to occur. This self-evident notion is so frequently ignored that it warrants discussion. Raw specimens are not freely porous objects. Fluids of any sort take time to diffuse into the mass. If there are numerous intercellular channels, as in lymph nodes, movement is faster than if cells are tightly adherent to one another, but penetration still is not instantaneous. Most specimens present membrane barriers that must be crossed each time the fluid moves into the next cell. Because membranes have fatty interiors, aqueous fixatives penetrate poorly. Alcoholic versions of common fixatives (alcoholic formalin, alcoholic zinc formalin, and alcoholic glyoxal) are able to penetrate much faster.

In most cases fixation increases permeability, but some fixing agents (e.g. mercuric salts) create such tight intermolecular bonds that diffusion may be impeded, and the fixative cannot penetrate all the way into the specimen. While alcoholic solutions of aldehyde fixatives do not seem to affect permeability adversely, plain alcohol used for dehydration certainly does.

Rule (3) and **(4)** dictate that adequate time be given for the fixation process (penetration + chemical reaction). Beyond that, no physical encumbrances should be introduced during the handling of the specimen. Squeezing with forceps introduces localized artifacts because penetration is hindered at the sites of tissue damage. More commonly, forcing oversized chunks of tissue into a cassette inhibits or prevents penetration by any fluid and may render processing an exercise in futility. The tissue will remain unfixed, processing fluids will not dehydrate or clear, and the block will not section. If such a disaster is then trimmed thinner and reprocessed, sections may be possible, but the tissue will be rotten. There is no excuse for overly thick specimens (Richard W. Brown. 2009).

TABLE (3-1): (Drury and Wallington, 1980).

Target	Fixative of Choice	Fixative to Avoid
Proteins	10% NBF	Osmium Tetroxide
Enzymes	Frozen Sections	Chemical Fixatives
Lipids	Frozen Sections* Glutraldehyde Osmium Tetroxide	Alcoholic fixatives 10% NBF
Nucleic Acids	Alcoholic fixatives	Aldehyde fixatives
Mucopolysaccharides	Frozen Sections	Chemical fixatives
Biogenic Amines	10% NBF	Bouin's,
Glycogen	Alcoholic based fixatives	Osmium Tetroxide

TABLE (3:2): Starting points for processing and post-fixation requirements (Geoffrey Rolls. 2012).

Fixative	Post-fixation treatment required	Commence processing in	Comment
10% NBF	None	Additional fixation in buffered formalin if required, otherwise 70% ethanol.	Placing specimens in alcohol concentrations greater than 70% may cause precipitation of phosphate from the buffer solution.
Formal calcium	None	70% ethanol	
Formal saline	None	Additional fixation in formal saline if required, otherwise 70% ethanol	
Zinc formalin (unbuffered)	Brief rinse in water	Additional fixation in formalin if required, otherwise 70% ethanol.	Rinse removes excess zinc salts which may be corrosive. If phosphate buffered formalin is used in station 1, residual zinc salts can form a precipitate.
Zenker's fixative	Wash in water	70% ethanol	Rinse removes chromate which can otherwise form an insoluble precipitate. Sections must be treated to remove mercury pigment prior to staining.
Helly's fixative	Wash in water	70% ethanol	Rinse removes chromate which can otherwise form an insoluble precipitate. Sections must be treated to remove mercury pigment prior to staining.
B-5 fixative	After fixation store in 70% ethanol prior to processing	70% ethanol	Sections must be treated to remove mercury pigment prior to staining.
Bouin's solution	After fixation store in 70% ethanol prior to processing	70% ethanol	Water washing after Bouin fixation may remove some soluble picrates. These are insoluble after alcohol treatment.
Hollande's solution	Brief wash in water	Additional fixation in buffered formalin if required, other-	Water wash required. If phosphate buffered formalin is used in station 1, residual salts can form an insoluble phosphate precipitate.

		wise 70% ethanol.	
Gendre's solution	Wash with 80% alcohol to remove excess picric acid	80% alcohol	Residual picric acid can adversely affect staining.
Clarke's solution	None	80% ethanol	
Carnoy's solution	None	Absolute ethanol	Fixation should not be prolonged as excessive hardening will result.
Methacarn	None	Absolute ethanol	Fixation should not be prolonged as excessive hardening will result.
Alcoholic formalin	None	Absolute ethanol	
Formol acetic alcohol	None	Absolute ethanol	

Further reading:

- Ainley CD, Ironside JW. Microwave technology in diagnostic neuropathology. J Neurosci Methods1994;55;183-190.
- Buesa RJ. Haven't you calibrated your microwave oven yet? J Histotechnol 2002;25;39-43.
- Chan J K C. Tumor of lymphoreticular system, diagnostic Histopathology of tumors, Churchill living stone 2001; 2:1101-1103.
- Drury R B and Wallington E A. Carleton Histological Techniques, fifth edition, Oxoford University press, London 1980; pp 36-44.
- Eltoum I, Fredenburgh J, Myers RB, et al: Introduction to the theory and practice of fixation of tissues. J Histotechnol 24: 173–190, 2001.
- Eltoum I, Fredenburgh J, Myers RB, et al: Introduction to the theory and practice of fixation of tissues. J Histotechnol 24:173–190, 2001.
- Fox P C, Johnson F B, Whiting J, Roller P P. Formaldehyde fixation. J Histochem Cytochem 1985; 33: 845-853.
- http://www.leicabiosystems.com/pathologyleaders/fixation-and-fixatives-5-practical-procedures-to-optimise-quality-the-effects-of-heat-and-microwaves/c22952.06-March-2012.
- Grizzle, W.E., Fredenburgh, J., 2001. Avoiding biohazards in medical, veterinary and research laboratories. Biotechnic and Histochemistry 76, 183–206.
- Hesse G. Chemistry of aldehyde fixation. J Acta Histochem 1973; 46: 253-266.
- http://www.nsh.org/what is histotechnology
- Kok LP, Boon ME. Microwave cookbook for microscopists. Leiden: Coulomb Press Leiden, 1992.
- Lemire TD. Microwave irradiated canine and feline tissues: Part 1. Morphologic evaluation. J Histotechnol 2000;23;113-120.
- Leong AS. Microwave fixation and rapid processing in a large through put histopathology laboratory. Pathol 1991;23;271-273.
- Leong AS-Y. Fixation and fixatives. In Woods AE and Ellis RC eds. Laboratory histopathology. New York: Churchill Livingstone, 1994;4.1-1 - 4.1-26.

- Mayers CP. Histological fixation by microwave heating. J Clin Pathol 1970;23;273-275.
- Puchtler H and Meloan S N. On the chemistry of formaldehyde fixation and its effects on immunohistochemical reaction. J Histochemistry 1996; 82: 201-204.
- Richard W. Brown. Histologic Preparations: Common Problems and Their Solutions, Paperback, first edition, 2009.
- Ruijter ET, Miller GJ, Aalders TW et al. Rapid microwave-stimulated fixation of entire prostatectomy specimens. Biomed-II MPC Study Group. J Pathol 1997;183;369-375.
- Ryter A. Contribution of new cryomethods to a better knowledge of bacterial anatomy. Ann Inst Pasteur Microbiol 1988; 139(1): 33-44.

Decalcification defined as removal of inorganic calcium from bone and pathologically calcified tissues to make them flexible to allow sectioning, although preparation of section of undecalcified (mineralized) bones and teeth is possible with special methods and equipments. In more technical terms, it is the dissolution of the hydroxyapatite complex, $Ca_{10}(PO_4)_6(OH)_2$, and can be represented by the following equation:

$$Ca_{10}(PO_4)_6(OH)_2 + 8H+ \leftrightarrow 10Ca^{+2} + 6HPO_4^{-2} + 2H_2O.$$

Before decalcification, it is essential that bone should swan into thin slices in order to allow penetration of fixative and to reduce time required for fixation & decalcification (Yuehuei H. & Kylie L. 2003).

Slices of bone, 3-5 mm in thickness, obtained by a fine tooth fret-saw or more easily by band saw. Saw dust may be produced, and small fragments of bone will deposit on cut surface or deeply in specimen (bone dust artifact) especially cancellous bone when a specimen is cut with a band saw prior to fixation. This artifact should not be misinterpreted as the dystrophic calcium commonly seen in a bone infarct. To minimize this artifact, bone specimens can be gently brushed under running water before being placed into fixative.

A satisfactory decalcification procedure should insure the following:

- Complete removal of calcium salts.
- Lack of distortion of cells & tissues.
- Lack of harm full effects on staining (Scharticles. 2014).

Fixation of bone:

In order to protect the cellular and fibrous elements of bone from damage caused by the acids used as decalcifying agents, it is particularly important to thoroughly fix these specimens prior to decalcification (Moore RJ.1994 & Carson FL.2007). Poorly-fixed specimens become macerated during decalcification and stain poorly afterwards. This is very noticeable in areas containing bone marrow. It is therefore common practice for laboratories to extend fixation times for bone specimens before commencing decalcification. It is important to provide ready access for the fixative to penetrate the bone, so skin and soft tissue should be removed from large specimens if practicable. Bone specimens should be sawn into thin slices as soon as possible to enhance fixation and an adequate volume of fixative provided. High-quality fine tooth saws should be used to prepare bone slices. Coarse saws can cause considerable mechanical damage and force bone fragments into the soft tissues present in the specimen. Buffered formalin is a satisfactory fixative for bone but where the preservation of bone marrow is important some laboratories will use alternatives such as one of the Zinc formalin mixtures, B5, formal acetic alcohol (Davidson's fixative), or Bouin (GeoffreyRolls. 2012).

METHODS OF DECALCIFICATION:

There are four common methods for decalcification.

ACIDS:

An acid will act to release the calcium from its combination with the anions (hydroxyapatite) and effect an ion exchange to give a soluble calcium salt (Kiernan 2015).

$$Ca_{10}(PO_4)_6(OH)_2 + 20H^+ + 20Cl^- \longrightarrow 10Ca^{2+} + 20Cl^- + 6H_3PO_4 + 2H_2O$$

$$Ca_{10}(PO_4)_6(OH)_2 + 20H^+ + 20NO_3^- \longrightarrow 10Ca^{2+} + 20NO_3^- + 6H_3PO_4 + 2H_2O$$

$$Ca_{10}(PO_4)_6(OH)_2 + 20HCOOH \longrightarrow 10Ca^{2+} + 20HCOO^- + 6H_3PO_4 + 2H_2O$$

Also, these acids serve as a source of hydrogen ions which the latter removing the hydroxide ions liberated as a result of dissolution of the hydroxyapatite (Kiernan 2015).

$$Ca_{10}(PO_4)_6(OH)_2 \rightleftharpoons 10Ca^{2+} + 6PO_4^{3-} + 2OH^-$$

Continuous removal of hydroxide ions from the solution will prevent the system from reaching equilibrium, therefore the reaction will proceed from left to right until all the hydroxyapatite has dissolved (Kiernan 2015).

$$H^+ + OH^- \rightleftharpoons H_2O$$

The acids used for decalcification are either inorganic acids (hydrochloric and nitric) or organic acids (formic and acetic). Formic acid is very commonly used because it is fairly slow and gentle to the tissue. Staining is usually very strong, even after prolonged exposure. The inorganic acids remove calcium faster. When the end point is carefully controlled, they are more compatible with immunohistochemistry procedures. The calcium ions that have been removed can saturate the solution around the specimen and prevent further decalcification if the solution is not agitated and changed regularly. Vacuum will facilitate infiltration and remove carbon dioxide bubbles that formed on the specimen surfaces.

Nitric acid:
- Used for rapid decalcification (maximum 48 hours).
- Sometimes causes tissue damage and inhibit nuclear staining in prolong incubation.
- Used in concentration 5% – 10% in D.W.
- Tissue transferred directly to 70% alcohol.

Formic acid:
- Slower than nitric acid (2 – 20 days).
- Less harmful effect on tissue structure & staining (Nuclear staining is better).

- Sometimes prevent reliable assessment of end point.

Perenyi's fluid:

10% nitric acid	40.0ml
Absolute alcohol	30.0 ml
0.5% chromic acid.	30.0 ml.

All these ingredients may be kept in stock and should be mixed immediately before use. This solution may acquire blue violet tinge after a short time without effect in the decalcifying property. It is slow for decalcifying hard bone but excellent fluid for small deposits of calcium e.g. calcified arteries, coin lesions and calcified glands. Also, good for human globe, which contains calcium due to pathological conditions. There is little hardening of tissue, but excellent morphologic detail is preserved.

Gooding and Stelwart's fluid:

90% formic acid	5-10 ml.
Formalin	5 ml
Distilled water to 100 ml.	

Evans and Krajian fluid:

20% aqueous trisodium citrate	65 ml
90% formic acid	35 ml

This solution has a pH of 2-3.

Formic acid sodium citrate method:
Procedure:
1. Place calcified specimen in large quantities of formic acid-sodium citrate solution until decalcification is complete (change solution daily for best results).
2. Wash in running water for 4-8 hours
3. Dehydrate, clear and impregnate with paraffin or process as desired.
This technique gives better staining results than the nitric acid method, since formic acid and sodium citrate are less harsh on the cellular properties. Therefore, even with over exposure of tissue in this solution after decalcification

has been complete, causes little loss of staining qualities.

Formalin Nitric acid:

Formalin   10 ml
Distilled water   80 ml
Nitric acid   10ml

Nitric acid causes serious deterioration of nuclear stainability which partially inhibited by formaldehyde. Old nitric acid also tends to develop yellow discolouration which may be prevented by stabilization with 1% urea.

Tricholoracetic acid:
- Recommended for teeth.
- Good staining results.

ION EXCHANGE RESIN WITH ACID DECALCIFYING:

Ion exchange resins in decalcifying fluids are used to remove calcium ion from the fluid. Therefore, ensuring a rapid rate of solubility of calcium from tissue and reduction in time of decalcification. The resins used is ammonium form of sulfonated polysterene resin along with various concentrations of formic acid. Ammonium ions from the resin are exchanged for calcium ions, so this keeps the solution free from calcium ions and speeds up the reaction (Carson 2007).

The resin is layered on the bottom of a container to a depth of half inch, the specimen is allowed to rest in it. After use, the resin may be regenerated by washing twice with dilute N/10 HCL followed by three washes in distilled water. Use of ion exchange resin has properties of:
- Quick and efficient decalcification.
- Does not improve staining result.
- Impossible assessment of decalcification end point.

ELECTROLYTIC DECALCIFICATION:

This is based on the principle of attracting calcium ions in the electrolyte solution to a negative electrode by the use of an electric currant. Materials used in this method include a durable glass jar containing the electrolyte (mixture of formic acid and hydrochloric acid), the electrodes (brass plate as negative electrode and platinum wire as positive electrode) thermometer and power unit.

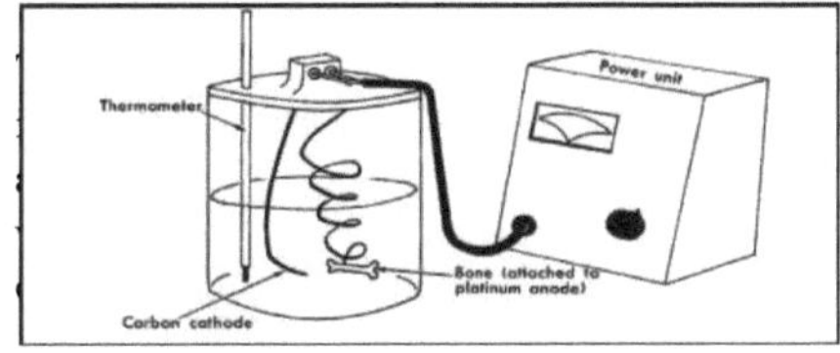

CHELATORS:

A chelator is an organic chemical that bonds with and removes free metal ions from solutions. Chelating agents sometimes referred to in the older literature as "complexing agents" react with one of the ionic species, derived from the substance to be dissolved, and form a stable complex with the substance, so reducing the concentration of the free ions in the solution to the point where the target substance dissolves. Ethylene diamine tetra acetic acid (EDTA) is a chelating agent that reacts with the ionized calcium on the outer side of the hydroxyapatite as below equation (Kiernan 2015).

$$[EDTA]^{2-} + Ca^{2+} \longrightarrow [CaEDTA]^{2-} + 2H^{+}$$

It is the most widely used chelator for decalcification in concentrations of up to 14%. This is a slow process (4 – 40 days) but has little or no effect on other tissue elements. Some enzymes are still active after EDTA decalcification (Drury & Wallington, 1980).

DETERMINATION OF DECALCIFICATION END POINT:

If high-quality results are to be obtained it is important to determine the point at which all the calcium has been removed, because, from this point on, tissue damage seems to occur at an increasing rate.

Over-decalcification, particularly with the strong acid decalcifiers, spoils the staining of basophilic elements such as cell nuclei and in some circumstances can cause maceration of the softer tissue elements. On the other hand, specimens that are incompletely decalcified may be difficult or impossible to section (GeoffreyRoll. 2013).The following methods can be used for determination of decalcification end point.

Flexibility method *(Manipulation, Probing and Bending)*:

Probing or bending is generally the most commonly described method for end point determination. This may be a misnomer, as it is actually a method to determine whether the specimen is soft enough. This method is adequate for determining when a sample is ready to be sectioned, but by the time the sample is deemed pliable enough for sectioning, it can be well past the optimal end point for staining. At the opposite end of the spectrum, samples containing large percentages of dense cortical bone may be flexible, but still harbor centralized areas of undecalcified material. Probing with a sharp object, such as a needle or a scalpel blade, can leave undesirable artifacts.

Radiography (X-RAY):

Radiography can determine whether the calcium has been removed from a specimen. It is described by Carson's as "the most accurate method of determining the completeness of decalcification." But in order to ensure this, a pre-decalcification exposure to establish baseline readings and relative settings is suggested to maximize this accuracy.

This additional step and the process of developing the film makes it time-consuming. In addition to the costs of the generating unit and developer plus chemicals, the price of the film puts the cost of mere end point determination beyond the reach of most laboratories unless it is incorporated into a study data collection or an overall documentation regime.

Timed Immersion:

Timed immersion can be relatively successful with like-kind samples. For example, a manufacturer may state that the average bone marrow biopsy will be completely decalcified after x amount of time in 20 calcified tissue volumes of their product. Or your laboratory may establish its own protocol, as ours did: "a 5 mm slab of femoral head will be adequately decalcified to do full face sectioning after 24 hrs in 250 mL of a 1.35 N hydrochloric acid solution." Again, this will ensure adequate sectioning, but may provide less than optimal staining, depending on the density and the exact calcium content of the sample (Yuehuei H. & Kylie L. 2003).

Chemical test (calcium oxalate test):

Chemical testing for the presence of calcium in the acid decalcifying fluid by precipitation of insoluble calcium hydroxide or calcium oxalate, a negative result indicates completion of decalcification.

Daily testing is preferred with weak acid such as formic acid. Bancroft suggests weekly testing for EDTA. Not all acids and acid-chelator combinations are conducive to convenient chemical testing; thus, the choice of decalcifant can be a limiting factor in using this method.

Procedure (Bancroft J D and Cook H C. 2002):

- Take 5 ml^3 of used decalcifying fluid in test tube.
- Add a piece of litmus paper (indicator).
- Add ammonia hydroxide (strong ammonia); drop by drop, shacking after each drop until litmus paper indicates solution is neutral, if a white calcium hydroxide forms immediately after adding ammonia hydroxide, a large quantity of calcium is present, so decalcification should repeat. If this step is negative (clear) then go to next step.
- Add 5 ml^3 saturated ammonium oxalate & shack well.
- Allow solution to stand for 30 min. If precipitation occur repeat the process or if the solution remains clear it is safe to assume decalcification is complete.

$$Ca^{2+} + C_2O_4^{2-} + H_2O \longrightarrow CaC_2O_4.H_2O(s)$$

FACTORS INFLUENCING THE RATE OF DECALCIFICATION:

Concentration: The concentration of active agent will affect the rate at which calcium is removed. Published formulations for decalcifying solutions strike a balance between speed and degree of tissue damage. It must be remembered that the concentration of active agent will be depleted as it combines with calcium, and so it is wise to use a large volume of decalcifier and renew it several times during the decalcification process.

Temperature: Increased temperature will speed up the decalcification rate but will also increase the rate of tissue damage, so must be employed with great care (Page KM. 1996).

Agitation: Although agitation of any decalcifant will prevent the stagnation of ion transport into the surrounding solution, studies reported by Brain and Bancroft indicate that agitation does not significantly increase the diffusion of the calcium ions through the bone to the outside fluid. So, with large samples, as the surface and "outer core" of calcium is eliminated, the rate of decalcification of the "inner core" is then governed by the diffusion rate. Thus, with large samples, the ultimate gain in turnaround time is not significant. With this in mind, the minimum daily agitation is recommended to be "manually, two to three times a day" (Bancroft JD, Stevens A.1996 & Brain EB 1966).

SURFACE DECALCIFICATION:

Surface decalcification and water softening can be very useful to solve the most common problem in decalcified tissue sectioning: a hard cutting surface resulting from incomplete decalcification and/or incomplete dehydration or clearing of the specimens. When cutting a tissue block, the feeling of scraping and tears seen in the section may mean incomplete decalcification. This also damages the knife's cutting edge. A hard cutting surface makes satisfactory sectioning impossible. Surface decalcification may be used to deal with this problem. One method is the use of a pad of cotton or sponge soaked with decalcifying solution (1% hydrochloric acid solution in 70% ethanol, or 10% formic acid) placed over the surface of the block face for 10 min (Brown GG, 1969). Another method of surface decalcification is to simply immerse the block in one of the decalcifying solutions for 30–60 min. These steps may result in progressive decalcification and tissue softening, with little or no adverse effect on subsequent staining. Often, even a well-decalcified bone may still need some "surface decalcification" before each round of a serial cuting. Water also has a softening effect. An exposure of 15–30 min to water (attaching a wet sponge or placing in water) allows water to enter the exposed tissue, often softening it for a depth of up to 500 µm (Kiernan JA. 1990).

Keratin and chitin are softened by use of concentrated sulphuric acid and with the aid of heat keratin is completely dissolved from the tissue sections. But much tissue distortion will also occur. For softening of chitin, the following procedure gives a satisfactory result.

i. Fix the specimen in fixative of choice.
ii. Place the specimen in following solution until completely dechitinized.

Mercuric chloride	4 g m
Chromic acid	0.5 gm
Nitric acid (Conc.)	10.0 ml
Ethyl alcohol 95%	50.0 ml
Distilled water	200.ml

Change the solution every two days for best results.

ii. Wash in running water for 3 hours
v. Dehydrate, clear and impregnate with paraffin.

TREATMENT FOLLOWING DE-CALCIFICATION AND PRIOR TO PROCESSING:

Various methods for neutralizing residual acid decalcifier before processing have been published, including extensive washing in tap water or the application of alkaline solutions. Generally, a short, effective wash in tap water should be sufficient as any remaining acid will be removed during processing (Callis G & Sterchi D.1998).
It is important to remove the bulk of the decalcifier to avoid contaminating the processing reagents and the processor with acid.

Choosing a suitable schedule for decalcified bone or other decalcified tissues:

Once the mineral has been removed, a standard processing schedule can be used. It must be borne in mind that despite complete decalcification, bone, particularly compact bone, will contain dense areas that require thorough processing. It is better to use a schedule which is too long than too short. Your choice will depend on the nature and size of the specimen. Application of vacuum during wax infiltration should improve the quality of the finished blocks.

Conclusion:

- Decalcification is a straightforward process, but to be successful requires:
  - A careful preliminary assessment of the specimen.
  - Preparation of slices of reasonable thickness for fixation and processing.
  - The choice of a suitable decalcifier and adequate volume, changed regularly.
  - A careful determination of the end-point.
  - Thorough processing using a suitable schedule.
- If you believe the decalcification end-point is close, and you wish to slow the process down to avoid over-decalcification and consequent tissue damage, as might be the case when your laboratory is unoccupied during a weekend, specimens can be removed from decalcifier, rinsed and placed back into formalin (important if hydrochloric acid is being used). Decalcification can then be resumed when convenient (Callis G, Sterchi D. 1998). An alternative is to refrigerate the specimen at 4°C in its decalcifier to slow down the process (Page KM. 1996).
- It is important to carefully consider the nature of any bone specimen received for processing because the relative amounts of cortical and cancellous bone are important and will determine the

time required for decalcification and processing. For example, the iliac crest trephine specimen consists of a rim of cortical bone overlying a cylinder of cancellous bone. The cortical bone will be the last to give up its calcium salts during decalcification and unless it is completely decalcified difficulty will be experienced in obtaining decent sections.

PREPARATION OF UNDECALCIFIED BONE (Calcified):

Sections of undecalcified bone are required for the following:

- Study of normal bone structure and distribution of bone mineral.
- Examination of microradiographs.
- Techniques based on the discovery of antibiotics (Tetracycline) administered, which are localized in areas of bone growth that can be demonstrated by fluorescence microscopy.

Undecalcified embedding and sectioning are specialized procedures used for the evaluation of osseous tissues (bone or calcified tissues), dental tissues and especially specimens containing metal implants.

With this technique, specimens are embedded in plastics or resins such as glycol methacrylate, methyl methacrylate (MMA) or Spurr's resin. In choosing a plastic embedding medium, the goal is to match the hardness of the embedding medium to the hardness of the bone or cartilage in order to produce successful sections. Embedding in plastic offers many advantages in hard-tissue histology. Generally, there is no need for decalcification. Using a sliding or heavy-duty rotary microtome, thin sections can be made due to the better support given by the media to cellular components. There are some differences between plastic embedding and paraffin embedding in terms of tissue processing and sectioning. The time required for each step is much longer for plastic embedding; no dehydration is needed; clearing is not always used; and more choices of sectioning methods exist for plastic-embedded specimens.

There are three major sectioning methods for plastic embedded specimens: direct sectioning using a heavy-duty microtome, "sawing-grinding," and sawing only.

Sectioning with Microtomes:

Small undecalcified bone specimens embedded in glycol methacrylate or MMA can be cut using automatic rotary microtomes such as the Leica with a tungsten carbide blade (for MMA or glycol methacrylate) or with a large glass blade (for glycol methacrylate). Larger undecalcified specimens can be cut using a sliding microtome (Yuehuei H. & Kylie L. 2003).

Sawing-Grinding Methods:

"Sawing-grinding" is the traditional method used for plastic-embedded specimens. The specimen is sectioned with a diamond-coated wafering saw (e.g., Buehler Isomet 2000, Struers Accutome-5, or Leco VC-50) into 0.2–1.0-mm-thick slices. The slices are then glued onto a Plexi glass slide and ground on a grinding machine (such as the Buehler Ecomet 3, Struers Dap-V, or Leco VP-160) to produce 30–100-μm-thick sections. In patient and skilled hands, the thickness of the ground sections can be less than 50 μm. The process is tedious and time-consuming (Pazzaglia UE, *et al.* 1994).

Sawing Methods:

Two systems are available for sawing hard tissues embedded in plastics and resins. One is the modified inner circular sawing technique (Fijnmetaal Techniek Amsterdam, The Netherlands) originally reported by van der Lubbe and Klein (Klein CP, *et al.*1994). This without grinding. Another sawing system is a diamond-coated wire saw unit, Well model 3241 or 4240. According to my experience and that of others,12 small sections as thin as 75 μm can be cut using this method, in a matter of minutes. The

39

sections are then glued onto slides, stained, and coverslipped. Due to their simplicity, efficiency, and relatively lower cost compared to the Exakt system, these saws are becoming more popular for the sectioning of undecalcified or implant-containing specimens. The advantage of these two techniques is that they are capable of sectioning hard tissues or implant containing specimens without grinding (Burr DB, *et al.*1990).

Further reading:

- Bancroft J D and Cook H C. Manual of histological technique and their diagnostic application, fifth edition, Churchill living stone, London 2002.
- Bancroft JD, Stevens A: *Theory and Practice of Histological Techniques, 4th ed.* Churchill Livingstone, New York, NY, 1996:314–320.
- Brain EB: The Preparation of Decalcified Sections. Charles C. Thomas, Springfield, IL,1966:69–143.
- Brown GG: Primer of Histopathologic Techniques. Appleton-Century-Crofts, New York, NY, 1969:38–51.
- Burr DB, Milgrom C, Boyd RD, et al: Experimental stress fractures of the tibia. Biological and mechanical aetiology in rabbits. *J Bone Joint Surg [Br]* 72:370–375, 1990.
- Callis G, Sterchi D. Decalcification of Bone: Literature Review and Practical Study of Various Decalcifying Agents, Methods, and Their Effects on Bone Histology. *The Journal of Histotechnology* 1998;**21**;49-58.
- Carson FL. *Histotechnology*. 2nd ed. Chicago: ASCP Press, 1997.
- Drury R A B and Wallington E A. Carleton Histological Techniques, fifth edition, Oxoford University press, London 1980; 3:
- http://www.leicabiosystems.com/pathologyleaders/fixation-and-fixatives-5-practical-procedures-to-optimise-quality-the effects-of-heat-and-microwaves/c22952.06-March-2012.
- Kiernan JA: Histological and Histochemical Methods: Theory and Practice. Pergamon Press, Oxford, UK, 1990:32–35.
- Klein CP, Sauren YM, Modderman WE, et al: A new saw technique improves preparation of bone sections for light and electorn microscopy. *J Appl Biomater* 5:369–373, 1994.
- Moore RJ. Bone. In Woods AE and Ellis RC eds. *Laboratory histopathology*. New York: Churchill Livingstone, 1994;7.2-10.
- Page KM. Bone. In Bancroft JD and Stevens, A eds. *Theory and Practice of Histological Techniques*. New York: Churchill Livingstone, 1996.
- Pazzaglia UE, Bernini F, Zatti G, et al: Histology of the metal-bone interface: interpretation of plastic embedded slides. *Biomaterials* 15:273–277, 1994. 50,104
- http://www.scharticles.com/effect-temperature-rate-decalcification/.
- Yuehuei H. An & Kylie L. Martin. Handbook of Histology Methods for Bone and Cartilage, first edition, Humana Press Inc, Suite 208.Totowa, New Jersey 07512, 2003.

Tissue processing is preparatory treatment of tissues, entailing impregnation of specimen with an embedding medium to provide support and suitable consistency for cutting (sectioning or microtomy).

Tissue specimens are "processed" through a series of solutions that takes them from fixation, which is typically an aqueous environment, into a non-aqueous support medium. The ultimate goal is to provide the specimen with internal and external support from a medium of like hardness so that the specimen can withstand microtomy without damage. The most common supporting medium is paraffin, but many other substances are also used. Standard paraffin processing procedures include exposure to chemical dehydration through graded alcohol solutions, then a transition solution (commonly referred to as a clearant) followed by infiltration and embedding in paraffin (http://docslide.us. 2015).

This process can be done manually or by using either open or enclosed automatic processing instrumentation. Microwave processing is rapidly gaining popularity. Microwave techniques generally utilize only absolute ethyl alcohol, isopropanol and paraffin. Graded alcohols are not necessary, and the use of clearants is eliminated because carry-over alcohol is evaporated during the final paraffin step. Processing in the microwave will not compromise the morphology or antigenicity of the specimen.

STEPS OF TISSUE PROCESSING:

DEHYDRATION:

Dehydration means the removal of water. The process is used in histotechnology during both processing and staining techniques. During processing procedures, dehydration is used to remove the free water molecules, and if performed correctly, leave the molecularly bound water. Dehydration is normally accomplished using alcohol solutions; most commonly ethyl, denatured or isopropyl; occasionally methyl; or butyl for plant and animal tissue. Other solutions such as acetone and various universal solvents can also be used. If specimens are improperly dehydrated and water is left in the specimen, the clearant and infiltration medium will not penetrate the tissue, and it will be soft and mushy. Excessive dehydration will remove the bound water, causing shrunken, hard, brittle specimens that require excessive soaking before sectioning. After fixation in aqueous solvent, the delicate tissue needs to be dehydrated progressively starting in 50% ethyl alcohol. The other routine tissue specimen may be put in 70% alcohol. A higher concentration of alcohol initially is inadvisable because this may cause very rapid removal of water, which may produce cell shrinkage. An exception to this is in the case of Heidenhain's Susa fixed tissue, where it may be placed directly in 95% alcohol. Tissue transferred from alcoholic based fixatives like Carnoy's fixative may be placed in higher grades of alcohol or even in absolute alcohol.

For routine biopsy and postmortem tissue of 4-7 mm thickness 70%, 90% and absolute alcohol (2-3 changes for 2-4 hours each) are sufficient to give reasonably satisfactory result (Carson FL. 2007).

Other dehydrating agent:

Acetone is clear, colourless, volatile and inflammable fluid. It has a rapid action in dehydrating the tissue but, produces shrinkage then distortion and subsequent brittleness to the tissue. Acetone is low cost, usually dehydrates within 20-30 minutes, but four changes of acetone should be used, it is preferable to use acetone after low strength of alcohol so that distortion of the tissue is less.

Dioxane dehydrates and clears at the same time without hardening or shrinkage. It is miscible with paraffin, water and alcohol, so tissues from dioxane can be transferred straight to paraffin. Dioxane is toxic to man and more expensive than alcohol.

Isopropyl alcohol is miscible with water and other organic solvents, it does not harden the tissue like alcohol, but it is expensive.

Additives for dehydrating agent:

Anhydrous copper sulphate is used in higher grade of dehydrating alcohols. A layer 2.5 cm thick is placed at the bottom of a dehydrating vessel or beaker and is covered with 2 or 3 filter papers to prevent contamination of the tissues. Anhydrous copper sulphate is white, it removes water from alcohol which in turn has been diluted upon absorption of water from the tissues. The change of copper sulphate colour from white to blue indicates that both alcohol and water should be changed. Usage of copper sulphate enhances the process of dehydration and also prolongs the life of alcohol.

Also, phenol acts as a softening agent for hard tissues such as tendon, nail, and dense fibrous tissue and keratin masses. Phenol (4%) should be added to each of the 95% ethanol stations. Alternatively, hard tissue can be immersed in a glycerol/alcohol mixture (S. Kim Suvarna, *et al.* 2012).

CLEARING:

Clearing is the transition step between dehydration and infiltration with the embedding medium. Many dehydrants are immiscible with paraffin wax, and a solvent (transition solvent, ante medium, or clearant) miscible with both the dehydrant and the embedding medium is used to facilitate the transition between dehydration and infiltration steps. Shrinkage occurs when tissues are transferred from the dehydrant to the transition solvent, and from transition solvent to wax. In the final stage, shrinkage may result from the extraction of fat by the transition solvent.

The term clearing arises because some solvents have high refractive indices (approaching that of dehydrated fixed tissue protein) and, on immersion, anhydrous tissues are rendered transparent or clear. This property is used to ascertain the endpoint and duration of the clearing step. The presence of opaque areas indicates incomplete dehydration.

Criteria for choosing clearing agent:
- Speedy Removal of dehydrating agent.
- The type of tissues to be processed, and the type of processing to be undertaken.
- The processor system to be used.
- Intended processing conditions such as temperature, vacuum and pressure.
- Safety factors.
- Cost and convenience.

Common clearing agent:
- *Xylene*: Rapid in action, render tissue transparent and readily eliminated. Xylene is highly inflammable.
- *Chloroform*: It is more expensive, heavy non-inflammable, inconvenient to handle and little hardening (used for brain).
- *Toluene*: Similar to Xylene, recommended for general purposes.
- *Cedar wood oil*: Gentle action, little hardening eliminated slowly. It produces needle like crystal artifact in the presence of acetic acid, which prevented by adding Xylene.

IMPREGNATION (Infiltration or Interpenetration):

It is the saturation of tissue cavities and cells by a supporting substance which is generally, but not always, the medium in which they are finally embedded. Tissues are infiltrated by immersion in a substance such as a wax, which is fluid when hot and solid when cold. Alternatively, tissues can be infiltrated with a solution of a substance dissolved in a solvent, for example nitrocellulose in alcohol-ether, which solidifies on evaporation of the solvent to provide a firm mass suitable for sectioning.

Vacuum impregnation:

It is the impregnation of tissues by a molten medium under reduced pressure. The procedure assists the complete and rapid impregnation of tissues with wax and reduces the time. It facilitates complete removal of transition solvents, and prolongs the life of wax by reducing solvent contamination. Vacuum infiltration requires a vacuum infiltrator or embedding oven, consisting of wax baths, fluid trap and vacuum gauge, to which a vacuum of up to 760 mm Hg is applied using a water or mechanical pump. Modern tissue processors are equipped to deliver vacuum, or vacuum and pressure to all or some reagent stations during the processing cycle. Tissues which benefit vacuum impregnation are lungs, muscles, spleen, decalcified bone, skin & tissues from CNS (Carson FL. 2007).

Factors influencing the rate of impregnation:

When a tissue immersed in a fluid, interchanges occurs between tissue fluids and surrounding fluid. The process is continuing through all stages of processing, from fixation to final impregnation.

*Agitation:*Tissue placed in liquid is agitated so that the fluid immediately in contact with the surface of tissue which is mixed by tissue fluid is replaced by the fresh immersing liquid. This can be achieved by a pumping system which removes and replaces fluid at selected intervals or by rotation and vertical oscillation method. Efficient agitation reduces the processing time by 25-30%, with improved impregnation of the tissue.

Temperature: At low temperatures, structural elements of tissues are stabilized against the destructive effects of solvent changes. This is possibly because of the stiffening and strengthening effect of cold upon biopolymers, resulting from diminution in thermal disruption of secondary bonds of the tissue constituents. Unfortunately, at low temperatures reagent viscosities increase and diffusion rates decrease, resulting in prolonged processing times. Isothermally processed mammalian tissues show finer details and fewer artifacts than those processed by the more practicable, common an isothermic techniques. Heat increases the kinetic energy of molecules and rate of diffusion, with a corresponding decrease in solution viscosity.The application of mild heat within the range 37°C to 45°C, during the dehydration and clearing steps considerably reduces processing times, but may concomitantly increase shrinkage. Tissue shrinkage during infiltration in paraffin wax results mainly from the effect of heat on collagen.

High infiltration temperatures cause marked tissue shrinkage and hardening, which can be avoided by maintaining embedding waxes 2-3°C above their melting points. Prolonged immersion in paraffin wax at the correct temperature results in only slight tissue shrinkage, though tissues such as blood, muscle and yolk sac may harden and become brittle. The extent to which tissues are affected during paraffin wax infiltration depends upon the combination of fixative, dehydrant and transition (clearing) solvent used as well as the tissue type. Microwave stimulated processing involves complex molecular interactions, the key element of which is internal heating, with stimulation of diffusion and concomitant reduction in the duration of tissue processing (Carson FL. 2007).

Viscosity: The higher viscosity slows the rate of penetration.

Ultrasonic: Use of ultrasound (sonication) increases the penetration rate. In ultrasonic stimulated processing, tissues and fluids are subjected to high frequency agitation and the phenomena is associated with simultaneous reduction in processing time.

Pressure and Vacuum: High pressure facilitates infiltration of dense specimens with viscous resinous embedding media at the block forming stage, but is rarely employed for biological specimens. Positive pressures for fluid transfer that are encountered in closed system processors are probably too low to have a significant influence on tissue infiltration. Vacuum applied during dehydration, clearing and infiltration stages improves the quality of processing. Tissues, particularly lung, are de-aerated, and the solvent boiling point is reduced, thus facilitating evaporation of the reagent from the molten infiltration medium. Duration of wax infiltration is dependent upon viscosity and is not reduced by the application of vacuum (John Crocker & David Burnett. 2005).

EMBEDDING:

It is the process by which tissues are surrounded by a medium such as agar, gelatin or wax which when solidified will provide sufficient external support during sectioning. This step is carried out using an "embedding center" where a mould is filled with molten wax and the specimen placed into it. The specimen is very carefully orientated in the mould because its placement will determine the "plane of section", an important consideration in both diagnostic and research histology. A cassette is placed on top of the mould, topped up with more wax and the whole thing is placed on a cold plate to solidify. When this is completed, the block with its attached cassette can be removed from the mould and is ready for microtomy. It should be noted that, if tissue processing is properly carried out, the wax blocks containing the tissue specimens are very stable and represent an important source of archival material (www.leica biosystems.).

Techniques of casting (embedding):

1. Open cassette to view tissue sample and choose a mold that best corresponds to the size of the tissue. A margin of at least 2 mm of paraffin surrounding all sides of the tissue gives best cutting support. Discard cassette lid.
2. Put small amount of molten paraffin in mold, dispensing from paraffin reservoir.
3. Using warm forceps, transfer tissue into mold, placing cut side down, as it was placed in the cassette.
4. Transfer mold to cold plate, and gently press tissue flat. Paraffin will solidify in a thin layer which holds the tissue in position.
5. When the tissue is in the desired orientation add the labeled tissue cassette on top of the mold as a backing. Press firmly.
6. Hot paraffin is added to the mold from the paraffin dispenser. Be sure there is enough paraffin to cover the face of the plastic cassette.
7. If necessary, fill cassette with paraffin while cooling, keeping the mold full until solid.
8. Paraffin should solidify in 30 minutes. When the wax is completely cooled and hardened (30 minutes) the paraffin block can be easily popped out of the mold; the wax blocks should not stick. If the wax cracks or the tissues are not aligned well, simply melt them again and start over.

The following points must be taken carefully during casting.

- Paraffin should not be allowed to cool around the tissue to be blocked so before introducing the tissue in the mould it should be kept in heated wax or in cassette placed over thermostatic hot plate.

- To prevent excess of wax solidifying on the bottom of the block during winter pre-warmed moulds may be used.
- The cutting surface of the tissue should be facing at the bottom of the mould.
- If two or more tissues have to be cast remember to keep them both at the same depth.
- If small biopsy fragments have to be cast, the largest piece should be first blocked and other pieces should be as near as possible.
- All four corners of the block should be in one horizontal plane.
- The tissue should have at least 2 mm wax around its edges.
- Smear mineral or machine oil on the inner surface of the mould for facilitating easy removal of block.
- Whitish areas around tissue in block denote crystallization which may be due to moisture or due to incomplete removal of clearing agent.
- Specimen orientation is very important for the demonstration of proper morphology. Incorrect orientation may result in diagnostic tissue elements being damaged during microscopy or not being evident for pathology review. Most tissue sections are cut from the largest area, but some tissue needs special mention.

Orientation of tissues:

Products are available that help ensure proper orientation: marking systems, tattoo dyes, biopsy bags, sponges, and papers. Orientation of the tissue should offer the least resistance of the tissue against the knife during sectioning. A margin of embedding medium around the tissue assures support of the tissue. Tissues requiring special orientation include:

- Tubular structures: cross-section of the wall and lumen should be visible; arteries, veins, fallopian tube and vas deferens samples.
- Skin biopsies; shave punch or excisions, cross-section of the epidermis, dermis and subcutaneous layers must be visible.
- Intestine, gallbladder, and other epithelial biopsies: cut in a plane at right angles to the surface, and oriented, so the epithelial surface is cut last, minimizing compression and distortion of the epithelial layer.
- Muscle biopsies: sections containing both transverse and longitudinal planes.
- Multiple pieces of a tissue are oriented side by side with the epithelial surface facing in the same direction (S. Kim Suvarna. 2012).

Summary of some embedding media.	
Paraffin wax (p. wax)	- Most widely used (routine). - Reasonable speed of processing. - Sections ribboning & blocks are durable. - Wide range of section thickness (1- 60) μm. - Not suitable for hard & multi layer tissues (bone – brain).
Ester wax	- Soluble in alcohol & Xylene. - Lower melting point & harder than P. wax. - Suitable for cutting thin sections (2-3) μm. - Minimal shrinkage & suitable for bone & smooth materials (insect). - No special condition for block storage. - More expensive than P. wax.

Water soluble wax (solid polyethylene glycols)	. Tissue directly impregnated (no need for dehydration & clearing). . Reduced tissue shrinkage and preserve lipid. . Blocks solidified at room temperature (time consuming). . Blocks stored away from moisture; or coated with P. wax.
Cellulose nitrate (celloidin & low viscosity nitro cellulose)	· Suitable for hard & multi layer tissues (bone – brain). · Reduce shrinkage. · Time consuming requiring several weeks for complete impregnation. · Difficult to cut thin sections (less than 10 µm). · Non ribboning medium. · Difficult storage (in jars of alcohol) so it is space consuming. · High flammability.
Celloidin –Paraffin (double embedding)	· Improve cohesion of layers. · Facility of cutting ribbons. · Durable blocks. · Useful with bone, brain & muscle.
Synthetic resins (acrylic, polyester & epoxy resins)	· Used particularly to prepare sections for EM (0.5-2) µm. Also may used to prepare sections of undecalcified bone. · Superior preservation of tissue structure and lack of tissue distortion.
Paraplast mixture of highly purified paraffin and several plastic polymers.	· It has greater elasticity than normal paraffin wax, therefore, the results are superior. · It ribbons well allowing almost wrinkle free serial sections to be cut with ease at 4-micron thickness. · It should not be used for thin walled structures as it prevents complete expansion of the specimen.
Bioloid	· Good embedding medium in which thin walled structures can be sectioned satisfactorily.
Gelatin.	· Supporting tissues to be cut on freezing microtome.

PROCESSORS:

Transferring the tissue mechanically from one reagent to another. It reduces processing time by the action of continuous agitation, thus eliminates the possibility of human errors of leaving the tissue for long time in one solution due to forget fulness. There are two types of Automatic tissue processor:

Tissue transfer processors:

These processors are characterized by the transfer of tissues, contained within a basket, through a series of stationary reagents arranged in-line or in a circular carousel plan. The rotary or carousel is the most common model of automatic tissue processor, and was invented by Ar endt in 1909. It is provided with 9-10 reagent and 2-3 wax positions, with a capacity of 30-110 cassettes depending upon the model. Fluid agitation is achieved by vertical oscillation or rotary motion of the tissue basket. Processing schedules are card-notched, pin or touchpad programmed. Tissue-transfer processors allow maximum flexibility in the choice of reagents and schedules that can be run on them, in particular, metal-corrosive fixatives, a wide range of solvents, and relatively viscous nitrocellulose solutions can all be accommodated. These machines have a rapid turn-around time for day/night processing. In more recent models the tissue basket is enclosed within an integrated fume hood during agitation and transfer cycles, thus overcoming the disadvantages of earlier styles (www.coursehero.com.).

Fluid transfer processors:

In fluid-transfer units, processing fluids are pumped to and from a retort in which the tissues remain stationary. There are 10-12 reagent stations with temperatures adjustable between 30-45°C, 3-4 paraffin wax stations with variable temperature settings between 48-68°C, and vacuum-pressure options for each station. Depending upon the model, these machines can process 100-300 cassettes at any one time. Agitation is achieved by tidal action. Schedules are microprocessor programmed and controlled. Vacuum-pressure cycles coupled with heated reagents allow effective reductions in processing times and improved infiltration of dense tissues.

Fluid-transfer processors overcome the main drawbacks of the tissue-transfer machines. Tissues are unable to dry out within the sealed retort, and reagent vapors are vented through filters or retained in a closed-loop system. Processors are provided with alert systems and diagnostic programs for troubleshooting and maintenance. Some models are unable to accept mercury or dichromate-based fixatives, certain solvents, for example chloroform, or wax additives such as Piccolyte (www.coursehero.com. 2015).

Notes:
- Fluid and wax beakers must be filled up to appropriate mark and located in their correct position in the machine.
- Any spillage of the fluid should be wiped away.
- Accumulations of wax must be removed from beaker, covers, lids and surrounding areas.
- Wax bath thermostats should be set at satisfactory levels usually 2-3°C above the melting point of wax.
- Particular attention should be paid to fastening the processing baskets on the carousel type of machines; if the baskets are shed they will remain in one particular regent for a long period till it gets noticed.
- Timing should be set with uptmost care when loading the machine.
- Paraffin wax baths should be checked to ensure that the wax is molten.

Automated routine tissue processing schedule:(Drury & Wallington. 1980).

10% buffered formalin	2 hrs
70 percent alcohol	3 hrs.
90 percent alcohol	3 hrs.
Absolute alcohol	1 hrs.
Absolute alcohol	1 hrs.
Absolute alcohol	2 hrs.
Absolute alcohol	2 hrs.
Xylene	2 hrs.
Xylene	2 hrs.
Wax bath	3 hrs.
Wax bath	3 hrs.

Note: there are many protocols for tissue processing differs according to the tissue nature, techniques to be applied and diagnostic purposes.

MANUAL TISSUE PROCESSING:

Manual tissue processing is usually undertaken for the following reasons:
- Power failure or breakdown of a tissue processor.
- A requirement for a non-standard processing schedule as for rapid processing of an urgent specimen.
- Delicate material.
- Very large or thick tissue blocks.
- Hard, dense tissues (nitrocellulose methods).
- Special diagnostic, teaching or research applications.
- Small scale processing requirements.

· Resin embedding.

The main advantage of manual processing over automated methods lies in the flexibility of reagent selection, conditions and schedule design to provide optimum processing for small batches of tissues. Exposure of tissues to the deleterious effects of some reagents can be carefully monitored and regulated through observation and precise timing. There is usually considerable latitude in the processing times given in schedules, although maximum rather than minimum times should be used, as it is better to extend processing rather than risk of under processed tissue problems. Manual processing is accelerated using microwave ovens or ultrasonics.

Universal solvents with particularly favorable attributes, normally precluded from routine machine processing because of budgetary or safety constraints, can be successfully used in small volumes under controlled conditions for manual processing.

Nonetheless, manual processing can be time-consuming and inconvenient. Care must be exercised so that tissues are left overnight in reagents that will cause minimal harm effects. A permanent series of solutions in wash bottles simplifies processing small single specimens. Tissues are processed in tubes and agitated on a rotor. Reagents are pipetted, or decanted through a fine sieve. Multiple specimens or large blocks are economically processed in large lidded jars of processing fluids. The specimen to reagent volume ratio should be at least 1:50. Agitation is provided by a magnetic-stirrer.

Dehydrated tissues float on the surface when transferred to higher density transition solvents such as chloroform or cedar wood oil. However, if placed in lower density mixtures of dehydrant-transition solvent before finally transferring to pure transition solvent, tissues will remain submerged throughout the clearing stage. An alternative approach is to carefully layer the dehydrant onto the transition solvent and introduce the tissue into the upper layer. The tissue sinks as the dehydrant gradually replaces the transition solvent. Reagents are carefully decanted, and the specimen placed in a fresh change of transition solvent.

Rapid manual tissue processing schedule: (Drury and Wallington. 1980).

· Fix the specimen in Carnoy's fluid for 45 min.
· Dehydrate in absolute ethyl alcohol for15 min.
· Clear in xylene 1 for 10 min.
· Clear in xylene 2 for 15 min. (or until clear).
· Impregnate in paraffin wax 1 for 20 min.
· Impregnate in paraffin wax 2 for 45 min

POSSIBLE ARTIFACTS DURING TISSUE PROCESSING:

The purpose of dehydrating agents is to remove the water from specimens prior to infiltration with paraffin. The most common dehydrating agent is alcohol. Artifacts induced during dehydration account for the vast majority of all processing artifacts. There are two possible outcomes from improper dehydration: inadequate dehydration and excessive dehydration.

Typically, the absolute alcohol contains residual water. If the percentage of water in the absolute alcohol exceeds 2 percent, the tissue will not be properly desiccated. When the free water persists, the tissue cannot be properly infiltrated with paraffin and, therefore, will be unsuitable for sectioning. In these cases, the tissue must be reprocessed to the alcohol stage and then properly dehydrated.

If tissue specimens are excessively dehydrated, on the other hand, the tissue will become brittle and not section properly. Some tissue types are prone to excessive dehydration, including liver and spleen. Tissue dehydrated with Acetone is especially prone to excessive dehydration.

Clearing agents function is to remove the alcohol from tissue specimens to facilitate infiltration of paraffin. The most popular clearing agents, xylene and toluene, are aromatic hydrocarbons and have a number of potential problems associated with them. Excessive treatment with xylene, for example, can harden tissues and make them brittle. In addition, xylene and toluene are flammable and toxic. To address these drawbacks, a number of commercially available xylene substitutes have been developed, including Americlear (Allegiance Healthcare Corp., McGaw Park, IL) and SafeClear (CMS/Fisher Healthcare, Houston).

Since 1869, paraffin has been used in the histologic preparation of tissue samples. The infiltration of specimens with wax provides the physical support necessary for sectioning. Since hot molten paraffin is used to infiltrate tissue specimens, a number of artifacts are introduced during the heating process. These include the denaturation and coagulation of proteins and the shrinkage and hardening of tissue. Factors that influence how well the material is infiltrated are:

- Temperature. The temperature of the paraffin is determined by its melting point. The most common paraffin used in labs has a melting point of approximately 58°C. There are a number of points to consider when selecting a temperature range for the paraffin used in the laboratory. For example, paraffins with higher melting points provide increased support in hard tissues but can produce more brittle tissues than those embedded with low melting point paraffins. Secondly, the size of the crystalline structure is influenced by the speed at which the paraffin cools. The faster the paraffin cools, the better quality sections are produced. And finally, although low melting point paraffins are commercially available that reduce the loss of immunoreactivity seen with higher melting point paraffins, current antigen retrieval methods limit their utility.
- Time. Since molten paraffin is used for infiltration, this step should be as short as possible. This is especially true when working with small biopsy specimens that are more likely to show shrinkage artifacts or cut poorly in response to being "overcooked."
- Quality of Paraffin. Recent advances in paraffin manufacturing have improved the quality of paraffin compared to that of 100 years ago. Today, most commercially available paraffins include additives that influence the rate of infiltration, melting point and cutting characteristics. These products vary widely in quality; comparative studies should be done by individual labs to ensure quality results.

Artifacts Seen Using Automated Tissue Processors:

Automated tissue processors must be monitored to insure quality. While instrument performance is critical, the most commonly encountered artifacts result from failure to change solutions on a regular basis. Each processing run contaminates the alcohols, xylenes and paraffins. Failure to change reagents on a regular basis leads to improper processing. All labs should have quality control standards in place that require them to rotate their reagents based on the number of specimens processed.

Since automated tissue processing is a batch process, there's a tendency to process all samples, regardless of size, in the same run. Small biopsy specimens clearly require shorter incubation times and reduced exposure to heat. When biopsy specimens are processed using standard schedules, the specimens have the tendency to become over-processed and brittle.

Dedicated programs need to be implemented to insure proper handling of small tissue samples.

A related problem with automated tissue processors involves samples being exposed to the wrong solvent. This fault is seen in cases of instrument failure or is secondary to human error when a reagent is placed in the wrong container. In these situations, the tissue must be reprocessed.

The over packing of the processing chamber can limit the circulation of solvents, leading to poor fixation. A related problem is seen when processing baskets are used without securing the lid. This may result in cassettes floating on the surface of the chamber, limiting exposure to processing solutions.

TISSUE REPROCESSING:

In spite of great care to prepare quality specimens, some are not properly fixed or processed. To fix this problem, however, the tissue can be reprocessed. To reprocess tissue specimens, the tissue is removed from the paraffin by immersing the sample in multiple changes of xylene. The paraffin-cleared tissue is then hydrated through a descending alcohol series and refixed in formalin. The tissue is reprocessed and embedded.

While this is a labor-intensive process, it's an important technique that can be used to save a specimen that has not been properly handled. A new automated tissue-reprocessing feature (patent pending) has been developed for use on the Ventana Renaissance Tissue Processor that automates this manual method.

RESTORATION OF TISSUE DRIED DURING PROCESSING:

Despite precautions taken during processing, technical or mechanical malfunctions and human error may occur, resulting in tissue drying out prior to paraffin wax impregnation. The tissue will never be regarded as normal, but the following treatment may help provide slides of adequate diagnostic quality.

Tissue restoration solution:

70% ethanol	70 ml
Glycerol	30 ml
Dithionite	1 g

Tissues remain in the solution for several hours or overnight. Processing begins with the dehydrating solutions and continues to completion. Tissue may be difficult to section; coated or plus slides should be used.

The table below provides some troubleshooting tips for poor processing:		
Problem	**Possible Causes**	**Corrections**
Tissue feels soft or mushy during embedding	· Tissue may have been grossed in too thick · Tissue may have been processed on a program that was too short for that tissue type · Processing reagents may be saturated with water · Paraffin may be saturated with xylene or isopropanol	· Reprocess tissue on proper program · Reprocess tissue on correct processing protocol · Change reagents and reprocess tissue · Change paraffin and reprocess tissue
Tissue bounces out of paraffin block during microtomy or tissue	Poor dehydration and paraffin infiltration due to water left in the tissue	Change reagents and reprocess tissue on proper processing protocol

does not adhere to block or slides (Commonly experienced with uterus and prostate tissue, as well as dense organ core samples)		
Tissue looks greasy and "explodes" or separates rapidly when ribbon is placed on water bath	· If the temperature of the water bath is between 45-50° C, then the tissue is under-processed · Tissue may have been grossed in too thick · Tissue may have been processed on a program that was too short for that tissue type · Processing reagents may be saturated with water · Paraffin may be saturated with xylene or isopropanol	· Reprocess tissue on correct processing protocol · Reprocess on proper program · Reprocess tissue on correct processing protocol · Change reagents and reprocess · Change paraffin and reprocess tissue
Tissue does not adhere to slide or falls off easily	· If tissue slides are placed in oven prior to deparaffinization in xylene, tissue is under-processed · Reagents saturated with water or contaminated with the preceding reagent	· Reprocess tissue on correct processing protocol · Change reagents and paraffin and reprocess tissue on proper processing protocol
Hematoxylin and eosin (H&E) stained tissue section shows uneven nuclear staining and "blue blobs" lacking distinct chromatin patterns	If tissue was fixed properly, then sample was improperly dehydrated and infiltrated with paraffin	Change reagents and reprocess tissue on proper processing protocol

Further reading:

· Carson FL. Histotechnology. 2nd ed. Chicago: ASCP Press, 1997.
· Drury R B and Wallington E A. Carleton Histological Techniques, fifth edition, Oxoford University press, London 1980; 3:
· http://docslide.us/documents/tissue-processing-55844e3ff0ea0.html.
· http://www.leicabiosystems.com/pathologyleaders/an-introduction-to-specimen-processing/.
· https://www.coursehero.com/file/p3fi5av/Automated-tissueprocessing.
· John Crocker & David Burnett. The Sciences of Laboratory Diagnosis, second edition, John Wiley & Sons Ltd, The Atrium, Southern Gate, Chichester, West Sussex PO19 8SQ, England 2005, pp 27-30.
· S. Kim Suvarna, Christopher Layton and John D. Bancroft. Theory and Practice of Histological Techniques. Seven edition, Churchill Livingstone, china presses 2012.pp 107,108.

Microtome: (From the Greek *mikros*, meaning "small", and *temnein*, meaning "to cut"). It is a sectioning instrument that allows the cutting of extremely thin slices (sections). Microtomy is a method for the preparation of thin sections from materials such as bones, minerals and teeth, with section thickness between 0.05 and 100 µm. Today, the majority of Microtomes are a knife-block design with a changeable knife, a specimen holder and an advancement mechanism. In most devices, the cutting of the sample begins by moving the sample over the knife, where the advancement mechanism automatically moves forward such that the next cut for a chosen thickness can be made. The section thickness is controlled by an adjustment mechanism, allowing for precise control.

Applications of microtomes:

Traditional histology technique; tissues are hardened by replacing water with paraffin. The tissue is then cut in the microtome at thicknesses varying from 1 to 60 µm (micrometers) thick. From there the tissue can be mounted on a microscope slide, stained with appropriate aqueous dye(s) after prior removal of the paraffin, and examined using a light microscope.

Cryosectioning: water-rich tissues are hardened by freezing and cut in the frozen state with a *freezing* microtome or microtome-*cryostat (Cryomicrotome);* sections are stained and examined with a light microscope. This technique is much faster than traditional histology (5 minutes Vs 16 hours) and is used in conjunction with medical procedures to achieve a quick diagnosis. Cryosections can also be used in immunohistochemistry as freezing tissue stops degradation of tissue faster than using a fixative and does not alter or mask its chemical composition as much.

Electron microscopy; after embedding tissues in *epoxy resin*, a microtome equipped with a *glass* or gem grade *diamond* knife is used to cut very thin sections (typically 60 to 100 nanometers). Sections are stained with an aqueous solution of an appropriate heavy metal salt and examined with a transmission electron microscope. This instrument is often called an ultra microtome. The ultra microtome is also used with its *glass* knife or an industrial grade *diamond* knife to cut survey sections prior to thin sectioning. These survey sections are generally 0.5 to 1 micrometer thick and are mounted on a glass slide and stained to locate areas of interest.

Botanical microtomy; hard materials like wood, bone and leather require a *sledge* microtome. These microtomes have heavier blades and cannot cut as thin as a regular microtome (www.coursehero.2015).

MICROTOME TYPES:

Rotary microtome:

This instrument is a common microtome design. This device operates a staged rotary action such that the actual cutting is part of the rotary motion. In a rotary microtome, the knife is typically fixed in a horizontal position.The flywheel in many microtomes can be operated by hand. This has the advantage that a clean cut can be made, as the relatively large mass of the flywheel prevents the sample from being stopped during the sample cut. The flywheel in newer models is often integrated inside the microtome casing. The typical cut thickness for a rotary microtome is between 1 and 60 µm.

For hard materials, such as a sample embedded in a synthetic resin, this design of microtome can give well "Semi-thin" sections with a thickness of as low as 0.5 µm. Rotary microtome is good general purpose instrument used mainly for paraffin wax but may be used in some cellulose models (www.liquisearch.com. 2015).

Sled microtome:

A sledge microtome is a device where the sample is placed into a fixed holder (shuttle), which then moves backwards and forwards across a knife. Modern sled microtomes have the sled placed upon a linear bearing, a design that allows for the microtome to readily cut many coarse sections.

By adjusting the angles between the sample and the microtome knife, the pressure applied to the sample during the cut can be reduced. Typical applications for this design of microtome are of the preparation of large samples, such as those embedded in cellulose nitrate. Typical cut thickness achievable on a sled microtome is between 1 and 60 µm.

Cryomicrotome:

For the cutting of frozen samples, many rotary microtomes can be adapted to cut in a liquid nitrogen chamber, in a so-called cryomicrotome setup. The reduced temperature increases the hardness of the sample, such as by undergoing a glass transition, which allows the preparation of semi-thin samples. However, the sample temperature and the knife temperature must be controlled in order to optimize the resultant sample thickness.

Ultra microtome:

An ultra microtome used for the preparation of extremely thin sections, with the device functioning in the same manner as a rotational microtome, but with very tight tolerances on the mechanical construction. As a result of the care-ful mechanical construction, the linear thermal expansion of the mounting is used to provide very fine control of the thickness.

Vibrating microtome:

The vibrating microtome operates by cutting using a vibrating blade, allowing the resultant cut to be made with less pressure than would be required for a stationary blade. The vibrating microtome is usually used for difficult biological samples. The cut thickness is usually around 30-500 µm for live tissue and 10-500 µm for fixed tissue.

Saw microtome:

The saw microtome is especially for hard materials such as teeth or bones. The microtome of this type has a recessed rotating saw, which slices through the sample. The minimal cut thickness is approximately 30 µm, and can be made for comparatively large samples.

Laser microtome:

The laser microtome is an instrument for contact free slicing. Prior preparation of the sample through embedding, freezing or chemical fixation is not required, thereby minimizing the artifacts from preparation methods. Alternately this design of microtome can also be used for very hard materials, such as bones or teeth as well as some ceramics. Dependent upon the properties of the sample material, the thickness achievable is between 10 and 100 µm.

The device operates using a cutting action of an infra-red laser. As the laser emits a radiation in the near infra-red, in this wavelength regime the laser can interact with biological materials. Through a sharp focussing on the probe within the sample, a focal point of very high intensity can be achieved. Through the non-linear interaction the so-called optical penetration, which the focal region introduces a material separation in a process known as photodisruption. Through the application of very short laser pulse durations on the order of femtoseconds a pulse of very small energy in the target region be deposited, allowing for precise control of the energy imparted into the sample, limiting the interaction zone of the cut to under a micrometer. External to this zone, the ultra-short beam application time introduces minimal to no thermal damage to the remainder of the sample.

The laser radiation is directed onto a fast scanning mirror based optical system which allows for three-dimensional positioning of the beam crossover, whilst allowing for beam traversal to the desired region of interest. The combination of high power with a high faster rate allows the scanner to cut large areas of sample in a short time. In the laser microtome the laser-microdissection of internal areas in tissues, cellular structures, and other types of small features is also possible.

Rocking microtome:

- Small lightweight instrument.
- Suitable for class work.
- Suitable for P-wax.
- Easy to operate & maintain.

Freezing microtome:

- Designed to prepare frozen sections.
- Knife moves horizontally across the surface of specimen.
- Possible to produce ribbons.
- Difficult to produce serial section.

Microtomes use steel, glass, or diamond blades *depending* upon the specimen being sliced and the desired thickness of the sections being cut.

Steel blades are used to prepare sections of animal or plant tissues for light microscopy histology.

Glass knives are used to slice sections for light microscopy and to slice very thin sections for electron microscopy. *Industrial grade diamond* knives are used to slice hard materials such as bone, teeth and plant matter for both light microscopy and for electron microscopy.

Gem quality diamond knives are used for slicing thin sections for electron microscopy.

Generally, knives are characterized by the profile, which falls under the categories of planar concave, wedge shaped or chisel shaped designs.

Planar concave microtome knives are extremely sharp, but are also very delicate and are therefore only used with very soft samples.

The wedge profile knives are somewhat more stable and used for moderately hard materials, such as in epoxy or cryogenic sample cutting.

The chisel profile with its blunt edge raises the stability of the knife, whilst requiring significantly more force to achieve the cut (www.coursehero.com. 2015).

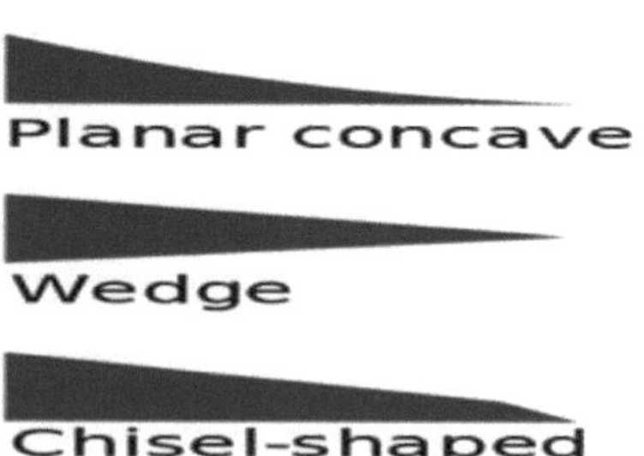

PARAFFIN SECTION CUTTING:

Equipment required:
- Microtome.
- Water bath preferably thermostatically controlled for paraffin wax of melting point 56°C, a water temperature of 45°C is sufficient ordinary distilled water is satisfactory; addition of a trace of detergent to water is beneficial in flattening of sections.
- Hot plate or drying oven thermostatically controlled for drying of sections at around the melting point of wax is satisfactory.
- Fine pointed forceps.
- Small hairbrush.
- Seeker.
- Scalpel.
- Clear cloth or paper towel.
- Slide rack.
- Clean glass slides a 76 x 25 x 1.2 mm slide is suitable.
- Section adhesive.
- Fluff less blotting paper.
- Ice cubes.
- Diamond marker pencil to write the identification details (S Ramakrishnan & KN Sulochana. 2012).

Fixing of block:

To fix the block in the block holder on the microtome, the block may be fixed directly or it may be fixed to a metal carrier which in turn is fixed to the microtome.

Insert the appropriate knife in the knife holder and screw it tightly in position. Adjust if required. The clearance angle should be set at 3-4 degree and angle of slope should be set permanently at 90 degrees. It is important to tighten the knife clamp screw securely, and block clamp screws most also be firm.

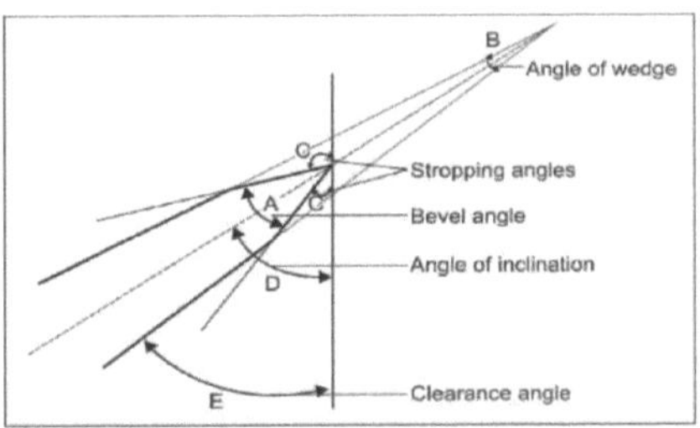

Move the block holder forward and upward until the paraffin wax is almost touching the knife edge Ensure, that the whole surface of the block will move parallel to the edge of the knife.

The exposed ends of the knife must all the times be protected by magnetic or clip on knife guards to avoid any accidents.

Trimming of tissue block:

Move the block forward until the wax block is almost touching the knife. To trim away any surplus wax and to expose a suitable area of tissue for sectioning, the section thickness during trimming is set at 10-30 micrometers according to the sample size.

Cutting (sectioning):

After exposing a suitable area of tissue, the section thickness is set to the appropriate level for routine purposes to 4-6 micrometers. Apply ice to the surface of the block for a few seconds and wipe the surface of the block free of water. This step is optional, but makes sections cut easily.

Ensure that the whole surface of the block will move parallel to the edge of the knife in order to ensure a straight ribbon of sections. The microtome is now moved in an easy rhythm, with the right hand operating the microtome and left hand holding the sections away from the knife. The ribbon is formed due to the slight heat generated during cutting, which causes the edges of the sections to adhere. If difficulty is experienced in forming the ribbon, it is sometimes overcome by rubbing one of the edges of the block with a finger.

During cutting, the paraffin wax embedded sections become slightly compressed and creased. Before being attached to slides, the creases must be removed and the section flattened. This is achieved by **floating** them on warm water. Thermostatically controlled water baths are now available with the inside coated black. These baths are controlled at a temperature 4-6°C below the melting point of paraffin wax. It is easy to see creases if the inside of the water bath is black.

The action of floating out must be smooth with the trailing end of the ribbon making contact with water first to obtain flat sections with correct orientation, floating out with the shiny surface towards the water is essential. When the ribbon has come to rest on water, the remaining wrinkles and folds are removed by using forceps or seeker.

Picking up sections:

The ribbon of sections floating on water is split into individual or groups of sections by use of forceps or seekers. Picking up a section of the slide is achieved by immersing the slide lightly smeared with adhesive vertically to three fourths of its length, bringing the section in contact with the slide. On lifting the slide vertically from the water, the section will flatten on to the slide. The sections are then blotted lightly with moistened blotting paper to remove excess water and to increase contact between section and slide. For delicate tissues or when several ribbons of sections are placed on the slide, omit the blotting, instead keep the slide in upright position for several minutes to drain.

Drying of the section:

Sections are then kept in an incubator with a temperature 5-6°C above the melting point of

wax, i.e. at 60°C for 20-60 minutes. It is better to overheat than under heat. If the sections are not well dried, they may come off during staining. The sections should not be allowed to dry without a good contact with the slide, such sections will come off during staining (S. Ramakrishnan & KN. Sulochana. 2012).

Methods of removing bubbles trapped beneath the sections:

Bubbles may get trapped under a section while in the tissue flotation bath, and must be removed before the section is picked on the slide, this may be done by place the sections on the slide and run 2% alcohol under them. Any fold or bubbles are removed.

Notes:

If sections fragment due to large amount of blood in tissue, the block should be coated with celloidin between sections. The surface of the block should be wiped dry, and painted with a camel hairbrush which has been dipped in 1% Celloidin. After allowing few seconds for the Celloidin to dry, a section is cut in the usual way. It must be remembered that when floating the sections to remove the creases, the celloidin layer must be uppermost, and the water should be a little hotter than usual to counteract the effect of celloidin. Following drying in the usual way, the celloidin is removed with equal parts of ether and alcohol before removing wax with xylene (www.rmsc.nic. 2015).

Serial sectioning may be needed to study the track of some structures or to find the extent of a lesion. Sections are collected from the very first cut that includes any tissue. Ribbons of ten 1-10, 11-20 and 21-30 and so on are picked up and mounted on the slides. Step sectioning is an alternative for serial sections and for the same reason sections are taken at periodic level through the block.

As mentioned earlier, the tissue to be sectioned must be properly fixed and processed in order to achieve an optimal microtomy product. But successful microtomy also depends on factors associated with instrumentation as well as the working environment. We have all heard the saying that "the microtome is rarely the cause of poor sections, unless it is old or damaged." Let us consider the following factors that affect microtomy:

- **Stable work surface to prevent microtome vibration:** The bench must be able to withstand the weight of the microtome and flotation bath, as well as the movement of the microtome during sectioning. Benches must be secured to the floor and/or wall. Microtomes should never be used on carts, card tables, or tables on wheels. Microtome vibration will introduce artifacts into the sections, causing undulations, chatter, and thick/thin sections.

- **Properly maintained microtome:** Although the microtome may rarely be the cause of poor sections, it should be the priority when it comes to maintenance and service. A broken microtome may be the cause of many sectioning problems and should be one of the first considerations during troubleshooting when problems arise.

  Debris can often collect on the upper or lower edges of your wax block. This build up can make obtaining cohesive wax ribbons difficult. So be sure to regularly clear away debris with a paint brush or similar tool.

- **All microtome parts are clamped down and finger tight to prevent vibration:** Vibration is the most common cause of undulations (wash boarding) in tissue sections. This includes the blade clamp, knife holder base, and knife tilt. Also, the block holder adjustments should be tightened properly to prevent the block from moving during sectioning. Tighten all microtome parts if wash boarding is grossly seen on tissue sections.

- **Proper knife tilt (clearance angle 3-8°) dependent on blade or knife used:** Once the optimal knife tilt is obtained, this adjustment should rarely if ever be changed.

- **Nick-free blade or knife:** A new blade should be used after blocks have been faced. Also, tissue that is calcified or has a lot of hair will reduce the life of a blade tremendously. A blade should be changed as soon as streaks or tears are noticed in tissue sections on the flotation bath.

- **Consistent cutting speed (one revolution per second):** Faster cutting may introduce artifacts such as undulations (wash boarding) or thick and thin sections, while slower cutting may allow the tissue block to expand and create thick and thin sections. The same cutting speed should be used for all sections in one ribbon, or tissue sections will vary in thickness and sections may not form a complete ribbon. Do not ever stop and start a cut mid-way through a section. If you are new to sectioning, it is advisable that you spend some time developing your sectioning rhythm on practice blocks before attempting to cut valuable tissue.

- **Clean water bath at proper temperature (5-10° C below melting point of paraffin):** Use distilled water free of microbes and check the water temperature at least once per day. Floating sections on water helps remove wrinkles and allows for easy sorting. After briefly floating, place the sections onto microscope slides and then dry. Drying is best done at 37°C overnight.

  Note: Do not float sections any longer than needed to remove their wrinkled, as longer time may affect morphology.

- **Properly fixed, processed, and embedded blocks:** If any of these pre-microtomy steps are suboptimal, the final product may be compromised and the diagnosis may not be attained. In under-fixed and under-processed tissue, it may be difficult to get a complete section. Tissue that is not embedded completely flat or at the proper orientation will not allow the microtomist to cut a complete and representative section for diagnosis.
- **Chilled and hydrated blocks:** Most tissue samples are over-dehydrated and can benefit from ice-water. Trays of ice covered with distilled water cool the paraffin and tissue to make microtomy easier, especially in warm climates. It is not recommended that blocks be placed in the freezer, since the paraffin and tissue can crack. Freezing blocks will introduce artifacts to tissue sections. Blocks that have calcium deposits should have the exposed block surface decalcified prior to sectioning.
- **Work environment:** A room that is not too cold, hot, humid, or drafty is best. Although this ideal environment is difficult to find in most laboratories in Sudan, measures should be taken to prevent temperature extremes (+20 °C), as well as drafts. The room temperature controller can be used to control the cooling in an individual room. With only an approx 0.5 Kelvin switching temperature differential, it makes exact temperature setting possible between +5 °C and +30 °C. If necessary, a time clock can be connected for time-controlled changing over from day to night temperature.
- **Coordination of microtomist:** This skill takes patience and practice.

It is advisable to use an adhesive media to promote tissue attachment to the glass slides used in histological preparation. This is routinely achieved by the application of a smear of glycerin/albumen mixture to the slide before the section is mounted and dried. However, this does not always provide a strong enough bond and the section may become detached from the slide during the staining procedure. Sections mounted on slides coated by one of the following methods are much more likely to remain attached during the more "aggressive" histological techniques. It should be noted that gelatin gives a positive reaction with some methods and poly-l-lysine is expensive hence the routine use of glycerin/albumen. For very fragile sections and some methods, it may be necessary to coat the slide with a protective film of celloidin. There are occasions when sections may detach from the slide and using of adhesive media may be obligatory:

- Exposure to strong alkali solutions during staining.
- Cryostat sections for immunofluorescence, immunohistochemistry or intra-operative consultation.
- Central nervous system (CNS) tissues.
- Sections that are submitted to extreme temperatures.
- Tissues containing blood and decalcified tissues.

Preparation of *POLY - L - LYSINE* coated slides:

1. Put the slides in racks and wash thoroughly in soapy water, rinse in tap water and finally rinse in distilled water.
2. Dilute poly - l - lysine 1:10 in distilled water or allow previously prepared solution to reach room temperature. (See 5.)
3. Place racks of slides in the solution for 5 minutes.
4. Drain slide racks on blotting paper and either dry at 60oC for 1 hour (use photographic drying cabinet), or leave to dry for 18 hours at room temperature covered with foil to keep off dust.

5. Filter the used poly - 1 - lysine solution and store at 4C° for future use. (It is stable for several months. Discard the solution upon any sign of mould growth). Bring to room temperature before use.

Preparation of **GELATIN** slides:

1. Put the slides in rack and wash thoroughly in soapy water, rinse in tap water and finally rinse in distilled water.
2. Immerse the slide rack in hot gelatin solution (0.5% gelatin in distilled water at 60-80°C). Leave for a few seconds for slides to warm up.
3. Drain the slide rack on blotting paper and remove excess gelatin solution by tipping the rack and allowing it to run off the slides.
4. Dry overnight at 37°C.
5. Store at room temperature.

3-aminopropyl triethoxysilane (AES) slides:

1. Put the slides in rack and wash thoroughly in soapy water, rinse in tap water and finally rinse in distilled water.
2. Allow the slides to dry completely.
3. Prepare a 2% solution of *3-aminopropyltriethoxysilane* (AES) in acetone in a dry staining dish.
4. Immerse the slides in the AES solution for 2 minutes.
5. Rinse the slides in two changes of distilled water.
6. Dry the slides at 37°C for 2 hours.
7. Slides may be stored at room temperature.

Note: AES slides can often be used in place of poly-l-lysine treated slides and are less expensive to prepare.

Charged or plus slides:

Laboratories often use slides that have been manufactured with a permanent positive charge. Placing a positive charge on the slides is accomplished by coating the slide with a basic polymer in which a chemical reaction occurs, leaving the amino groups linked by covalent bonds to the silicon atoms of the glass. These slides have proven to be superior in their resistance to cell and tissue loss during staining or pre-treatments such as enzyme and antigen retrieval (immunohistochemistry).

Cellodinization of sections:

1. Prepare a 1% solution of celloidin in a mixture of equal parts of ethanol and ether.
2. Dewax the sections and rinse in alcohol.
3. Place the slides in a coplin jar of the celloidin solution and leave for 5 minutes.
4. Remove the slides; wipe the backs to remove excess celloidin and place immediately in 80% alcohol for 5 minutes.
5. Rinse briefly in water and continue with the chosen technique.

The celloidin film will slowly dissolve in the dehydrating alcohol step at the end of the method. If the film proves difficult to remove, use a mixture of equal parts of ethanol and ether.

Troubleshooting for poor sections (summary) (Bancroft & Gamble. 2002).		
Faults in cutting		
Faulty	**The causes**	**Remedy**
Tear or scratch across the section or splitting of ribbon.	Jagged knife edge. Dirt or hair on knife edge.	Sharpen the knife. Clean the knife.
Tear or scratch across part of section.	Calcium, Carbon, or Suture etc., in the tissue or wax.	Examine block under magnifying glass. If calcium is present, decalcify block. Remove suture

		from the tissue with scalpel point. If dust is in wax Re-embed.
Holes in the section.	Air bubbles in the tissue or wax. A piece of hard material in tissue. A soft piece of tissue in block.	Re-embed. Remove hard material if possible. Reprocess specimen.
Cracks across the section parallel to knife.	A blunt knife. Knife tilt too small. Block too hard for thickness of specimen.	Sharpen knife. Adjust tilt. Warm block slightly or re-embed in soft wax.
Section shows thin and thick horizontal lines (chatters).	A loose knife. A loose block. A blunt knife. Extremely hard tissue	Tighten knife and/or block. Sharpen the knife. Soften the tissue if possible or rembed in harden wax.
Section cut thick and thin alternatively.	Knife tilt is too great and is compressing the block.	Adjust tilt.
Section compress at one end.	Blunt spot on the knife. A soft spot in the wax, due to presence of clearing agent.	Move block along the knife or sharp knife. Re infiltrate tissue and re-embed
Section curves to one end.	Edge of block is not parallel to knife. A dull spot on knife.	Trim edges. Move block along knife or sharpen knife.
Sections curl as they are cut.	Blunt knife. Sections too thick. Too much tilt to knife.	Sharpen knife. Adjust microtome. Correct the tilt.
Sections lift from knife on upward travel of block.	Blunt knife Too much tilt to knife. A build up of wax debris behind knife. A greasy knife.	Sharpen knife. Correct the tilt. Clean the knife
Knife bites deeply into block.	A loose knife. A loose block	Tighten the knife and block
The block no longer feeds towards knife.	Forward feed mechanism had expired	Release the safety locking catch, man back off feed mechanism and readjust knife holder
Sections crumble on cutting. .	Knife is blunt. Wax is too soft; has crystallized due to slow cooling or contamination with water or clearing agent. Defective processing e.g. incomplete fixation, dehydration, clearing or embedding.	Sharpen knife. Re-embed and block with fresh wax. Reprocess
Failure of block to ribbon.	Block not parallel to ribbon. Paraffin too hard. Knife tilted too much. Sections too thick.	Correct the alignment. Re-embed. Correct the tilt. Adjust the section thickness.

Faults due to poor processing		
Faulty	**The causes**	**Remedy**
The tissue is shrunken away from wax:	Insufficient dehydration.	Reprocess.
The tissue is too soft when block is	Insufficient fixation.	Reprocess.

trimmed.		
Specimen crumbles and drops out of the wax leaving a rim of wax as a section.	Insufficient infiltration. Overheated paraffin bath causing tissue to become hard and brittle.	Reinfiltrate and re-embed. Service the paraffin bath.
Tissue is dried out or mummified.	Mechanical failure of tissue processing machine or a basket was out of balance and hung up.	Place the specimen in the following rehydration solution for 18-24 hrs. Sodium Carbonate - 1.0 gm Dist. Water - 70.0 ml Absolute ethyl alcohol - 30.0 ml. Rehydrate the reprocess.

Further readings:

- Bancroft J D and Gamble M. Theory and practice of histological technique, fifth edition, Churchill living stone, London 2002.
- Drury R B and Wallington E A. Carleton Histological Techniques, fifth edition, Oxoford University press, London 1980.
- http://www.liquisearch.com/microtome/microtome_types/rotary_microtome.
- http://www.rmsc.nic.in/RHSDP%20Training%20Modules/Doc1.pdf..
- https://www.coursehero.com/file/11722332/Lesson-092).
- S Ramakrishnan &KN Sulochana. Manual of Medical Laboratory Techniques. JP Medical Ltd, 2012. Pp 394 – 400.

It is important to stain the tissue to see the different parts of the tissue components in contrasting color because if tissue examined directly after sectioning it will appear dull and uninteresting under microscope due to refractive index and color similarity between the fixed materials. Dyes are the most common way that done for staining. Hematoxylin and eosin is commonest routine contrasting stain in histology by which the nuclei stained by hematoxylin and cytoplasm with eosin. Also special stains other than H&E are use to impart color to specific tissue constituent.

Dye structure:

Dye is an organic ion or molecule that can absorb visible light (and so is seen as colored), that can attach to and impart color to other materials. Absorption of light is due to the chemical bonds forming an extended conjugated system.

Conjugated system:

It is a chain of atoms linked by alternating single and double covalent bonds in which spatial localization of all the bonding electrons is not possible. For instance, the benzene carbon skeleton is conventionally drawn as comprising three carbons–carbon single bonds plus three carbons–carbon double bonds. Because the double bonds are conjugated (alternating), all six bonds are identical, due to the delocalized π-electrons. Such delocalized electrons are mobile, and electrical influences are readily propagated from one part a conjugated molecule to another,   enhancing dipoles and polarizability, and favoring van der Waals forces.

Color production

Dyes have a conjugated system in its molecular structure, so the energy difference between the bonding and antibonding molecular orbitals is large enough to allow absorption in the visible spectrum then the dyes will be colored.

Dye nomenclature:

The Colour Index (CI) contains information on a wide range of dyes concerned with industrial dyeing. It was set up in an attempt to overcome all the confusion related with dyes naming. It introduced by the Society of Dyers and Colourists and the American Association of Textile Chemists and Colorists. In the color index the dyes are arranged according to their structure, with the most important feature being their chromophoric group and designated by a 5-digit number, C.I. number and specially constructed name. For example, CI 26125 or Solvent red 27 is the dye commonly known as oil red O.

Classification of stains

- *Depending on applications:*

Fluorescent probes:

This is coloring of living tissues either by using dissociation in staining fluid (supravital) or by injection of the dye into the living organism (intravital). Vital stains demonstrate cytoplasmic structure only through phagocytosis, thus staining of nucleus indicate cell death.

Lysochrome:

Stain is soluble in tissue fluids. Aqueous stains are unsuitable because water is widely distributed through cells and the staining would be too diffuse. Lysochromes are lipid-soluble, so they used in histology for demonstration of lipids.

Histochemical:

The stain chemically reacts with tissue components to produce coloured substance, either true dye such as (PAS) or coloured chemical products that are not dye as in Perls Prussian Blue reaction and enzyme histochemical reaction.

Metallic impregnation:

The commonest metal to use in light microscopy is silver, which produces a dense, black, fine deposit of silver and silver oxide where the silver ions have been reduced. Silver impregnation can be described as:

The argentaffin reaction:

In the argentaffin reaction, the tissue contains reducing groups that are sufficiently strong and present in sufficient quantity to give a visible deposit without added reducing agents.

The argyrophil reaction:

Some tissue groups are able to absorb silver, but small amounts are reduced to silver atoms. These silver atoms are too small to be visible, so the external reducer e.g. formaldehyde is required to produce visible black deposit.

Immunofluorescent:

More than one molecule of a fluorochrome (a dye or other stain exhibiting fluorescence when present in solution, cells or tissues, e.g., (acridine orange) can be conjugated with an antibody molecule. The resulting emitted light stands out against a dark unstained background. Absorption and emission spectra of different fluorochromes are exploited when two or more labeled antibodies are applied to the same preparation.

Immunostaining

This utilizes antibody-antigen rection in which a labelled antibody to be visualized at site of reaction. Now, immunohistochemistry is one of most popular diagnostic tools in histopatholgy.

- ***Depending on tissue affinity***

Acid dye

It is a dye in which the colored component is an anion, e.g. Congo red and eosin Y.

Basic dye

It is a dye with a cationic colored component, e.g. alcian blue, hemalum, or neutral red.

Neutral dye

It is an old name for an ionic dye whose anion and cation are both themselves colored dyes. Romanowsky stains provide an example, in which one key component is an azure B cation and the other is an eosin Y anion.

Amphoteric dye

Amphoteric describes a compound which can act as an acid (and donate protons) or a base (and accept protons) depending on the pH of the local environment. Amphoteric dyes exist in multiple ionic forms, e.g. neutral red has both cationic and non-ionic species, where as rhodamine B has cationic and zwitter ionic species. pH indicators are amphoteric dyes whose different ionic species are of markedly different colors; examples include indicators used to check the pH of solutions (e.g., indigocarmine) and those used for vital staining to assess the pH of cellular compartments (e.g., Carboxy-SNARF 1).

- *Depending on the source of stain*

Natural dyes

It is a dye, or dye precursor, synthesized by a plant or animal. Examples include hematoxylin from the logwood tree Haematoxylum campechianum and carminic acid from the cochineal insect Coccus cacti.

Hematoxylin is a phenolic compound extracted from logwood (Haematoxylum campechianum L.), a tree originally from Central America, now growing in many tropical and subtropical regions. The name "hematoxylin" is commonly applied to solutions for which hemalum would be more appropriate; examples are Delafield's hematoxylin, Gill hematoxylin, Harris hematoxylin.

Carminic acid is a red anthraquinone natural dye derived from cochineal, which can form metal coordination complexes. Some of these, especially with aluminum or iron, are used as biological stains, in particular for chromosomes.

Synthetic dyes

It is a colorant synthesized by humans, from organic precursor compounds derived originally from coal tar, but currently from crude petroleum. Synthetic dyes are subclassification based on the structure of chromophoric systems into:

Azo dyes: These dyes contain $-N=N-$ chromophore group. Many of the azo dyes used as microscopic stains are acid dyes like orange G and Congo red.

Nitro dyes: They have the nitro group $-NO_2$ chromophore, e.g. picric acid, martius yellow.

Thiazine dyes: These have $-C-N=C-$ and $-C-S=C$ chromophore group. This group contains important metachromatic dyes, like toluidine blue and methylene blue.

Diphenylmethanes: They contain $-NH$ chromophore group, such as auramine.

Triphenylmethanes: they have $=N-$ chromophore group, like light green and malachite green.

Azin dyes: These dyes contain $C-O=C$ and $C-N=C$ chromophore. Celestine blue and Nile blue sulphate are examples.

Xanthenes: The planar skeleton of the oxygen containing heterocyclic compound xanthene is chromophore of these dyes as eosin and xanthene.

Acridine: dyes the structure of acridine resembles that of xanthene except that the heteroatom is nitrogen instead of oxygen.R. Example: acridine orange.

Oxazine dyes: They contain $C-O=C$ chromophore group. Most oxazine dyes used in biology or medicine are either colored cations or metal-binding phenolic compounds such as cresyl violet and Celestine blue.

Anthraquinone dyes: These dyes are containing anthraquinonethe ring in middle of the three fused rings like carminic acid.

Mechanism of staining

We shall discuss below theory of mechanism of staining. First, however, it is important to look at the chemical bonding (attractive forces or intermolecular atrractions) involved between the dye and tissue components as follows:

Ionic bonds

These are the most important form of bonds in histological staining. Ionic bonds occur due to electrostatic attraction between oppositely charged ions present in the tissues and in the dye. So-called acid dyes are negatively charged (i.e. are anions) whilst so-called basic dyes are positively charged (i.e. anions). Acid dyes will therefore preferentially bind with tissue components containing positive charges (e.g. proteins at low pH) while basic dyes bind preferentially to tissue sites with negatively charged entities such as nucleic acids and glycosaminoglycans.

Hydrogen bonds

Hydrogen bonds are weak bonds only form if the two interacting groups are brought sufficiently close together. They are form between a hydrogen atom in one molecule and a small atom of high electronegativity (O, N or F.) in another molecule. Hydrogen bonds are not affected by pH or salt concentration, but are affected by urea and water. They are important in amyloid staining by congo red.

Van der Waals forces

They are weak force, and can act only between molecules that are very close together. They occur in molecules that contain dipoles or induced dipoles, which later defined as a molecule or an atom have uneven distribution of charge across it. Van Der Waals forces are divided into three types:
- **Dipole-dipole forces (Keesom forces):** which are between dipoles and dipoles.
- **Dipole-induced dipole forces (Debye forces):** which exist between dipoles and induced dipoles.
- **Dispersion forces (London forces):** which present between induced dipoles and induced dipoles.

Covalent bonds

They are very strong bonds in which two electrically neutral atoms share an electron with each other to satisfy the outer shell's required number. They are stable bonds so, cannot be washed out of a section or not easily broken once formed. Furthermore, they are important in some histochemical techniques like Feulgen reaction.

Hydrophobic bonding

This describes the tendency of hydrophobic molecules or groupings originally dispersed within an aqueous environment to come together. Phenomena driven by hydrophobic bonding include folding of polypeptide chains, where hydrophobic amino acid residues come together in the core of the protein; and the use of a hydrophobic dye to stain a hydrophobic tissue substrate such as suberin or lipid.

The chemical bonding that we have described above may individually be too weak. The actual bonding that causing the true stable coloring may be result of a combination of these bonds together. In addition to physical properties of dye and tissue can also contribute to accumulation of dye in tissue sites.

Throughout the history of dyeing, there have been opposing theories on its mechanism. One is the physical theory which depends upon simple solubility like fat stains for lipids (lipids are more soluble in the 70% alcohol or other solvent in which it may be dissolved) and adsorption phenomenon (a large body attracts to itself minute particles from a surrounding media). The other is the chemical theories in which a radical of dye binds to the pertinent chemical substance of the tissue. Acid dyeing is the uptake of the anion of an acid dye (A dye in which the colored component is an anion, e.g. Congo red and eosin Y) into those cell and tissue structures. Where biopolymers that are cationic predominate, typically proteins. These are cationic if acid dyeing is carried out at low pH, when amines are present as NH_3^+ and carboxylic acids as non-ionized free acids (i.e. $-COOH$) while Basic dyeing is the uptake of the cation of a basic dye (A dye with a cationic colored component, e.g. alcian blue, hemalum, or neutral red.) into those cell and tissue structures where biopolymers which are anionic predominate. These biopolymers are most commonly DNA and RNA (with phosphate anions), or glycosaminoglycans and polysaccharides (with sulfate anions and, at higher pH, carboxylate anions). Between these two theories Mann (1902) and Conn (1925) take a much broader view of the whole staining mechanism, and they include both physical and chemical forces of bonding which assumely known as dye-tissue attractive forces.

The attractive forces for long time considered as the only main sources of tissue staining until Horobin (1982,1988) changed this concept to include the total staining system (solvent-dye-tissue).

Stain-tissue interactions:
- Ionic bonding
- Hydrogen bonding
- Covalent bonding
- Van der Waals forces
Solvent-solvent interaction:
The hydrophobic effect
Stain-stain interaction:
The metachromatic reaction.

Metachromasia:

Metachromasia is a staining phenomenon when the tissue is stained in different colours from the original dye colour. Many of the metachromatic dyes used in microscopic staining are thiazines while Substances like mucins, especially the sulphated mucins can be stained in this metachromatic way are called chromotropes.

This phenomenon occurs as a resuilt of dye polymerization due to the ionic binding of the cationic dye molecules with tissue polyanions and van der Waals force between the nonpolar aromatic rings of the dye. The depolymerization of dye causes colour absorption shifts to shorter wavelengths, leaving only the longer wavelengths to be seen.

The degree of polymerization (monomer, dimer, trimer and polymer) increases the metachromasia reaction as seen in thiazine dyes:
- The monomeric form (alpha): the color blue remains the same.
- The di, and trimeric form (beta): the dye gives purple color.
- The polymeric form (gamma): the dye produces red color.
-

Direct and indirect staining

Direct staining
The dye stains tissue directly when placed in its simple or alcoholic solution, such as methylene blue.

Indirect staining
Some dyes utilize an intermediate substance called a mordant to link with tissue, like hematoxylin.

Mordants
Mordants are the salt of the divalent and trivalent metals that able to mediate a dye–tissue interaction. The mordant combines with the dye by covalent or co-ordinate bonding known as dye lake. Oxygen containing (e.g. in phenols, carboxyls and quinones) or nitrogen containing (in amine, azo and nitro groups) are mainly groups on the dye that forming the dye lake. Sulfate of alumminium, iron and chromium are most often salts that used in histological stains. Sometimes the mordant can be applied before dye is used (pre-mordanting), sometimes it is mixed with dye (meta-mordanting) or sometimes applied after dye (post-mordanting).

Progressive and Regressive Staining

Progressive staining

The dye is allowed to interact with the target tissue structure until the desired density of colour is reached. This type of staining needs checks at frequent intervals to prevent overstaining or to have light staining and influences by pH of the dye solution, thickness of tissue, concentration of dye, etc.

Regressive staining

This involves the staining of all or most tissue components, with stain then removed by differentiation process from some tissue elements, leaving the "target" entities stained.

Differentiation

It is procedure by which the dye removing from undesired tissue in regressive staining. It carries out by Acid in basic dye or base in acid dye, like 1% acid alcohol.

Accentuators

Accentuators are generally simply used to control pH, e.g. potassium hydroxide in Löffler's methylene blue and phenol in carbol fuchsin. They are neither form any dye lake nor take part in any chemical reaction.

Accelerators

When an accentuators used in neurological techniques it has known as Accelerators like veronal buffer in Cajal method for axis cylinders and chloral hydrate in Cajal method for motors end-plates.

Trapping agenta

A trapping agent prevents the escape of dye that entered the tissue entity. For example, the use of iodine to trap the violet dye inside the relatively impermeable wall of gram positive bacteria, whilst it can be removed from the more permeable gram negative bacteria.

Further reading:

Baker, J.R. (1958). Principles of Biological Microtechnique. London: Methuen.
Conn, H. J.(1925). Biological Stains. The Williams and Wilkins Company, Baltimore, Md.
Horobin, R.W. (1980). Structure–staining relationships in histochemistry and biological staining. I. Theoretical background and a general account of correlation of histochemical staining with the chemical structure of the reagents used. Journal of Microscopy119: 345–355.
Horobin, R.W. (1982). Histochemistry: An Explanatory Outline of Histochemistry and Biophysical Staining.Stuttgart: Gustav Fischer.
Horobin, R.W. (1988). Understanding Histochemistry: Selection, Evaluation and Design of Biological Stains.Chichester: Ellis Horwood.
Kiernan, J.A. (2015) Histological and Histochemical Methods: Theory and Practice. 5th edition, Scion Publishing.
Mann, G. (1902). Physiological Histology. Methods and Theory. Oxford: Clarendon Press.

STAINING PROCEDURE

The most common method of histological study is to prepare thin sections (3-5 micron) from paraffin embedded tissues. These are then suitably stained and mounted in a medium of proper refractive index for study and storage. Commonest mountants used are resinous substances of refractive index close to that of glass. These are soluble in xylene. Hence sections are dehydrated and cleared in xylene and mounted. Mounting in aqueous mounting media is done directly after staining for sections which cannot be subjected to dehydrating and clearing agents. The basic steps in staining and mounting paraffin sections are as follows:

- Deparaffinization.
- Hydration.
- Removal of mercury pigments wherever needed.
- Staining.
- Dehydration and clearing.
- Mounting.

Deparaffinization:

Removal of wax is done with xylene. It is essential to remove the wax completely; otherwise subsequent stages will not be possible. At least 2 to 3 changes in xylene are given for suitable length of time. Sections of this stage should appear clear and transparent. Presence of any patches indicates the presence of wax and sections should be kept longer in the xylene.

Hydration:

Most of the stains used are aqueous or dilute alcoholic solutions. Hence it is essential to bring the section to water before the stains are applied. The hydration is done with graded alcohols from higher concentration to lower concentration. Alcohol and acetone are miscible with xylene. First change is made to absolute alcohol or acetone followed by 90%, 70% alcohol and finally distilled water. Sections now should appear opaque. Presence of any clear areas is indicative of the presence of xylene. To remove this xylene sections should be returned to absolute alcohol and rehydrated.

Removal of mercury pigments whenever needed:

In case mercury containing fixatives e.g. Zenker, Susa etc are used, mercury pigments are precipitated on the sections. It has to be removed before staining is done. This is brought about by treatment with iodine solutions which changes mercury to an iodine compound. This in turn is converted to tetrathionate by thiosulphate, which is readily soluble in water. The slides are placed in running water to wash out all extraneous chemicals.

Staining:

Various staining procedures are applied from this hydrated stage. The most common stain applied for histological study is Hematoxylin and Eosin. Various types of hematoxylin formulations are used, certain of these stains use strong chemicals e.g. ammonia. Sections tend to float off the slides in such stains. This can be prevented by coating the sections by a thin layer of celloidin. For this sections are returned to absolute alcohol and then dipped in a dilute solution of celloidin and finally hardened in 70% alcohol. Washing and rinsing of tissue sections is a necessary part of most staining techniques. It eliminates carrying over of one dye solution to the next. Excess dye, mordants, or other reagents might react unfavorably or precipitate when placed in the fluid employed in the next step. Alum Hematoxylin stains nuclei and red color, which is converted to blue black color, when the section is washed in weak alkaline tap water.There are many formulations for preparing hematoxylin stains. Use of many is a matter of personal preference of whether progressive or regressive staining is being used. In situations where hematoxylin staining is followed by acidic stains, Iron hematoxylin is preferred as it resists decolourization by these counter stains. Various formulations differ mainly in regards to mordant and the shorter oxidizer used.

Dehydration and clearing:

Dehydration is done is graded alcohols or acetones from 70% to absolute alcohol or acetone. Dehydrating alcohol and acetones can remove some of the stains. Time has to be suitably modified to minimize fading of stains. Since alcohol and acetone are miscible in xylene, it is used for clearing the sections. Any sections from which water has not been completely removed would give a milky appearance after the first xylene. Such sections should be returned to absolute alcohol and the process repeated. Mounting is done after 2nd or 3rd xylene.

Cover slipping and mounting:

Make quite sure that the sections are quite clear. Do not let the section go dry before mounting.
- Hold the slide between the thumb and the forefinger of one hand and wipe with a clean cloth both ends of the slides. Look for the engraved number to make sure the side the sections are present.
- Clean carefully around the section and lay on a clean blotting paper with section up-

permost along with appropriate coverslip which has already been polished.
- Place a drop of mountant on the slide over coverslip. Amount of mountant should be just enough. Invert the slide over the coverslip and lower it so that it just adheres to the cover slip quickly turn the slide over, then lay it on a flat surface to allow the mountant to spread. Do not press or push the slide at all. It can damage the section.
- After the mountant has spread to the edge of the coverslip wipe around it for neatness. If proper care has been taken there should be no air bubbles. If many are present, slide should be returned to the xylene to remove the coverslip. It will slip off and remounting is done. No attempt should be made to pull the coverslip. Slight warming of the slide from below will make the small air bubbles to escape from the slide of the coverslip. Coverslip should be in the center of the slide with neatly written label on one slide.
- A good knowledge of various mountants and the coverslips is necessary for proper selection of the procedure (Cook, DJ. 2006).

- Preparation date must be written on all bottles.
- Keep all stains and solutions covered when are not in use.
- After the slides are removed from oven should be cooled before being put in xylene.
- Filter all stains before use.
- Once the slides have been put in the xylene to remove paraffin they should not be allowed to dry out. Particular care must be taken not to let the sections dry at the time of mounting as the xylene easily evaporates and if the section dried be-

fore mounting preparation would become useless.

- Care should be taken that level of any solution used during staining is such as to cover the slides.
- Drain the slides well and blot the bottom on filter paper before putting into the next solution. This is particularly necessary in transferring from 95% to absolute alcohol and absolute alcohol to xylene.
- If bluing is done by alkali *e.g.* ammonia, it should be well washed out. Failure to do that will lead to disagreeably hazy blue colour of nuclei.
- Xylene used to remove paraffin should not get mixed up with the clearing xylene. It also should be frequently changed as it tends to get saturated.

AUTOMATED STAINING SYSTEM:

Automated processing of tissues is widely accepted and a similar automation is possible with staining. The same general principles apply to both situations. Automation frees staff from a routine task that is relatively straightforward and allows them to do more demanding tasks. The use of an absolutely regular procedure ensures that there is little variation in results, so that direct comparisons are valid from one batch of stained sections to the next. This accuracy and reproducibility are crucial in some applications such as diagnostic and exfoliative cytology where the colour of the cytoplasm is an important diagnostic feature.

The disadvantage is that there is less flexibility. All of the sections will be given the same treatment, regardless of their requirements. It is also only feasible for techniques that are carried out for a large number of samples.

Machines are fine for doing hundreds of haematoxylin and eosin stains, but it is not reasonable to use a machine for stains where the technique is only required for two or three slides each day.

It also does not lend itself to situations where different results are needed; for example, when photographing at low magnifications, an over stained section will give better results than the usual staining intensity. An ordinary stain will give insufficient contrast for the film's recording capabilities but a more-intense stain will give stronger differences between the tissue components.

Automated staining also demands reproducible reagents. If there is a change in a reagent's staining properties, the machine will not recognize this and compensate for the change in the way that a person would. Most histologists can easily compensate for gradual changes in reagents as they age or for sudden alterations from a new batch of stain without too many problems. Machines only follow the program and cannot tell that there is any need to change. Any alterations result in machines needing to be reprogrammed, for example, if a different batch of reagent is prepared. This inflexibility may also result in reagents being discarded sooner than they would be for manual staining in order to maintain a standard program. Automated staining machines are also less flexible in producing single stains, even when they are already programmed for that stain. Thus, producing a single slide may hold up some types of machine; these machines must go through the full cycle before another section can even begin since the steps are uneven. These machines are inefficient for staining single sections.

An alternative strategy is to have all the steps the same length (e.g. 1 min) so that sections can be added at any time and will follow the same path.

The difficulty here is that, if a longer time is needed, then several baths of the same reagent are required. These machines often cannot cope with large numbers of sections in a short space of time. Automated staining machines are very useful for absolute regularity with large numbers of sections needing the same treatment at the same time. They have found a significant role in two main areas:

1. Haematoxylin and eosin staining in histology, Papanicolaou staining in cytology and blood-film staining in haematology. This is because the sheer numbers needing staining make it worthwhile.

2. Immunohistochemistry, nucleic acid hybridization and similar techniques. Here the actual numbers are smaller but the need for absolute consistency is greater, so these techniques have moved to more automation. The use of automatic coverslipping machines is often linked to automated staining. The process of mounting sections is very mundane, so automation is possible. There are fewer requirements for variety in mounting, so provided they are working well these machines are a useful addition to the laboratory (Cook, DJ. 2006).

MAOUNTANTS:

The mounting medium should have a high refractive index (RI). Most tissues have an RI of between 1.5 and 1.55, so a mounting medium with an RI in this range will give maximum clarity. There is no single mounting medium that is suitable for all specimens and stains. There are two major types of mounting media used and the difference is in the solvent. The commonest types are the *resinous mounting* media, which are based on hydrophobic organic solvents, usually xylene, and which need the section to be dehydrated and cleared before mounting. Water-based (*Aqueous*) mounting media will accept tissues straight from distilled water and are used when a xylene based medium would not be appropriate, e.g. if the dye or histochemical reaction product is soluble in xylene.

The properties that need to be considered in a mounting medium are:

. Refractive index: If the RI is much lower than 1.5, then tissues will not be completely transparent and diffraction will occur. This is usually a disadvantage as it reduces clarity but it can sometimes be an advantage as it will give some contrast to even unstained tissues.

. Clarity under normal conditions of use. Some media can become opaque as they dry out and are not suitable for long-term preservation.

. Effects on the stain itself: Some mounting media will cause fading. This is most common with acidic mounting materials, which will cause significant fading, especially in the light. Some media may also act as solvents for the dyes and as a consequence the dye diffuses or leaches out into the mountant. This will gradually obscure the tissues.

. Fluorescence: This is really only critical for fluorescence microscopy but it is generally a useful characteristic for a general mounting medium since it eliminates the need to use a special mountant when fluorescence is being used.

. Setting: The ability of a mountant to dry or set quickly and hold the coverslip in place is very useful. Many aqueous-based media fail to harden sufficiently and the coverslip will need 'ringing' to preserve the section (Cook, DJ. 2006).

.

Resinous mounting media:

Canada balsam:

This was the original resinous mounting medium used in histology. Canada balsam is derived from the *Abies balsamea* fir tree and is available as a dried, brittle, yellow solid. It will melt at high temperature and is soluble in xylene. Approximately 60 g in 100 ml of xylene gives a good working mountant, although it takes a few days to dissolve completely. The yellow colour of the mountant hardly seems to matter when viewed through the microscope. The mountant is usually significantly acid and will cause fading, especially of basic dyes. It is relatively expensive and is mainly of historical importance rather than being a common mountant.

DPX and BPS:

DPX (Distrene, Plasticiser, Xylene) and **BPS** (Butylphthalate Plasticised Styrene) are two synthetic mounting media based on polystyrene. *Distrene* is a trade name for the polystyrene produced by the Distrene Company. Polystyrene is a common plastic used to make foam cups, packing material, plastic cutlery *etc*. By itself, polystyrene is not elastic enough and requires a plasticiser to make it usable as a mounting medium. In DPX the plasticiser is tricresyl phosphate, and in BPS the plasticiser is dibutylphthalate, which the authors considered to be more effective than tricresyl phosphate.

These two mounting media have been extensively used and have proven themselves as very suitable replacements for Canada balsam. They have the further advantage that excess mounting medium may be stripped from slides very easily once the medium has dried. Simply cut around the coverslip with a scalpel blade, and then gently lift the excess medium from the glass. It will easily peel away.

Kirkpatrick and Lendrum specified a particular polystyrene for DPX, Distrene-80, which has a molecular weight of about 80,000. Due to commercial changes in manufacture and distribution, they specified Dow Chemical Company's *Natural Styron 686E*. The same product has been sold in the UK by the name *Styron 27/66-7* (1972) and, by a different distributor, *Polystyrene SA99/W Crystal* (1977). When DPX is ordered, BPS may be supplied as little distinction is made in practice.

To make any of the three variations of DPX, mix the plasticiser and xylene together then add the polystyrene. Mix periodically until completely dissolved and of consistent viscosity. Adjust the viscosity if necessary by adding xylene to make thinner or by evaporation of the xylene to make thicker. The concentrations of polystyrene and plasticiser vary a little in formulas given by various authors.

<table>
<tr><td colspan="3">DPX, Kirkpatrick and Lendrum (1939)</td></tr>
<tr><td>Polystyrene</td><td>10</td><td>g</td></tr>
<tr><td>Xylene</td><td>80</td><td>mL</td></tr>
<tr><td>Tricresyl phosphate</td><td>15</td><td>mL</td></tr>
<tr><td colspan="3">• Distrene-80 MW about 80,000 was specified.</td></tr>
</table>

<table>
<tr><td colspan="3">BPS, Kirkpatrick and Lendrum (1941)</td></tr>
<tr><td>Polystyrene</td><td>20</td><td>g</td></tr>
<tr><td>Xylene</td><td>70</td><td>mL</td></tr>
<tr><td>Dibutylphthalate</td><td>10</td><td>mL</td></tr>
<tr><td colspan="3">• Distrene-80 MW about 80,000 was specified.</td></tr>
</table>

<table>
<tr><td colspan="3">BPS, Lendrum's recommendation (1972, 1977)</td></tr>
<tr><td>Polystyrene</td><td>24</td><td>g</td></tr>
<tr><td>Xylene</td><td>80</td><td>mL</td></tr>
<tr><td>Dibutylphthalate</td><td>8</td><td>mL</td></tr>
<tr><td colspan="3">• Dow Chemical's Natural Styron 686E, also known as Polystyrene SA99/W Crystal and Styron 27/66-7, was recommended as suitable.</td></tr>
</table>

Other resins:

Some other resins have also been recommended for use in mounting media, but it is sometimes difficult to be sure of what compound is meant. One such is "coumarone resin", a polymer of benzofuran. Other than that, little information is given with regard to the molecular weight, or whether a polymer of benzofuran and indene is meant. One such formula specifies the resin under a trade name of *Clarite* or *Nevillite I*, and suggests a 60% solution of the resin in xylene (Groat). Polyvinyl acetate has also been suggested. None of these resins have gained popularity.

Aqueous mounting media:

There is no fully satisfactory aqueous medium and several different ones are used for different purposes. They differ in the way in which the RI of water (1.33) is raised sufficiently to give a clear image. Most are best considered as temporary mounts and need ringing to hold the coverslip in place and prevent drying out. Tissues do not need any treatment before mounting and can be mounted directly from water or buffer.

Glycerol:

Glycerol is a trihydric alcohol with a high RI. It can be used alone or with the addition of a buffer to control the pH. It is a useful medium for fluorescent staining, for example, for immunofluorescent antibody techniques. The addition of *p*-phenylenediamine is said to retard the fading of fluorescence. It neither hardens nor dries out and is usually used as a very short-term mountant, although it can be ringed for slightly longer use (Cook, DJ. 2006).

Glycerol jelly:

This uses the addition of gelatin (up to 12% in some formulations) to allow the medium to set. The usual formulation has a lower RI (1.42) than most mounting media, so the clarity is reduced and some unstained structures will be visible. It is solid at room temperature and needs to be melted in a water bath before use. It is very easy to get air bubbles trapped in this medium, so it is convenient to melt it and get rid of any air bubbles by warming it in a vacuum-embedding oven. Glycerol jelly is quite a good growth medium for some bacteria and fungi, so there is usually an antibacterial addi-

tive (e.g. phenol), but it still does not keep well. Sections may also allow the growth of organisms in storage, so it is best thought of as a temporary mount.

Apathy's medium:

This uses a gum (gum arabic or gum acacia) and sucrose to raise the RI. It has an RI of around 1.5, so it can give nicely transparent preparations. It has a tendency to crystallize in storage and can set by drying but this is quite slow. Again, it may need the addition of an antibacterial agent to help preserve it.

Polyvinyl alcohol or polyvinylpyrollidone media:

These are synthetic and less liable to bacterial contamination than the organic-based mountants, although the addition of phenol is still advisable. They dissolve in water or buffer but need constant stirring. They solidify slowly by evaporation but specimens can be ringed to prevent this. These are more permanent than the other water-based mounting media, but are still not as good as a resinous medium.

Temporary mounts (ringing):

Ringing is the term used for sealing the edges of a coverslip when the mounting medium does not set. Ringing was originally so called because the coverslips were round and so there being a ring of the sealant round the coverslip. Ringing was done on a turntable to give a nice neat finish. Originally it used a gold size followed by a black asphaltum varnish. This produced a very neat finish and some commercial suppliers of prepared slides still finish many of their preparations in a similar way as it looks good. Most laboratories have dropped this and ringing is now just a temporary expedient rather than an aesthetic requirement.

Good temporary ringing can be achieved in a number of ways. Ordinary nail varnish works quite well and comes in a bottle with its own brush, which makes it convenient and simple. The only drawback is that it is dissolved in acetone, which may affect some materials, although I have never found this to be a problem. Many styrene-based types of cement can also be used and again are convenient as they come in tubes ready to squeeze out around the coverslip. Again the solvent is a theoretical problem but I have not had problems. These cements can often be semi-permanent. Paraffin wax can also be used. A piece of warmed metal (such as the flat end of a broad spatula) is used to apply a layer of molten wax, which immediately sets. Provided the slide is dry, this is quick and easy but is easily broken and will not store well (Cook, DJ. 2006).

Further reading:

- Baker, J.R. (1958). Principles of Biological Microtechnique. London: Methuen.
- Carson, F.L. (1997) Histotechnology. A Self-Instructional Text, 2nd edn. Chicago: American Society of Clinical Pathologists Press.
- Bancroft, J.D. and Gamble, M. (eds) (2008). *Theory and Practice of Histological Techniques*, 6th edn. London: Churchill-Livingstone.
- Cook, DJ. Cellular Pathology: An Introduction to Techniques and Applications, 2nd edition. Scion Publishing Ltd. July, 2006, chapter 6 Staining theory. pp68 – *103*.
- Drury R B and Wallington E A. Carleton Histological Techniques, fifth edition, Oxford University press, London 1980
-

Background:

Hematoxylin is the most important used dye in the medical laboratory, being able to differentiate malignant cells from non- malignant cells makes it an excellent tool in the diagnosis of diseases affecting tissues. Its ability to stain several intracellular and extracellular substances in shades of blue to black also makes it very useful in histochemistry and histopathology.

Hematoxylin

Hematoxylin is a natural dye extracted from the heartwood of the tree Haematoxylum campechianum, although histotechnologists are more familiar with the name as Hematoxylon campechianum. The genus names Hematoxylum and Hematoxylon are derived from two Greek words: *haimatos* that means blood, and *xylon* that means wood. The two words together mean "wood of blood" or "blood wood", a reference to the colour of the tree's heartwood from which hematoxylin is extracted. The hematoxylin is extracted from heartwood of the blood wood tree with hot water (the orange-red solution is formed which turns into a black solution on cooling), and then precipitated out from the aqueous solution using urea or ether to obtain a brownish tan powder. Depending on the genetic line of the tree, hematoxylin content ranges from 0% - 10% (Godwin Avwioro. 2011).

This dyestuff may be referred to as haematoxylin or hematoxylin, with spellings of haematein or hematein for the oxidation product. Both spellings are valid, being merely the British and American regional variants, respectively. In this document, hematoxylin and hematein will be used. Although it is common practice to use

hematoxylin, it is not itself the dye. During the preparation of staining solutions, hematoxylin is converted into hematein. This is usually accomplished with chemical oxidizing agents, but is sometimes accomplished by atmospheric oxygen over time.

Oxidation:

Hematoxylin itself is not a dye, and it has to be oxidized to hematein, which is a dye, before it can be used (Horobin and Kiernan, 2002). The oxidation process, produces several oxidized derivatives of hematein, renged from monoxyhematein to pentoxyhematein. Simple alcoholic or aqueous solutions made with hematoxylin are usually pale yellow brown in colour. On oxidation, the colour changes to a deep, mahogany brown. When combined with an aluminum salt such as aluminum potassium sulphate, the colours are pale, transparent violet (unripened) and deep opaque purple (ripened). They may also be combined with iron salts. In these, the colour is deeper, usually a very dark violet. This process is called ripening, and can be accomplished in two distinct ways.

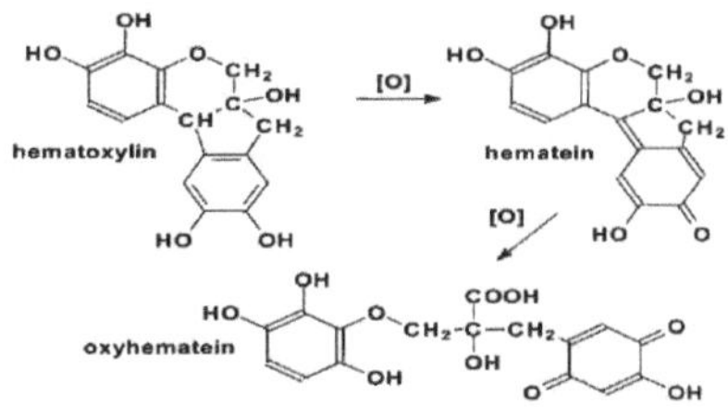

Natural oxidation:

This is done by atmospheric oxygen by putting the hematoxylin solution in an oversize flask, so it can be shaken, with the top plugged loosely with cotton batting, allowing air to enter. This is left in a warm, light and airy place (a window sill) for oxidation to take place. Oxidation may take several months, and is determined by testing the solution from time to time.

Chemical oxidation:

This is done by chemical oxidizing agents like hydrogen peroxide, mercuric oxide and sodium iodate. The latter is the most common type. Concentrations of sodium iodate typically are based upon the amount of hematoxylin and usually about 217 mg for each gram of hematoxylin (Kumar and Kiernan, 2010).

Others oxidizers have also been suggested for particular formulas, but sodium iodate can be substituted for all of them if used at the stated amount.

Oxidant per gram of hematoxylin:

Oxidizing agent	Formula	Maximum	Recommended
Sodium iodate	$NaIO_3$	200 mg	40-150 mg
Mercuric oxide	HgO	500 mg	100 mg
Potassium permanganate	$KMnO_4$	177 mg	175 mg
Potassium periodate	KIO_4	50 mg	50 mg
Hydrogen peroxide USP	H_2O_2	2.0 mL	2.0 mL

Mordant

Hematein is anionic and has weak affinity to combine with nucleic acid. But when hematein combined with a metallic salts (mordant) such as aluminum (as ammonium or potassium alum), or iron (ferric chloride or iron alum) a cationic dye-metal complex is formed that behaves as a basic dye and combines with nucleic acid. The Adjacent hydroxyl and carbonyl-groups of hematein facilitate the formation of coordination complexes with metals including, but not limited to, aluminum (Bryan D Llewellyn. 2013).

Reaction with nucleus:

Nuclear molecules that have been proposed to bind hematein-Al complexes include basic (positively charged) proteins such as histones, as well as deoxyribonucleic acid (DNA).
The attraction or binding of hematein-Al^{+3} to DNA is likely due to the electrostatic attraction of the cationic hematein-Al^{+3} complexes for the phosphate groups, as these groups carry a negative charge at staining conditions.

Because most alum hematoxylin formulae are fairly acid, the nuclei will at first be stained the purplish\ brown color of the acid dye. Changing their color to blue gives a much better contrast with the usual red counterstain (eosin).

Spectrophotometric investigations of Bettinger and Zimmerman (1992) found several colored complexes in hemalum solutions, and the inter-convertibility of these compounds with change in pH probably causes 'blueing' of nuclei when specimens stained in a hemalum are washed in slightly alkaline water. This "blueing" converts the red Hm-Al complex ions to blue polymers that are insoluble in water and organic solvents and also are remarkably resistant to fading (Kumar and Kiernan, 2010).

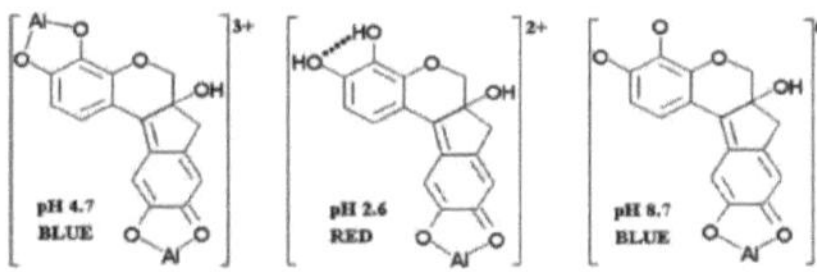

When the endpoint has been reached by either progressive or regressive methods, nuclear color can be changed by one of the following alkaline vapors or solutions.

a) Ammonia vapor for a few seconds.
b) 5% ammonium hydroxide for 2 minutes.
c) Running tap water for 10 minutes.
d) Scott's tap water substitute (TWS) for 2 minutes.

Differentiation

The common way of staining with hematoxylin solutions is to over stain (both chromatin and cytoplasm) and then removes, or differentiates, the excess. This is the essence of regressivestaining. Differentiation is usually done with acid-alcohol, which is 70% or 95% ethanol with 1% v/v concentrated HCl. The other way is progressive staining in which hematoxylin stains color primarily chromatin and to a much less extent cytoplasm to the desired optical density, regardless of the length of staining time.

Hematoxylin categorized according to the mordant used into many types

ALUM HEMATOXYLIN:

Alum hematoxylin solutions contain potassium alum or ammonium alum as the mordant. They include Ehrlich's (Ehrlich P. 1886), Mayer's, Cole's (Cole E C. 1943), Harris (Papanicolaou GN. 1942), Delafield's, Gill's (Gill GW, *et al.* 1974) and Carazzi's hematoxylin. Alum hematoxylins are used when the counter stain does not contain an acid. Acidic counter stains such as van Gieson rapidly remove alum hematoxylin from sections; therefore, they are not used on tissues, which have been stained with an alum hematoxylin (Weigert K & Eine Kleine, 1904).

Ehrlich's hematoxylin:

Ehrlich's hematoxylin is a regressive stain requiring differentiation with 1% acid alcohol. It has a staining time of 5-30 minutes depending on the extent of oxidation of hematoxylin and previous treatment of tissue such as fixation. When counterstained with eosin, Ehrlich's hematoxylin is used for the demonstration of general tissue structures where they stain various tissue structures in shades of blue, pink and red. It also stains mucopolysaccharides and cement lines of bone. The glycerin content helps to stabilize the stain and prevent over oxidation. It also slows down the rate of evaporation. The acetic acid in Ehrlich's hematoxylin reduces the pH and sharpens nuclear staining (Lillie RD. 1977).

Staining time 10-15 minutes	
Constituents	
6g	Hematoxylin
300ml	Absolute alcohol
300ml	Distilled water
300ml	Glycerol
30ml	Glacial acetic acid

Add excess potassium or ammonium alum until solution is saturated. Dissolve hematoxylin in the alcohol and add other reagents in the order given. The alum should be added until the solution is saturated. The prepared solution should be covered with a loose cotton wool or gauze and exposed to light for 4 to 6 weeks to enable it to oxidize or ripen. Solution lasts more than a year (**Ehrlich**, P. 1886).

Harris hematoxylin:

Harris hematoxylin is a powerful nuclear stain, which may be used regressively and progressively. In view of its improved selectivity of nuclear staining, it is generally used in exfoliative cytology for the demonstration of malignant and non- malignant cells. Staining time is 2-5 minutes. Harris hematoxylin contains mercuric oxide, which oxidizes hematoxylin to hematein making it possible for the solution to be used almost immediately (Harris HR. 1900).

Staining time 5 minutes	
Constituents	
2.5g	Hematoxylin
50ml	Absolute alcohol
50g	Ammonium or potassium alum
500ml	Distilled water
1.5g	Mercuric oxide
20ml	Glacial acetic acid

Dissolve the hematoxylin in absolute alcohol, and the alum in distilled water. Where necessary, heat may be applied. Then, mix the two solutions. Boil solution in a large flask, add mercuric oxide and mix. Cool immediately in cold water and add glacial acetic acid. The stain can be used immediately. It lasts for about three months.

Mayer's hematoxylin:

Mayer's hematoxylin is a more powerful stain than Ehrlich's hematoxylin and a precise nuclear stain which is used progressively, although, it may be used regressively with a staining time of 40-60 minutes. Mayer's haemalum, unlike Ehrlich's hematoxylin does not stain mucopolysaccharides. Therefore, it is used as a nuclear counter stain for the demonstration of glycogen, amyloid and Mucicarmine. Nuclei of microfilaria and amoebae in sections and smears are well demonstrated with this stain. Mayer's haemalum is also used in the Celestine blue-haemalum nuclear stain. Mayer's haemalum contains sodium iodate, which oxidizes hematoxylin to haematein; therefore, the stain may be used immediately after preparation. Chloral hydrate in Mayer's hematoxylin acts as a preservative, while the citric acid sharpens nuclear staining. Potassium alum or ammonium alum is the mordant in Mayer's hematoxylin. Staining time as a progressive stain is 5-10 minutes, while as a regressive stain is 40-60 minutes.

Constituents	
1g	Hematoxylin
1000ml	Distilled water
50g	Potassium alum or Ammonium alum
0.2g	Sodium iodate
1g	Citric acid
50g	Chloral hydrate

Reagents are added in the order given, making sure that each addition dissolves before the next is added. Heat may be applied where necessary. The stain may be used immediately and lasts 3-4 months (Mayer, P. 1891).

Cole's hematoxylin:

Cole's hematoxylin can be used as a progressive stain, and it can also be used regressively as a routine stain similar to Ehrlich's hematoxylin with a staining time of about 5 -10 minutes. Cole's hematoxylin may be used in place of Mayer's hemalum in the Celestine blue haemalum nuclear stain. It contains iodine, which oxidizes hematoxylin to hematein making it possible for the solution to be used immediately (Cole EC. 1943).

Staining time 5 minutes **Constituents**	
1.5g	Hematoxylin
50ml	1% iodine in 95% alcohol
700ml	Saturated aqueous ammonium or potassium alum
250ml	Distilled water

Heat distilled water until it boils and dissolve hematoxylin in it. Then add iodine and alum. Cool and filter. Stain lasts about 3 months.

Gill's hematoxylin (Gill GW, *et al.* 1974):

Solution	
730ml	Distilled water
250ml	Ethylene glycol
2g	Hematoxylin
0.2g	Sodium iodate
17.6g	Aluminium sulphate
20ml	Glacial acetic acid

Combine the reagents in the order given and mix for 1 hour at room temperature. The stain can be used immediately.

Carazzi's hematoxylin (Carazzi D. 1911)***:***

Solution	
0.5g	Hematoxylin
0.01g	Potassium iodate
25g	Potassium alum
100ml	Glycerol
400ml	Distilled water

Add the hematoxylin to the glycerol. Dissolve the potassium iodate in about 25ml of the water and prepare the alum using the remainder. Mix the hematoxylin and alum solutions and then carefully add the potassium iodate.

IRON HEMATOXYLIN:

The mordant in these solutions are ferric chloride or ferric ammonium sulphate. These ferric compounds in addition to being mordants also oxidize hematoxylin to hematein causing over oxidation of prepared and stored hematoxylin. For the latter reason, iron hematoxylin solutions are prepared just before use, but simple alcoholic and aqueous solutions of hematoxylin must be prepared and kept for 4-6 weeks as stock solutions to enable ripening or oxidation before use. The solutions of hematoxylin and the iron alum are either mixed immediately before use as in Weigert's and Verhoeff's hematoxylins or tissue sections are mordanted in the iron alum before application of the hematoxylin solution as in Heidenhain's hematoxylin. Iron hematoxylins are used when an acidic counter stain such as van Gieson is to be applied to a section because iron hematoxylins are not quickly decolorized by acidic stains.

Heidenhain's iron hematoxylin:

Heidenhain's iron hematoxylin is a regressive cytological stain which stains tissue jet black, and by careful selective differentiation, many tissue and cell components can be revealed in shades of black and grey (Bancroft JD & Stevens A, 1975). This makes it useful for photomicrography. In the technique, iron alum is also used as a differentiating agent and as an oxidising agent, which oxidises hematoxylin to hematein, the active staining component. Being a cytological stain, tissue sections must be very thin to enable easy demonstration of cell constituents. Staining time is 30-45 minutes at 56^0C. Heidenhain's iron hematoxylin will demonstrate mitochondria, chromatin, chromosomes, nucleoli, centrioles, nuclear membrane, cross-striations of muscle fibers and myelin. Red blood cells are stained black. Heidenhain's iron hematoxylin is usually not counterstained, but it may be counterstained with a connective tissue stain such as van Gieson. Staining time 30-45 minutes at 60^0C or 12-24 hours at room temperature (Bryan D Llewellyn. 2013).

Constituents 5% Iron alum (mordant and differentiator)	
5g	Ferric ammonium sulphate
100ml	Distilled water

0.5% hematoxylin in 10% alcohol	
0.5g	Hematoxylin
10ml	Absolute alcohol
90ml	Distilled water

Dissolve hematoxylin in alcohol before adding water. The solution should be allowed to ripe for 4-6 weeks before use.

METHOD (Gray, Peter. 1954):

1. Dewax in xylene 3 changes for 3 minutes in each stage.
2. Take sections to 90% alcohol through absolute alcohol.
3. Mordant in 5% iron alum solution -30-45 minutes at 60^0C or 12-24 hours at room temperature.
4. Rinse very briefly in water.
5. Stain in 0.5% hematoxylin - for the same time and temperature as in 5% alum.
6. Rinse briefly in water.
7. Differentiate in 2-5% iron alum. (2% iron alum is easier to control) **OR** Saturated alcoholic picric acid diluted 2 to 3 (6%) is slower, easier to control and differentiates muscle striations better.
8. Wash in running water to remove iron alum - 5 minutes.
9. Dehydrate through 90% to absolute alcohol, clear in xylene and mount.

Results	
Shades of grey and black depending on degree of differentiation.	Mitochondria, chromosomes, chromatin, nucleoli, centrioles, nuclear membrane, ground cytoplasm, cross striations of muscle fibres.

Weigert's iron hematoxylin:

Weigert's iron hematoxylin is used for the staining of cell nuclei when subsequent staining reagents contain acid such as in van Gieson stain which will decolourise nuclear staining if stained previously with a solution of hematoxylin which contains potassium alum or ammonium alum as the mordant. The Weigert's hematoxylin, which is 1% alcoholic hematoxylin, is stored separately from the mordant, which is acidified ferric chloride. Equal volumes are mixed immediately before use. The resulting colour should be purplish black with a staining time of 20-30 minutes. Weigert's iron hematoxylin is used for the staining of cell nuclei when demonstrating collagen and muscle with the van Gieson stain and the trichrome connective tissue stains (Weigert K & Eine Kleine, 1904).

Constituents:

Solutions A and B

Solution A
1% alcoholic hematoxylin (not less than 5 days old to enable ripening)

Solution B	
4ml	30% aqueous ferric chloride
100ml	Distilled water
7ml	Hydrochloric acid

Mix equal volumes of solutions A and B just before use. The mixed solution lasts about 24 hours, depending on the age of the hematoxylin.

1% acid alcohol (differentiator)	
70ml	Absolute alcohol
29ml	Distilled water
1ml	Hydrochloric acid

METHOD:

1- Dewax in xylene 3 changes for 3 minutes in each stage and rehydrate through absolute alcohol, 90%, and 70% to distilled water for 3 minutes in each stage.
2- Stain with Weigert's Hematoxylin for 15-30 minutes (equal volumes of solutions A and B).
3- Wash in water.
4- Differentiate in 1% acid alcohol.
5- Rinse in water.
6- Counter stain with eosin for 1-3 minutes.
7- Wash in water.
8- Dehydrate in absolute alcohol, clear in xylene and mount.

Verhoeff's iron hematoxylin (Verhoeff FH. 1908)*:*

Verhoeff's iron hematoxylin is an elastic tissue stain. The constituents, 5% alcoholic hematoxylin, 10% ferric chloride and strong iodine are prepared separately and mixed immediately before use. This is because prepared Verhoeff's hematoxylin does not keep because of its rapid over oxidation. The ferric chloride is acting as a mordant, and it is also used as a differentiator. Staining time is 25-60 minutes.

Constituents:

Stock Solutions	
10ml	5% alcoholic hematoxylin
4ml	10% ferric chloride
4ml	Strong iodine.

- Strong iodine is prepared by dissolving 4g potassium iodide in 100ml distilled water. 2g iodine is then added to the solution.
- The solutions are prepared and kept separately as stock. They are mixed in the order and volumes given above immediately before use.
- Prepared solution does not last more than a few hours and at most one day depending on the age of the hematoxylin solution.

METHOD:

1-Bring section to water.
2-Stain section with Verhoef's solution for (15-20) min.
3-Wash with water.
4-Differentiate with 2% Fecl3 until Elastic fiber appears black color.
5-Wash in D.W.
6-Rinse in 95% Alcohol to remove iodine deposit from background.
7-Counter stain with eosin for (2-3) min.
8-Dehydrate, clear and mount.

Results	
Black	Elastic fibres
Brown	Nuclei

According to coun-ter stain	Cytoplasm and other con-nective tissue
If counter stained with van Gieson	
Red	Collagen
Yellow	Muscle fibres, red blood cells
Black	Elastic fibres

PHOSPHOTUNGSTIC ACID HEMATOX-YLIN (PTAH) MALLORY'S:

In many laboratories, PTAH has now become a routine stain for nervous tissue owing to its ability to stain astrocytes, fibroglia, myoglia, muscle striations, collagen, reticulin, fibrin, etc. in shades of blue and red. PTAH is a progressive stain with a staining time of 1-16 hours at room temperature or 1-2 hours at 60^0C. Tissue sections may be treated with Mallory bleach to suppress staining of myelin. The bleaching process involves treating sections with potassium permanganate and oxalic acid. The dehydrating alcohols rapidly remove the red staining from the sections; therefore, dehydration in alcohol should be very rapid. Staining time 3-24 hours (Mallory, FB. 1897).

Constituents	
1g	Hematoxylin
20g	Phosphotungestic acid
1000ml	Distilled water

The hematoxylin and phosphotungestic acid dissolved separately in distilled water, applying heat if necessary and mix the two solutions. Then make it up to 1000 ml with distilled water. Stain is ready for use after 24 hours. If hematoxylin is used in place of hematein, then the stain should be oxidized with 0.177 g potassium permanganate and used after 24 hours. Alternatively, the stain may be exposed to light and warmth for 5 to 6 weeks to allow for natural oxidation before use.

METHOD:

1. Dewax and hydrate
2. Oxidize in 0.25% potassium permanganate - 5 minutes.
3. Rinse in distilled water.
4. Bleach in 5% oxalic acid - 5 minutes.
5. Wash well in tap water.
6. Stain in PTAH solution at room temperature - 3-24 hours.
7. Dehydrate very rapidly through 95% alcohol and absolute alcohol because alcohol removes the red staining rapidly.
8. Clear in xylene and mount.

Results	
Shades of blue.	Nuclei, centrioles, fibrin, cross striations of muscle fibres, red blood cells, fibroglia fibres, myoglia, astrocytes
Yellow to brick red.	Collagen, reticulin fibres, ground fibres, ground substance of bone, cartilage

HEMATOXYLIN WITHOUT MORDANT:

Freshly prepared hematoxylin has been used to demonstrate various minerals in tissue sections. Now these methods suppressed by more specific techniques (Godwin Avwioro. 2011).

Eosin

This is not a single dye, but a variety of related dyes. All are derived from fluorescein, which is a useful fluorescent dye widely used to label antibodies but is useless for ordinary light microscopy. By substituting halogens or nitro groups for some hydrogens, a variety of shades of red can be produced from yellowish to bluish e.g. eosin Y (yellowish) changes to eosin B (bluish) if the bromine groups on positions 2′ and 7′ are changed to nitro groups.

The dyes are also fluorescent but are solely used as red dyes, although the parent dye fluorescein is widely used as a labeling compound in immunofluorescence. The sodium salts of the dyes are all freely soluble in water and fairly soluble in alcohol, but will precipitate as eosinic acid if the pH is very low. However, adding dilute acids will improve eosin staining but may over differentiate the nuclear stain.

Eosin is an anionic dye so attracted to cationic groups of tissue proteins (especially the ε-amino group of the side-chain of lysine and the guanidino group of arginine) by ionic forces, and then held in place by van der Waals forces (kiernan1990). Eosin is a very good cytoplasmic stain, as it gives several shades to the tissue. The range of shades can be extended even further if more than one dye is used in the solution. Some workers claim that up to seven different shades can be distinguished, although I have always found it difficult to distinguish more than about four. Eosin solutions keep reasonably well unless they become contaminated by fungi, when they will develop significant growth. This growth can be inhibited by adding a small amount of thymol to the solution, and this acidic material also enhances the staining.

Ethyl eosin is an ester rather than the more usual sodium salt and is only slightly soluble in water. It is used when eosin staining is needed from alcoholic solution. It must be differentiated in alcohol. Eosin is also an important component of Romanowsky stains, which are all eosinates of azure dyes. Its pre-eminent role in staining is shown by the fact that many structures are referred to as eosinophilic when they will stain equally well with other acid dyes. Eosin gives a good red cytoplasmic counterstain but if other colours are required than other dyes must be used.

The principles outlined for haematoxylin staining also apply to eosin Y or the other red counter stains, except that the endpoint is not quite as sharp. A good counter stain will not only contrast sharply with the blue nuclei, but it will allow the non-nuclear tissue components to be clearly differentiated from each other; smooth muscle from collagen, for example.

Eosin Y is normally dissolved in 95% ethanol. Therefore, an eosin-stained slide will be decolorized if it is left very long in 95% ethanol before coverslipping. Eosin solubility in 100% ethanol is considerably less, but here, too, stain can be lost slowly. To avoid these problems, slides should be run quickly from the eosin dish to the clearant dish. If you use a staining rack, you will find that 7-10 "sloshes" in 95% ethanol will probably be sufficient, before advancing into 100% ethanol, and then quickly into clearant to avoid any eosin loss. The shade of the red counter stain is important for optimum contrast with the blue nuclei. Eosin Y normally has a somewhat yellow-orange color, but adding a little acetic acid to the solution will cause it to become redder. That improves the contrast with the blue nuclei. Be careful not to add too much acid, however, as it can reduce or even eliminate the contrast due to intensity differences between tissues stained with eosin Y.

The density of the red color is important for differentiating the non-nuclear components. Too little color will make the slides look pale and washed out, and will cause a certain amount of glare. On the other hand, too much dye will blur the distinction between the non-nuclear tissue elements (Bryan D Llewellyn. 2013).

Eosin 1% stock

- Dissolve 1gm of eosin Y water- soluble in 20ml of distilled water and 80ml of 95% alcohol.

Eosin working solution:
- Stock Eosin - 1 Part
- Alcohol 80% - 3 Parts
- Add 0.5ml of acetic acid just before use per 100 ml.

RAPID HEMATOXYLIN AND EOSIN METHOD FOR FROZEN SECTIONS(Avwioro OG. 2010):

Solutions required *(Mayer's or Harris hematoxylin, 1% HCl in 70% alcohol, Scott's tap water substitute or ammonia vapour, 1% alcoholic eosin).*

METHOD:
1. Dewax in three changes of xylene for 3 minutes in each stage.
2. Hydrate in descending alcohol concentrations of 100% through 90% and 70% to distilled water for 3 minutes in each stage.
3. Stain in Harris or Mayer's hematoxylin - 2 to 5 minutes
4. Rinse in water
5. Differentiate in 1% HCl in 70% alcohol - 1 minute
6. Rinse in water
7. Blue in ammonia vapour for 5 to 10 seconds or in Scott's tap water substitute for 2 minutes
8. Counter stain with 1% eosin - 1 minute
9. Transfer to 70% alcohol eosin - 1 minute.
10. Complete dehydration in absolute alcohol for 1 minute.
11. clear through rinse in xylene and mount using DPX.

Results:
Nuclei Blue
Cytoplasm Pink
Red blood cells, Paneth cell granules, eosinophlic substances. Red

H&E FOR GENERAL TISSUE STRUCTURE (Avwioro OG. 2010).

Solutions required *(Erhlich's hematoxylin, 1% HCl in 70% alcohol, 1% eosin).*

METHOD:
1. Dewax in three changes of xylene for 3 minutes in each stage.
2. Hydrate in descending alcohol concentrations of 100% through 90% and 70% to distilled water for 3 minutes in each stage.
3. Stain in Erhlich's hematoxylin for 15 minutes
4. Rinse in water
5. Differentiate in 1% HCl in 70% alcohol 1 minute
6. Rinse in water
7. Blue in tap water 10 minutes or in Scott's tap water substitute 2 minutes
8. Counter stain with 1% eosin 1 minute
9. Rinse in water
10. Complete dehydration in absolute alcohol.
11. Clear through rinse in xylene and mount using DPX.

Results:
Nuclei Blue
karyosomes Dark blue
Cytoplasm Pink
Collagen and osteoid tissue Light pink
Cartilage, cement lines of bone, calcified bone Shades of blue.
Red blood cells, eosinophil granules, Paneth cell granules, keratin Red

Further reading:
- Avwioro OG. Histochemistry and tissue pathology, principles and techniques. Claverianum press, Nigeria. 2010.
- Bancroft JD, Stevens A. Histopathological stains and their diagnostic uses. Edinburgh: Churchill Livingstone, 1975.
- Bettinger C, Zimmermann HW (1992) New investigations on hematoxylin, hematein, and hematein-aluminium complexes. 2.

Hematein-aluminium complexes and hemalum staining. Histochemistry 96: 215–228.

· Bryan D Llewellyn. Hematoxylin Formulae. http://stainsfile.info. October 2013.

· Carazzi D: Eine neue Haematoxylinlbsung. Z Wiss Mikr 1911; 28:273-4.

· Cole EC. Studies on hematoxylin stains. Stain Technol. 1943; 18; 125-142.

· Cook, DJ. Cellular Pathology: An Introduction to Techniques and Applications, 2nd edition. Scion Publishing Ltd. July, 2006, chapter 6 Staining theory. pp68 – *103*.

· Ehrlich P. Hamatoxylinl osung. Z. Wiss. Micr. 1886; 3; 150.

· Gary W. Gill, (2010) H & E. in Dako Education Guide: Special Stains and H & E. Second Edition. North America, Carpinteria, California

· Gill GW, Frost JK, Miller KA. A new formula for a half-oxidised hematoxylin solution that neither overstains nor requires differentiation. Acta. Cytol. 1974; 18;300-311.

· Godwin Avwioro. Histochemical use of Haematoxylin – Areview. JPCS Vol (1). April- 2011.

· Gray, Peter. (1954). The Microtomist's Formulary and Guide. The Blakiston Co.

· Harris HR. On the rapid conversion of haematoxylin into haematein in staining reactions. J. Appl. Microsc. 1900; 3; 777-780.

· Heidenhain R. Eine neue Verwendung des haematoxylin. Arch. Mikr. Anat. 1885; 24; 468-470.

· Horobin R W & Kiernan J A, (2002). Conn's Biological Stains, 10th ed. BIOS Scientific Publishers, Oxford, UK

· Kirkpatrick, J. and Lendrum, A.C., (1939) Mounting Medium for microscopical preparations gives good preservation of colour. Journal of pathology and bacteriology. v. **49**, pp. 592-594. Geneva, NY, USA.

· Kirkpatrick, J. and Lendrum, A.C., (1941) Further observations on the use of synthetic resin as substitute for Canada balsam. Journal of pathology and bacteriology. v. **53**, pp. 441-443. Geneva, NY, USA.

· Kumar, G. and Kiernan, J. A. (2010) *Education Guide: Special Stains and H & E*. 2nd ed. Carpinteria, CA: Dako North America.

· Lendrum AC, McFarlane D. A controllable modification of Mallory's trichromic staining method. J. Pathol. Bact. 1940; 50; 381-4.

· Lendrum, A.C. (1977) Letter to the editor Journal of Clinical Pathology, v. **30**, pp. 1087. UK.

· Lendrum, A.C., Slidders, W. and Fraser, D.S., (1972) Renal hyaline: A study of amyloidosis and diabetic fibrinous vasculosis with new staining methods Journal of Clinical Pathology, v. **25**, pp. 373-396. UK.

· Lillie RD. HJ Conn's biological stains. 9th ed. Baltimore, MD: Williams and Wilkins, 1977.

· Mallory FB. On certain improvements in histological technique. J. Exp. Med. 1897; 2;529-533

· Mayer P. Ueber das Forben mit haematoxylin. Mitt Zool Stat Neapel 1891;10;170-186.

· Papanicolaou GN. A new procedure for staining vaginal smears. Science. 1942; 95; 438-439.

· Verhoeff FH. Some new staining methods of wide applicability. Including a rapid differential stain for elastic tissue. JAMA 1908; 50; 876-877.

· Weigert K. Eine Kleine Verbesserung der haematoxylin-van Gieson-Methode. Z Wiss Mikr 1904; 2; 1-5.

Carbohydrates are compounds of carbon, hydrogen and Oxygen, the latter two usually in the proportion of water. Chemically, they are ketones or aldehydes derivatives of polyhydroxy alcohols. Their general formula is $C_n (H_2O)_n$. Generally, carbohydrates are classified into two broad categories namely simple carbohydrates and glycoconjugates but can be divided into numerous subtypes based on their chemical structure as below.

Simple carbohydrates:

Monosaccharides: one sugar unit like glucose, mannose and galactose

Oligosaccharides: few sugar units (2-10) like sucrose and maltose

Polysaccharides: many sugar units such as glycogen and starch

Glycoconjugates:

Connective tissue glycoconjugates: proteoglycans, hyaluronic acid.

Mucins: neutral mucins, sialomucins, sulfomucins.

Other glycoproteins: Membrane proteins (receptors, cell adhesion molecules and blood group antigens).

Glycolipids: Cerebrosides and Gangliosides.

For the purposes of this chapter related to the staining of tissue carbohydrates, two main entities will be considered: glycogen and mucins.

GLYCOGEN

Glycogen is an intracytoplasmic biopolymer in which carbohydrates are stored in human. Greatest amounts found in liver, cardiac and skeletal muscles and significant amounts in hair follicle, endometrium gland, vaginal and ecto

cervical epithelium, megakaryocyte, Neutrophil, umbilical cord and mesothelial cells.

Liver glycogen maintains normal blood glucose concentration, especially during the early stage of fast (between meals).

After 12-18 hours fasting, liver glycogen is depleted. However, muscles glycogen acts as a source of energy within the muscle itself especially during muscle contractions.

Chemically glycogen consists of linear (straight) or branched chains of D-glucose of the same monosaccharide with an average chain length of approximately 8–12 glucose units and 2,000-60,000 residues per one molecule of glycogen.

Glucose units are linked together linearly by α-1-4 glycosidic bonds from one glucose to the next. Branches are linked to the chains from which they are branching off by α -1-6 glycosidic bonds between the first glucose of the new branch and a glucose on the stem chain.

There are two types of glycogen particles are distinguishable morphologically. Rosettes (alpha particles) comprised of varying numbers of 200 Å particles, with an aggregate diameter of 600 to 2,000 Å. And single granules (beta particles) 200 to 400 Å in diameter.

Glycogen may have diagnostic significance in several types of tumors, including:

- Carcinoma of: bladder, kidney, liver and pancreas.
- Adinocarcinoma of: lung and ovary.
- Ewing's sarcoma, seminoma, mesothelioma, and juvenile rhabdomyosarcoma (Bancroft and Gamble.2002).

Normal glycogen distribution patterns may be disrupted in diseases caused by carbohydrate metabolism enzyme deficiencies, such as von Gierke's disease and Pompe's disease.

Fixation and preservation:

Carbohydrates are hydrophilic, have abundant hydroxy and polar groups. Glycogen is soluble in water, but insoluble in alcohols. The hydroxy groups and the anionic, ester and amide side chains of carbohydrates do not react with formaldehyde, ethanol or other compounds used for fixation and tissue processing. Retention of mucosubstances in fixed animal tissues is due largely to insolubilization of associated proteins by coagulation or covalent cross-linking of nearby protein molecules. Histochemically the interesting parts of sugars are the anionic groups and diols which are unchanged in paraffin sections. Frequently, glycogen diffuses within the cells of the liver before being immobilized during fixation by an aqueous formaldehyde solution, giving rise to an artifact known as *polarization*. This artifact sometimes can, but not always, be avoided by using a non-aqueous fixative.

Fixatives containing alcohol or picric acid are generally favoured for glycogen (Bouns – Rossman – 80% alcohol). Suza and Zinker are contraindicated. For optimal preservation, freezing is used. Glycogen demonstration may have improved by giving formalin fixed tissues secondary fixation in Rossman for 24hours.

For *decalcification;* tricholoracetic acid is recommended when glycogen demonstratation is requested (Schumacher U, *etal.* 2005).

Glycogen staining:

There are three major approaches for tissue carbohydrates (mucosubstances) demonstration:

- *The ionized acidic groups* (anions of sialic acids and half-sulfate esters) can be detected with cationic dyes.
- *The hydroxy groups* (diols) can be selectively oxidized to aldehydes, which are then visualized by a chromogenic chemical reaction. The periodic Acid-Schiff (PAS) reaction is the example of this type.
- *Terminal monosaccharide or oligosaccharide saccharide units* may be labeled by virtue of their specific affinity for carbohydrate-binding proteins such as lectins, which are used in much the same way that labeled antibodies are used for immunohistochemistry.

The periodic Acid-Schiff (PAS)

In 1946, McManus first applied the PAS reaction in histology. The principle of the reaction is that periodic acid will bring about oxidative cleavage of carbon-to-carbon atom in 1,2- glycols or their amino or alkali amino derivatives producing dialdehydes fuchsin sulphoric acid, which combine with basic pararosanilin to form a magenta (red purple) coloured compound (Kasten 1960).

Periodic acid is the oxidant of choice. One of its superior properties is that it will not further oxidize the resulting aldehydes into carboxylic acid, which may give weekly or –ve PAS reaction. It used in concentration between 0.5% and 2.5% (preferably 1%). However, four important point must be considered when periodic acid is used:

- Oxidation time must be limited to a maximum of 10 minutes.

- Oxidation should not be carried out at more than 20°C.
- The periodic acid solution should have a pH of 3–5.
- Prepared solutions must be kept at 4°C in a refrigerator.

PAS technique

Periodic acid solution:

Periodic acid	1 g
Distilled water	200 ml

Schiff's reagent:

Dissolve 1 g basic fuchsin in 200 ml of boiling distilled water, removing the flask of water from the bunsen just before adding the basic fuchsin; this will avoid premature renovation of the laboratory in a deep magenta color. Allow the solution to cool to 50°C, and add 2 g Sodium metabisulfite with mixing. Allow to cool to room temperature then add 2 ml concentrated hydrochloric acid, mix, add 2 g activated charcoal and leave overnight in the dark at room temperature. Filter through a No.1 Whatman paper, when the solution should be either clear or a pale yellow colour. Store in a dark container at 4°C.

Method:

1. Dewax sections and bring to distilled water.
2. Treat with periodic acid, 5 min.
3. Wash well with several changes of distilled water.
4. Cover with Schiff's solution, 15 min.
5. Wash in running tap water, 5-10 min to intensify the colour
6. Stain nuclei with Harris's hematoxylin, differentiating as appropriate in acid-alcohol and blueing as usual.
7. Wash in water.
8. Rinse in absolute alcohol.
9. Clear in xylene and mount as desired.

Results:

Glycogen	magenta
Nuclei	blue.

Best's carmine method (Best 1906)

The staining of glycogen is accomplished by hydrogen bond formation between hydroxyl groups (OH) of the glycogen and hydrogen atom (H) of carminic acid. Fibrin, mast cell granules and neutral mucin stain weakly with this method, so this method is sensitive rather than specific for glycogen.

Carmine stock solution:

Add 2 g carmine, 1 g potassium carbonate and 5 g potassium chloride to 60 ml distilled water. Boil gently for 5 min, using a large flask to avoid spillage (the heating produces a carmine-metallic ion complex which is the active staining ingredient). Cool and add 20 ml of concentrated ammonia. Filter and store in a dark container at 4°C, where it should remain usable for several months.

Carmine working solutions:

Stock solution	5 ml
Concentrated ammonia	12.5 ml
Methanol	12.5 ml

Best's differentiator:

Methanol	40 ml
Ethanol	80 ml
Distilled water	100 ml

Method:

1. Dewax test and positive control sections and bring to water.
2. Stain the nuclei well (e.g. with an iron hematoxylin stain). Differentiate in acid-alcohol so that the background is clear, wash and blue.
3. Stain with carmine solution 5-15 min. The older the stock carmine used, the longer the staining time.

4. Wash well in either Best's differentiator or 74 O.P. industrial methylated spirit.
5. Rinse in fresh alcohol.
6. Clear in xylene and mount as desired.

Results:

Glycogen	deep red
Some mucin, fibrin	weak red
Nuclei	blue.

Diastase digestion (Lillie & Fulmer, 1976)

Diastase is a commonly used enzyme for glycogen digestion. It extracted from malt and contains both α and β amylases which depolymerize glycogen into smaller sugar units (maltose and glucose) that are washed out of the section.

Solutions:

Phosphate buffer

Monobasic sodium phosphate	1.97 g
Dibasic sodium phosphate	0.28 g
Distilled water	1000 ml

This solution may be kept in the refrigerator for several months.

Diastase solution:

Malt diastase	0.1 g
Phosphate buffer	100 ml

Method:

1. Dewax two serial sections in xylene and rehydrate through graded ethanol to water.
2. Place one slide in the diastase solution for 1 hour at 37C. The other slide is an untreated control and may remain in water for 1 hour.
3. Wash both slides in running tap water for 5–10 minutes.
4. Proceed with the PAS technique.

Results: (with PAS procedure)

Glycogen should demonstrate bright red/magenta staining in the untreated slide. Glycogen staining should be absent in the diastase treated slide.

MUCINS

Mucins are a family of high molecular weight ranging from 0.5 to 20 MDa, heavily extracellular glycosylated proteins (glycoconjugates) produced by epithelial tissues in most animals. Mucins key characteristic is their ability to form gels; therefore, they are a key component in most gel-like secretions.

Mucins are soluble in alkaline solution. Stain intensely with basic dyes and precipitated by acetic acid except, gastric mucins. They give metachromatic phenomenon with toluidine blue, thionine and azure A.

Mucins may function as lubricants or assist in cell adhesion or host defense. It has been found that mucins have an important function in defence against bacterial and fungal infections. It is the first barrier with which nutrients and enteric drugs must interact and diffuse through, in order to be absorbed and gain access to the circulatory system and their target end organs. Mucins are produced by many tumors including carcinoma, liposarcoma and mesothelioma. Abnormal systemic production of mucins is also found in diseases caused by enzyme deficiencies (Hurler disease, Schele disease, Hunter disease).

Most mature mucins are composed of two distinct regions:

- The amino- and carboxy-terminal regions are very lightly glycosylated, but rich in cysteines. The cysteine residues participate in establishing disulfide linkages within and among mucin monomers.
- A large central region formed of multiple tandem repeats of 10 to 80 residue sequences in which up to half of the amino acids are serine or threonine. This area becomes saturated with hundreds of O-linked oligosaccharides. N-linked oligosaccharides are also found on mucins, but in less abundance than O-linked sugars.

Mucins classification:

Mucins classification is a complex process, for purposes of this chapter here, be simply divided into neutral and acid mucins. Acid mucins further subdivided according to their origin (epithelial or connective tissue) and molecular structure (sulfated, carboxylated).

There no acidic reactive groups are present in this type of mucin, which consists of various hexosamines associated with free hexose groups. It is epithelial in type and is most abundant in Brunner's glands and gastric lining cells, in addition, it can usually be found to some degree in most alimentary and respiratory tract goblet cells and prostatic glands.

These contain hexosamine units like neutral mucins but are linked with glucuronic acid, iduronic acid or sialic acid in addition to sulphate radicals. Acid mucins are subdivided into two groups, (a) sulphated mucins (b) carboxylated mucins.

A. Sulphated mucins:

These are acid charged mucins in which carbohydrates have sulfate groups. The types are:

1. Strong sulfated mucins:
This type is subdividing into: strongly sulfated connective tissue mucins (proteoglycans) and strongly sulfated epithelial mucins

i. *Strongly sulfated connective tissue mucins (proteoglycans)*

These are connective tissue mucins, which are Alcian-blue-positive at pH 0.5 and below, PAS-negative or unreactive, at low pH values react with suitable cationic dyes and metachromatic at pH 1.0 and below with zure A. The subtypes are:

Chondroitin sulfate A:
Contains D-galactosamine and D-glucuronic acid and found in cartilage.

Chondroitin sulfate B: Similar in composition to type A, but also contains iduronic acid.

Present in aorta, heart valves and dermis of skin.

Chondroitin sulfate C: The chemical composition is similar to type A, but is sulfate-esterified. Found in cartilage, umbilical cord and dermis of skin.

Heparin/heparan sulfate: Both consist of N-Acetyl-D-glucosamine, N-sulfate-D-glucosamine and D-glucuronic acid. Found in aorta and cardiac connective tissues, and heparin in mast cells.

Keratan sulfate: consists of sulfate-esterified N-acetyl-glucosamine and galactose, but no uronic acids. Found in the cornea, nucleus pulposus of the intervertebral discs and in ageing cartilage.

Hyalurono sulfate (chondroitin): contains N-Acetyl-D-galactosamine and d-glucuronic acid and is found only in cornea.

ii. *Strongly sulfated epithelial mucins.*

This type of mucin is distinguished from those above, in being of epithelial origin.it reacts at low pH levels with cationic dyes similarly the strong sulfated connective tissue mucins, but differs in being PAS-positive. Seen in bronchial serous glands, lesser extent in intestinal goblet cells.

2. Weakly sulfated mucins
These are usually epithelial origin, consist of polysaccharide sulfate esters in which the sulfate radical is linked to various hexosamines such as glucosamine. They are PAS positive and stain with alcian blue at pH 1 and above. Present in wide variety of cell types and mucus glands.

B. Carboxylated mucins:

These are acid charged mucins in which carbohydrates have carboxylate groups. The types are:

a) Sialic acid-containing carboxylated mucins:

They are an acetylated derivative of neuranimic acid, contain no uronic acids and sulfate esters mucins and react with alcian blue at PH 2.5 and above and metachromatic at Ph 3.0 and above. They are subdividing according to sialidase activity into:

i. **Enzyme-labile:**

They are digested by enzyme sialidase, hence called labile. Examples are submandibular salivary glands, bronchial submucous glands, and goblet cells of small intestine.

ii. **Enzyme resistant:**

These are resistant to denaturatjon by the enzyme sialidase. Also, they are PAS-negative, unlike enzyme labile mucins. Examples are mucosal glands of large intestine, lesser estent in stomach and bronchus.

b) Uronic acid-containing carboxylated mucins:

They contain hyaluronic acid, react as an acid mucin by virtue of the carboxyl group on 0-glucuronic acid and is degraded by the enzyme hyaluronidase. Like other sulphated mucins (as far as alcian blue pH levels are concerned), they are metachromatic with Azure A and with toluidine blue but are negative to PAS.

Mucins demonstration

Fixation:

Formalin fixatives are good for mucins demonstration. Also, alcoholic fixatives can be used. For metachromatic staining, ideal fixative is mercuric chloride. Alkaline formalin should not be used because the mucins are soluble in alkaline solution. For decalcification EDTA, sodium citrate and formic acid can be used.

Methods of demonstration

The demonstration methods of mucins are classified into general, specific and differential methods.

General methods for mucins:

Southgate's mucicarmine (Mayer 1896, modified by Southgate 1927)

The active dye molecule used in the mucicarmine method is an anionic dye-metal complex of carminic acid and aluminium together with calcium.

The exact mechanism by which this method acts is unknown. It is believed that aluminium salts form a chelate complex with carminic acid, thus conferring an overall positive charge on the carmine complex and an attraction for polyanionic molecules like sialomucins and sulfomucins.

Preparation of stain

Grind 1 g carmine and place in a large (500 ml volume) conical flask. Add 100 ml of 50 per cent alcohol and mix. Add 1 g aluminium hydroxide, mix and add 0.5 g anhydrous aluminium chloride. Mix and boil gently for 2 h and 30 minutes. filter and store at 4°C.

Method:

1. Dewax sections and bring to water.

2. Stain the nuclei with one of the conventional alum hematoxylin solutions (not Ehrlich's
hematoxylin). Differentiate well, and blue.
3. Mucicarmine, 20 min.
4. Wash in water.
5. Rinse in absolute alcohol.
6. Clear in xylene and mount as desired.

Results;

Mucins	red
Nuclei	blue.

Specific methods for mucins:

These methods subdivided into methods for neutral mucins, acid mucin, sulphated mucins and sialomucins.

- **Methods for neutral mucins:**

Phenylhydrazine-PAS (Spicer 1961)

The tissue firstly treated by periodic acid to liberate aldehyde groups from both neutral and acid mucins, then preferential condensation by phenylhydrazine which the latter shows condensation with aldehydes formed from neutral mucins, as opposed to acid mucins which have negative charges able to repel the negatively charged phenylhydrazine molecule, so block the reactivity of neutral mucin, the subsequently staining by Schiff reagent colours acid mucins only as the PAS positivity of the acid mucosubstances is unchanged. In this way, it is possible to differentiate between neutral mucin and other (PAS +ve) mucins.

$$\text{TISSUE}-\overset{\overset{O}{\|}}{\underset{H}{C}} + H_2N-\overset{H}{N}-\text{C}_6H_5 \longrightarrow \text{TISSUE}-\underset{H}{C}=N-\overset{H}{N}-C_6H_5 + H_2O$$

Phenylhydrazine-PAS:

Solution:
Periodic acid solution (see page 88.)
5% aqueous phenylhydrazine hydrochloride
Schiff's reagent (see page 88.)
Method:
1. Dewax test and positive control sections and bring to distilled water.
2. Treat all sections with periodic acid, 5 min.
3. Wash well in several changes of distilled water.
4. Treat one positive control section and one each of the test sections with phenylhydrazine, 1 hour at room temperature. Duplicate sections are allowed to remain in distilled water during this period.
5. Wash sections in running water, 5 min. or so, then rinse well in distilled water.
6. Treat with Schiff's reagent, 15 min., followed by washing in running water, 5-10 min.
7. Stain the nuclei with Harris's hematoxylin, differentiate and blue.
8. Wash in water.
9. Rinse in absolute alcohol.
10. Clear in xylene and mount as desired.

Results:

Neutral mucin	negative
Acid mucins	magenta
Nuclei	blue.

- **Methods for acid mucins:**

Several methods have been used to detect acid mucins which include:

Alcian blue method (pH 2.5) (modified Mowry, 1956)

Alcian dyes are one of most dyes that used in carbohydrates histochemistry. They are a large dye containing the benzenoid rings of the copper phthalocyanine linked to four tetramethyl isothiouronium groups via thioether bonds.

Alcian blue is the most important type of it; but two other alcian dyes are alcian yellow and alcian green also used in some histochemical combination methods.

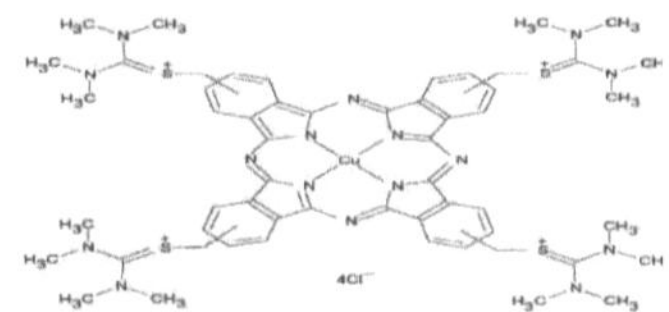

Staining mechanism, widely believed that the cationic isothiouronium groups bond via electrostatic linkages with polyanion molecules of mucins. The suitable pH in which acidest mucins ionized is 2.5 therefor is common for acid mucins.

Alcian blue pH 2.5(modified Mowry 1956)

Alcian blue solution

Alcian blue 8GX	1 g
3% acetic acid solution	100 ml

Nuclear fast red

Aluminum sulfate	5 g
Distilled water	100 ml
Nuclear fast red	0.1 g

Dissolve the aluminium sulfate in the water with heat. Add the nuclear fast red to water while still hot and filter.

Method

1. Dewax in xylene and rehydrate through graded ethanol to distilled water.
2. Stain in the alcian blue solution for 30 minutes.
3. Rinse in running tap water for 5 minutes.
4. Counterstain in nuclear fast red for 10 minutes.
5. Wash in running tap water for 1 minute.
6. Dehydrate in graded ethanol.
7. Clear in xylene and mount in a miscible medium.

Results

Acid mucins	blue
Nuclei	red.

Colloidal iron technique (modified Muller, 1955; Mowry, 1958)

This method is based upon the attraction of ferric cations in a colloidal ferric oxide solution for the negatively charged groups of acid mucins.

Then the tissue bound ferric ions are visualized by treatment with potassium ferrocyanide to form ferric ferrocyanide (Prussian blue).

$$4Fe^{3+} + 3[Fe(CN)_6]^{4-} \longrightarrow Fe_4[Fe(CN)_6]_3(s)$$

Colloidal iron technique (modified Muller 1955; Mowry 1958)

Stock colloidal iron solution

Bring 250 ml of distilled water to a boil and add 4.4 ml of a 29% ferric chloride solution (USP XI). Continue to boil until the solution turns dark red, at which time the solution should be removed from the heat and allowed to cool. This solution is stable for one year.

Colloidal iron working solution:

Stock colloidal iron solution	20 ml
Distilled water	15 ml
Glacial acetic acid	5 ml

Prepare just prior to use.

Acetic acid (12%) solution:

Glacial acetic acid	24 ml
Distilled water to make	200 ml

Potassium ferrocyanide (5%) solution:

Potassium ferrocyanide	5 g
Distilled water	100 ml

Hydrochloric acid (5%) solution:

Concentrated hydrochloric acid	5 ml
Distilled water	95 ml

Potassium ferrocyanide-hydrochloric acid

5% potassium ferrocyanide solution	50 ml
5% hydrochloric acid solution	50 ml

Mix just prior to use.

Acid fuchsin stock (1%):

Acid fuchsin	1 g
Distilled water	100 ml

Van Gieson working solution:

1% acid fuchsin stock	5 ml
Saturated picric acid	95 ml

Method

1.Dewax in xylene and rehydrate through graded ethanol to water.

2.Rinse in 12% acetic acid solution for 1 minute.

3.Cover the sections with the colloidal iron working solution for 1 hour.

4.Rinse in four changes of the 12% acetic acid solution (3 minutes each).

5.Place in the potassium ferrocyanide-hydrochloric acid solution for 20 minutes.

6.Rinse in running tap water for 5 minutes.

7.Rinse briefly in distilled water.

8.Stain with van Gieson working solution for 5 minutes.

9.Dehydrate the specimens in 95% ethanol and absolute ethanol, three changes each. Clear in xylene.

10.Coverslip using an appropriate mounting medium.

Results

Acidic mucins	bright blue
Collagen	red
Muscle and cytoplasm	yellow.

Metachromatic methods

Metachromasia is a specific form of dye aggregation defined by Pearse (1960) as the staining of tissue or tissue elements where the color of the tissue-bound dye complex differs from the original color of the dye complex, resulting in a marked contrast in color. It characterized by formation of new intermolecular bonds between adjacent dye molecules. These bonds occur only when the molecules are brought into proximity to one another.

Metachromatic dyes such as toluidine blue, thionin and azure A may be used to demonstrate acid mucins. These dyes have been used mainly for connective tissue acid mucins because the later have highly anionic proteoglycans with alternating sulfate and carboxylate groups which serves as a template to induce the formation of a polymeric dye structure in which the dye molecules likely bind to one another through hydrogen bonds or Van Dar Waal forces.

Azure A metachromatic technique (Hughesdon 1949)

Preparation of stain:

Azure A	0.2 g
Distilled water	100 ml

Method:

1. Dewax sections and bring to water.

2. Treat with 1 per cent aqueous potassium permanganate, 5 min.

3. Wash briefly in water.

4. Bleach with 5 per cent aqueous oxalic acid (approx. 30 sec).

5. Wash in running water, 3-5 min.

6. Azure A, 5 min.

7. Wash in water; differentiate with 0.2 per cent aqueous uranyl nitrate (usually 10-30 sec).

8. Wash in water and blot dry

9. Rinse in absolute alcohol.

10. Clear in xylene and mount in a DPX-type mountant.

Results:

Acid mucins	purple to red
Background	blue.

- **Methods for sulphated mucins:**

Some methods like alcian blue (pH 1.0) and methylation pre-treatment alcian blue or alcian blue combining with aldehyde fuchsin in addition to high iron diamine are selective for sulphated mucins.

Alcian blue method (pH 1.0) for sulphated mucins (Lev and Spicer, 1964)

Principle:

At this pH only sulphated acid mucins ionised, so the alcian blue stains it alone.

Preparation:

Alcian blue 1.0 g in 100 ml 0.1 N hydrochloric acid.

Method:

1. Bring sections to water
2. Stain in the Alcian blue solution for 10- 30 minutes.
3. Rinse briefly in 0.1 NHCL
4. Blot dry and dehydrate in alcohol
5. Clear in xylene and mount in resinous mountant

Results:

Sulphated mucins   blue.

'Mild' methylation-alcian blue method (Spicer, 1960)

Principle:

Firstly, tissue mild methylated to block acid carboxylated mucins.

TISSUE—C(O—H)(O) + HOCH₃ ⇌ TISSUE—C(O—CH₃)(O) + H₂O

Then, remaining sulphated acid mucins take alcain blue colour. The severe methylation blocks both sulphated and carboxylated acid mucins.

'Mild' methylation-alcian blue method (Spicer, 1960)

Solution:

Concentrated hydrochloric acid   0.8 ml
Methanol   99.2 ml

Method:

1. Dewax positive control and test sections and bring to distilled water.
2. Place sections in preheated methanol solution, 4 hours at 37°C. Duplicate sections are placed in distilled water for an equivalent time at 37°C.

3. Wash sections well in running water.
4. Stain all sections by the standard pH 2.5 alcian blue technique, counterstaining in neutral red.
5. Rinse in absolute alcohol.
6. Clear in xylene and mount as desired.

Results:

In the methylated sections only,
sulphated mucins   blue
Nuclei   red.

Combined aldehyde fuchsin-alcian blue method (Spicer & Meyer, 1960)

Principle:

As it known that, Schiff reagent (basic fuchsin + sulphur) becomes colored by aldehydes (basic fuchsin + sulphur + aldehyde) but with aldehyde fuchsin combination (basic fuchsin + aldehyde) becomes colored by sulphur (basic fuchsin + aldehyde + sulphur). Therefore, sulphated mucins take aldehyde fuchsin colour while alcain blue stains carboxylated mucins.

Aldehyde fuchsin solution:

Basic fuchsin   1 g
Paraldehyde   2 ml
Concentrated hydrochloric acid   1 ml
Ethanol   60 ml
Distilled water   40 ml

Dissolve the basic fuchsin in the alcohol-distilled water. Add the hydrochloric acid and the paraldehyde. Allow to 'ripen' 2-7 days at room temperature, then filter. Store at 4°C.

Alcian blue (pH 2.5) solution:

See p 92.

Method:

1. Dewax the test sections and a positive control section and bring to water. Rinse in 70 per cent alcohol.
2. Aldehyde fuchsin solution, 20 min.
3. Rinse well in 70 per cent alcohol, then in water.
4. Alcian blue solution, 5 min.
5. Rinse in water.

6. Dehydrate in absolute alcohol.
7. Clear in xylene and mount in a DPX-type mountant.

Results:

Sulfated mucins	purple.
Carboxylated mucins	blue.

High iron diamine (HID):

Spicer (1965) assumed that the two dye isomers (i.e. N,N-dimethyl-m-phenylene diamine dihydrochloride and N,N-dimethyl-p-phenylene diamine dihydrochloride) become oxidized by ferric chloride and form colored positively charged polymer. This cationic polymer reacts with sulfate and carboxylate groups of acid mucopolysaccharides.

The high iron percent makes the reaction special for sulphated acid mucins and that may be due to the oxidation of carboxylate acid mucins by or the lowering of pH (1.4) which carboxyl groups remain undissociated, so it takes alcian blue color as counterstain.

High iron diamine method (Spicer, 1965)

Solutions

High iron diamine solution

N, N-dimethyl-m-phenylenediamine $(HCl)_2$
        120 mg
N, N-dimethyl-p-phenylenediamine (HCl)
        20 mg

Distilled water	50 ml
Ferric chloride (60% solution)	1.4 ml

Dissolve the two diamine salts simultaneously in the distilled water, then add to the ferric chloride solution and mix. (This is conveniently made up in a Coplin jar.)

Method:

1. Dewax a positive control section and the test sections and bring to distilled water.
2. Treat all sections with the diamine solution 18-24 hours.
3. Wash well in running water.
4. Counterstain, if desired, with 1 per cent alcian blue in 3 per cent acetic acid, 5 min. Wash

and counterstain with 0.5 per cent aqueous neutral red, 2-3 min. Wash in water.
5- Rinse in absolute alcohol.
6. Clear in xylene and mount as desired.

Results:

Sulfated mucins	black-brown
Carboxylated mucins	blue
Nuclei	red.

- **Methods for carboxylated mucins:**

These methods demonstrate both labile and resistance sialomucins.

Combined high temperature methylation-saponification technique (Spicer & Lillie, 1959)

Firstly, the tissue section methylating at 60 C° to remove both sulphate and carboxylate groups basophilia of acid mucins.

$$\text{TISSUE}-C\!\!\begin{array}{c}O-H\\ \\ O\end{array} + HOCH_3 \rightleftharpoons \text{TISSUE}-C\!\!\begin{array}{c}O-CH_3\\ \\ O\end{array} + H_2O$$

$$\text{TISSUE}-OSO_3^- + H^+ + HOCH_3 \longrightarrow \text{TISSUE}-OH + H_3COSO_3H$$

Secondly, restore the basophilia of carboxylate acid mucins by saponification process while sulphated basophilia cannot restore.

$$R\text{-}C\text{-}COOCH_3 + KOH \longrightarrow R\text{-}C\text{-}COOK + CH_3OH$$

Finally, stain by alcian blue to detect remaining carboxylate acid mucins.

Combined high temperature methylation-saponification technique (Spicer & Lillie, 1959)

Methylation agent:

Concentrated hydrochloric acid	0.8 ml
Methanol	99.2 ml

Saponification agent:

Potassium hydroxide   1 g
Ethanol   70 ml
Distilled water   30 ml

Method:

1. Dewax three positive control sections arbitrarily labelled 'A', 'B' and 'C, also three sections of each test tissue similarly labelled and bring to distilled water; cover with a film of 0.5 per cent celloidin.

2. Place A and B sections in preheated methanol-hydrochloric acid solution 5 hours at 60°C. The C sections are placed in distilled water for the same time and temperature.

3. Wash all sections in running water for several minutes.

4. Treat the A sections only with the saponification agent for 30 min. at room temperature. The B and C sections are placed in 70 per cent alcohol for this period.

5. Wash all sections well in running water for approximately 5 min. and remove celloidin films by rinsing in absolute alcohol, then in equal parts of alcohol and ether. Wash again in water.

6. Stain with standard alcian blue solution (pH 2.5) for 5 min.

7. Wash in water.

8. Counterstain lightly with aqueous eosin, e.g. 0.1 per cent solution; 20-30 sec.

9. Wash in water.

10. Rinse in absolute alcohol.

11. Clear in xylene and mount as desired.

Results:

Section A: carboxylated mucinsonly blue

Section B: sulfated and carboxylated mucin negative

Section C: both sulfated and carboxylated mucins blue

Background pale pink.

Sialidase digestion technique (Spicer *et al.* 1962)

The sialidase (neuraminidase) is N-acetyl neuraminate glycohydrolase enzyme isolated from the bacterium vibrio cholera. This enzyme splits hydrolytically α-ketosidically-bound sialic acid (Drzeniek1973) therefore the loss of PAS or alcian blue staining following sialidase treatment is indicative of the presence of sialic acid in tissue specimen and if alcian blue-PAS method performed after sialidase we found sialomucins that normally would stain blue with alcian blue stain red with PAS.

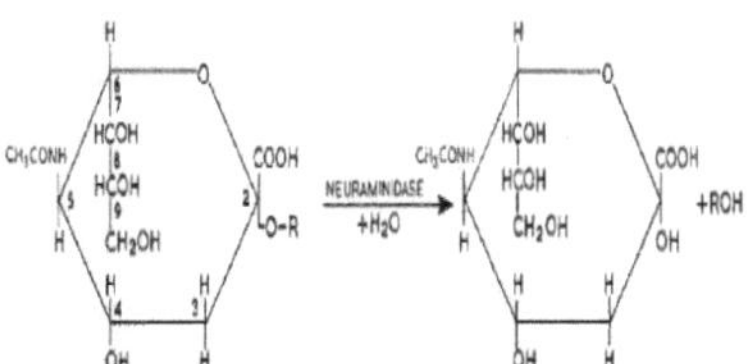

Sialidase digestion technique (Spicer *et al* . 1962)

Preparation of solution:

1 unit/ml sialidase (neuraminidase) ex. V cholera diluted to 1 in 5 with 0.2 M acetate buffer pH 5.5. Add 1 per cent calcium chloride w/v. The activity of the diluted enzyme will persist for a few weeks if stored at 4°C.

Method:

1 Dewax positive control and test sections and bring to water.

2. Rinse with buffer, then treat a positive control section and the test sections with sialidase solution, 16-24 hours at 37°C. Duplicate sections are treated with buffer only for the same period and temperature.

3. Wash all sections well in running water.

4. Either stain all sections with an alcian blue-neutral red sequence, or with the combined alcian blue-PAS technique.

5. Rinse in absolute alcohol.

6. Clear in xylene. Mount as desired.

Results:
Alcian blue—neutral red technique
Enzyme-treated sections containing sialidase-labile sialomucins will show a loss of alcian blue staining, when compared to the untreated sections.

Nuclei red.

Alcian blue—PAS technique
Enzyme-treated sections containing sialidase-labile sialomucins will show a loss of alcian blue staining, but a gain in magenta coloration, when compared to the untreated sections.

Nuclei blue.

Deacetylation-sialidase digestion technique (Ravetto 1968)

There is a class of sialomucins known as O-acetylated sialomucins which resistant to the digestive action of sialidase, so we need deacetylation step by alkaline aqueous alcohol solution of incorporation of O-acetyl groups in the polyhydroxy side chain in sialic acids.

$$R\text{-}CH(OCOCH_3) + KOH \longrightarrow R\text{-}CHOH + CH_3COOK$$

Deacetylation-sialidase digestion technique (from Ravetto 1968)

Deacetylating solution:

Concentrated ammonia	20 ml
Ethanol	70 ml
Distilled water	10 ml

Method:
1. Dewax positive control and test sections and bring to distilled water. Label one positive control and one of each test section A'; an equivalent set 'B' and a third set 'C'.
2. Treat the A sections with the deacetylating solution 24 hours at 37°C. The B and C sections should be placed in distilled water only, for the same time and temperature.
3. Wash the A sections well in running water and then rinse all sections in 0.2 M acetate buffer pH 5.5.
4. Treat A and B sections, only, with sialidase for 16-24 hours at 37°C. The C sections are placed in buffer only at this temperature.
5. Wash well in running water and stain all sections with the conventional alcian blue-neutral red sequence.
6. Rinse in absolute alcohol.
7. Clear in xylene and mount as desired.

Results:
Section A: both sialidase-labile and sialidase-resistant sialomucins will show loss of alcianophilia.
Section B: sialidase-labile sialomucins only will show loss of alcianophilia.
Section C: all acid mucins will stain normally.

Nuclei red.

Combined periodate borohydride saponification-PAS technique (modified from Culling *et al.* 1975)

Principle:
Following periodate oxidation, the aldehydes, which are formed from any normally PAS-positive carbohydrates present in the section, are blocked by sodium borohydride.

$$4RCHO + NaBH_4 \longrightarrow 4RCH_2OH + B(OH)_3 + Na^+ + OH^-$$

Subsequent saponification will break the masking O-acetyl bonds of any PAS-negative sialomucins present.

$$R\text{-}CH(OCOCH_3) + KOH \longrightarrow R\text{-}CHOH + CH_3COOK$$

Thus, exposing vie glycols which will react with PAS. So only the O-acetylated sialomucins will be stained magenta.

Combined periodate borohydride saponification PAS technique (modified from Culling *et al.* 1975)

Sodium borohydride solution:

Sodium borohydride	0.1 g
Disodium hydrogen phosphate (anhy)	1 g
Distilled water	100 ml

Dissolve the disodium hydrogen phosphate in the distilled water first, then the sodium borohydride; the working pH should be 9.4. Prepare fresh for use.

Saponification solution:

Potassium hydroxide	0.5 g
Ethanol	70 ml
Distilled water	30 ml

This solution does not need to be freshly prepared.

Method:

1. Dewax positive control and test sections and bring ta distilled water. Label ane positive control and one of each test section 'A'; an equivalent set 'B' and a third set 'C
2. Treat all sections (A, B, and C) with 1 per cent aqueous periodic acid, for 30 min.
3. Wash well in distilled water, then treat A and B sections only with the borohydride solution, 30 min.
4. Wash well in running water, then wash A sections in 70 per cent alcohol, followed by the alcoholic potassium hydroxide solution, 30 min. Finally, the A sections are washed in 70 per cent alcohol, then in distilled water, and treated with 1 per cent periodic acid, 5 min., followed by washing in distilled water.
5. Treat all sections A, B, and C, with Schiff's reagent, 15 min.
6. Wash in running water and stain cell nuclei as per the standard PAS technique.

Results:

Section A: only the O-acetylated (sialidase-resistant) sialomucins and glycogen, to a variable extent, will stain magenta.

Section B: there will be complete loss of PAS reactivity.

Section C: all normally PAS-positive carbohydrates will stain magenta.

▪ Differentiation methods

These methods differentiate between types of mucins in addition to differentiation between types of acid mucins.

- *Differentiation between neutral mucins and acid mucins:*

Alcian blue-PAS combination differentiate between neutral and acid mucins.

Combined alcian blue-PAS technique for acid and neutral mucins (Mowry 1956)

Principle:

The section is firstly stained with alcian blue to staining acid mucins and secondly by PAS to staining neutral mucins.

Preparation of stains:

Alcian blue

Alcian blue	1 g
3 per cent acetic acid	100 ml

Schiff's reagent (see page 88.)

Method:

1. Dewax sections and bring to water.
2. Alcian blue solution, 5 min.
3. Wash in water, then in distilled water.
4. 1 per cent aqueous periodic acid, 5 min.
5. Rinse well in distilled water.
6. Schiff's reagent, 15 min.
7. Wash in running tap water, 5-10 min.
8. Stain nuclei lightly with any of the usual hematoxylin solutions (not Ehrlich's); differentiate as appropriate and blue.
9. Wash in water.
10. Rinse in absolute alcohol.
11. Clear in xylene and mount as desired.

Results:

Acid mucins	blue
Neutral mucins	magenta
Nuclei	pale blue.

• *Differentiation between sulphated mucins and carboxylated mucins:*

Combined alcian blue-alcian yellow technique for differentiating strongly from weakly acidic mucins (Ravetto 1964)

Principle:
This method uses an alcian blue at low pH (0.5) to stain sulphated mucins and alcian yellow at pH (2.5) to stain carboxylated mucins.

Preparation of stains:

Solution a

Alcian blue	1 g
0.2 M hydrochloric acid	100 ml

Solution b

Alcian yellow	1 g
3 per cent acetic acid	100 ml

Method:
1. Dewax sections and bring to water. Rinse in 0.2 M HCI.
2. Alcian blue solution, 5 min.
3. Rinse in 0.2 M HCI then in water.
4. Alcian yellow solution, 5 min.
5. Wash in water.
6. Stain with 0.5 per cent aqueous neutral red, 2-3 min.
7. Rinse in water.
8. Dehydrate, clear in xylene and mount.

Results:

Sulfated mucins	blue
Carboxylated mucins	yellow
Mixtures of the above	green
Nuclei	red.

• *Between acid mucin subtypes:*
Acid mucins alcian blue reaction depends on pH and ion concentration of solution due to specify of each type.

Alcian blue technique involving critical electrolyte concentration (Scott & Dorling 1965)

Principle:
It is believed that electrolytes like magnesium chloride and sodium chloride can compete with alcian blue for tissue anions if the electrolyte in a sufficient quantity above a critical level of concentration and known as critical electrolyte concentration (CEC). The values given are obtained using 0.05 per cent alcian blue at pH 5.8.

0.06 M magnesium chloride: all acid mucins stain blue.

0.2-0.3 M magnesium chloride: only weakly and strongly sulphated stain blue.

0.5-0.6 M magnesium chloride: only strongly sulfated stain blue.

0.7-0.8 M magnesium chloride: only heparan/heparan sulfate and keratan sulfate stain blue.

0.9 M magnesium chloride: only keratin and above sulfate will stain blue.

Preparation:

Alcian blue	0 05 g
0.2 M acetate buffer pH 5.8	100 ml

Magnesium chloride ($MgCI_2$, $6H_2O$, M.W.= 203.30) to appropriate molarity required.

Method:
1. Dewax sections and bring to water.
2. Stain in the various molarities of alcian blue solution overnight at room temperature.
3. Wash in water and counterstain in 0.5 per cent aqueous neutral red, 2-3 min.
4. Rinse in absolute alcohol.
5. Clear in xylene and mount as desired.

Results:
Staining with alcian blue will be retained or lost according to the type of acid mucin present

Nuclei	red.

Alcian blue technique for acid mucins using varying pH of solution

Principle:
As it known, a tissue component is more intensely stained if the dye is used at the pH at which the reacting groups are fully ionized. So this property may be taken of this to use alcian blue solutions of varying pH to separate, and so

identify, the different acid mucins as shown below:

Strongly sulfated mucins: These react most consistently at low pH levels. Above pH 1.0, their staining reactions tend to be uncertain and will vary from a moderate positive to negative.

Weakly sulfated mucins: Much of this material will stain well from pH 2.5, down to 1.0 and often below this point.

Hyaluronic acid and N-acetyl sialomucin: These will stain well at pH levels ranging from 3.2 down to 1.7.

N-acetyl-O-acetyl sialomucin: Compared to N-acetyl sialomucin this substance will stain down to slightly lower pH values, i.e. to pH 1.5.

Solution:

Alcian blue	1 g
in either: 10 % sulfuric acid	100 ml

yielding a pH of 0.2
or 0.2 M hydrochloric acid	100 ml

yielding a pH of 0.5,
or 0.1 M hydrochloric acid	100 ml

yielding a pH of 1.0,
or 3 per cent acetic acid	100 ml

yielding a pH of 2.5,
or 0.5 per cent acetic acid	100 ml

yielding a pH of 3.2.

Method:
1. Dewax sections and bring to water. If the pH of stain employed is critical, rinse in the appropriate pH solution (e.g. the solvent for the dye).
2. Alcian blue, 5 min.
3. Wash in water or, if the pH of staining is critical, omit and blot dry instead.
4. Counterstain with 0.5 per cent aqueous neutral red, 2-3.min.
5. Wash in water.
6. Rinse in absolute alcohol.
7. Clear in xylene and mount as desired.

Results

Acid mucins	blue
Nuclei	red.

Further reading:

- Best, F. (1906) liber Karminfarbung des Clykogens und der Kerne. Zeitschrift fur wissen schaftliche Mikroskopic und fur mikroskopische Technik, 23: 319-322.
- Culling, C.F.A., Reid, P.F, Burton, J.D. and Dunn, W.L. (1975) A histochemical method of differentiating lower gastrointestinal tract mucin from other mucins in primary or metastatic tumours. Journal of Clinical Pathology. 28: 656-658.
- Drzeniek R. (1973) Substrate specificity of neuraminidases. Histochemical Journal 5:271-290.
- Hughesdon, P.E. (1949) Two uses of uranyl nitrate. I. Permanent metachromatic staining of mucin, journal of the Royal Microscopical Society. 69: 1-7.
- Kasten, F. H. 1960. The chemistry of Schiffs reagent. Int. Rev. Cytol*10:* 1-100.
- Lev, R., & Spicer, S. S. (1964). Specific staining of sulfate groups with alcian blue at low pH. *Journal of Histochemistry and Cytochemistry,12*, 309.
- Lillie, R. D., & Fulmer, H. M. (1976). *Histopathologic technique and practical histochemistry* (4th ed.). New York: McGraw-Hill.
- Mayer, P. (1896) Uber schleimfarbung. Mitteilungen aus der Zoologischen Station zU-Neapel. 12: 303.
- McManus, J.F.A. (1946) Histological demonstration of mucin after periodic acid, Nature.
- Mowry, R.W. (1956) Observations on the use of sulphuric ether for the sulphation of hydroxyl groups in tissue-sections. Journal of Histochemistry and Cytochemistry,4: 407.London), 158.202.

- Mowry, R.W. (1958) Alcian blue techniques for the histochemical study of acidic carbohydrates. Journal of Histochemistry and Cytochemistry. 6: 82.
- Muller, G. (1955). Übere inevereinfachung der reaction nach Hale. *ActaHistochemie, 2,* 68–70.
- Ravetto, C. (1964) Alcian blue-alcian yellow: a new method for the identification of different acidic groups, journal of Histochemistry and Cytochemistry. 12:44-45.
- Ravetto, C. (1968) Histochemical identification of N-acetyl-O-diacetylncuraminic acid resistant to neuraminidase. Journal of Histochemistry and Cytochemistry.16: 663.
- Scott, J.E. & Dorling, J. (1965) Differential staining of acid glycosaminoglycans (mucopolysaccharides) by alcian blue in salt solutions. Histochemie. 5: 221-2 3 3.
- Shariff S and Kaler A. Principles and Interpretation of Laboratory Practices in Surgical Pathology. Jaypee Brothers Medical Publishers (2016).
- Southgate, H. W. (1927). Note on preparing mucicarmine. *Journal of Pathology and Bacteriology, 30,* 729.
- Spicer, S.S. & Lillie, R.D. (1959) Saponification as a means of selectively reversing the methylation blockade of tissue basophilia. Journal of Histochemistry and Cytochemistry, 7: 123-125.
- Spicer, S.S. & Meyer, D.B. (1960) Histochemical differentiation of acid mucopolysaccharides by means of combined aldehyde fuchsin-alcian blue staining. American Journal of Clinical Pathology, 33: 453-460.
- Spicer, S.S. (1960) A correlative study of the histochemical properties of rodent acid mucopolysaccharides. Jounal of Histochemistry and Cytochemistry, 8: 18-35.
- Spicer, S.S. (1961) The use of cationic reagents in the histochemical differentiation of mucopolysaccharides. American journal of Clinical Pathology. 36: 39 3-407.
- Spicer, S.S. (1965) Diamine methods for differentiating mucopolysaccharides hislochemically. journal of Histochemistry and Cytochemistry, 13: 211.
- Spicer, S.S., Neubecker, R.D., Warren, I... & Henson, J.G. (1962) Epithelial mucins in lesions of the human breast. Journal of the National Cancer Institute, 29: 963-970.

Lipids are naturally occurring fat-like substances that are soluble in organic solvents but not in water.

Classification

- *According to their chemical structure into:*

Simple lipids

Are esters of fatty acids and alcohols. It include:
Neutral fats, triple esters of fatty acids and glycerol.
Ester waxes, esters of fatty acids and higher alcohols.

Compound lipids

Are simple lipids possessing a nitrogenous base and other compounds.
Phospholipids, lipid that contain a phosphoric acid radical.
Sphingolipids, lipid that contain sphingosine as nitrogenous base.

Derived lipids:

These are derivatives of simple or compound lipids by hydrolysis.
Fatty acids, derived from triglycerides.
Sterols, derived from ester waxes.

- *According to polar and nonpolar groups:*

Non-polar (Hydrophobic Lipids)

Unconjugated lipids: Fatty acids and cholesterol.
Esters: Cholesterol esters, mono-, di- and triglycerides waxes.

Polar (Hydrophilic lipids)

Phospholipids:

- *Glycerol-based:*

Phosphatidylcholine, (lecith ins), phosphatidyl serine, phosphatidyl ethanolamine (cephalins), phosphatidyl ethanolamine-based plasmalogens.
- *Sphingosine-based:* Sphingomyelins.

Glycolipids:
Cerebrosides, sulfatides, gangliosides.

Fixation:

The fresh frozen section is the best for demonstrating tissue lipids because the lipids are dissolved in xylene used in routine paraffin processing. Fixatives like osmium tetroxide and chrome acid are needed to prevent destructive and solvent effect of histochemical reagents. Formal calcium (10% formalin and 2% calcium) is the fixative of choice for lipid histochemistry.

Lipids Demonstration

The demonstration methods for lipids divide into two main groups, which are histophysical methods and histochemical methods.

Histophysical methods

These join fat stains and lipids birefringence.
- **Fat stains:**
A series of sudan dyes is the most popular reagent for detecting lipids, in spite of they demonstrate only those lipids that exist as fats at staining temperature, namely oily, greasy and hydrophobic lipids while that are in the solid or

crystalline state will remain unstained. Sudan III was the first fat stain but this and other sudan dyes like sudan I, II, brown, green and IV are also used. The sudan black B and oil red O are considered to be even more precise and sensitive than any of these dyes.

Many evidences have given to explain the staining mechanism: Firstly, the partition coefficient (Baker 1958) which applies to the stain in the presence of the two solvent, if the coefficient favours the fat the uptake will be strong. Secondly, the entropy effect (Horobin 1982) which means the tendency of a system to a charge spontaneously to maximize its disorder. Therefore, when fat stains cover the lipids section, it spontaneously moves from solution to lipids. Thirdly, the hydrophobic attraction (Dapson 2005) due to hydrophobic groups of fat stains and lipids. Finally, non-polar bonding (Prento 2001) because sudan dyes have no charged groups (auxochromes) in its structure.

Fat stains methods:

Sudan black B consists of two fractions: firstly, the blue-black fraction (SSBI) which its structure as 2,3-dihydro-2,2-dimethyl-4-[(4phenyl azo-1-naphthalenyl)-azo]-1H-perimidine that behaves like other fat stains and gives blue-black color to glycerol ester and unsaturated cholesterol (Pfuller 1977).

The other, is gray fraction (SSBII) its structure as 2,3-dihydro-2,2-dimethyl-6 - [(4-phenylazo-1-naphthalenyl)-azo]- 1H-perimidine that contains amino group and behaves like basic dyes to give gray color for phospholipids (Pfuller 1977).

Standard Sudan black B method for fats and phospholipids

Fixation and sections:
Cryostat sections post-fixed in formal-calcium; short fixed frozen sections; unfixed cryostat sections (preferred).

Method:
1. Rinse sections in 70% ethanol.
2. Stain for up to 2 hours in saturated Sudan black B in 70% ethanol.
3. Rinse in 70% ethanol to remove excess surface dye, and wash in tap water.
4. Counterstain nuclei with Kernechtrot for 2-5 minutes.
5. Wash well and mount in glycerine jelly.

Results:
unsaturated esters and triglycerides blue-black.
Some phospholipids appear gray, and those in myelin exhibit a bronze dichroism in polarized light.

The free fatty acids and lecithin extracted by ethanol during sudan black B method so Bayliss and Adams (1972) added bromination step before acetone extraction to preserve these compounds, also the bromine interacts with free cholesterol to forms compounds able to take sudan dye color.

Bromine Sudan black method for lipids (research) (Bayliss & Adams, 1972)

Fixation and sections:
Cryostat sections post-fixed for 1 hour in formal-calcium; short fixed frozen sections.

Method:
1. Mount sections onto slides and allow to dry.

2. Immerse sections in 2.5% aqueous bromine for 30 minutes at room temperature, inside a fume hood.
3. Wash in water and treat with 0.5% sodium-metabisulfite for 1 minute to remove excess bromine.
4. Wash thoroughly in distilled water and treat, together with an un-brominated section for the standard Sudan black method.

Bayliss (1981) inserted an acetone extraction step between bromination and staining to demonstrate only the acetone resistant phospholipids that remain in section.

Bromine-acetone Sudan black method for phospholipids (research) (Bayliss High 1981)

1. Treat sections with 2.5% aqueous bromine for 30 minutes at room temperature inside a fume cupboard.
2. Wash well and remove excess bromine with 0.5% sodium meta-bisulfite for 1 minute.
3. Wash thoroughly and allow slides to dry.
4. Extract neutral lipids with anhydrous acetone for 20 minutes at 4 CC.
5. Proceed with the standard Sudan black method outlined above.

Results:
Phospholipids   gray
Sphingomyelin bronze in polarized light.

The oil red O method localizes lipids more precisely and can be followed by a hemalum nuclear stain.

Oil red O in dextrin (Churukian method)

Fixation:
Fresh frozen or NBF, rinse, frozen
Solutions:
Oil red O solution
Oil Red O   0.5 g
Absolute isopropyl alcohol   100 ml
Allow to stand overnight.
Dextrin solution:

Dextrin   1 g
Distilled water   100 ml
Working solution:
Stock Oil Red O   60 ml
Dextrin   40 ml
OR
Oil red O solution:
Oil Red O   0.9 g
Absolute isopropyl alcohol   100 ml
Stir and leave overnight.
Dextrin solution:
Dextrin   1.2 g
Distilled water   120 ml
Working solution:
Oil Red O solution   180 ml
Dextrin solution   120 ml
Allow to stand for a day or more. Stable for months, filter before use.
Sections:
5 um mount on Super Frost/Plus slides, air dry.
Method:
1. Place slides directly into filtered 0.5% Oil Red O in Dextrin. Stain 20 minutes, rinse with running water briefly.
2. Counterstain with Gill II hematoxylin for 20-30 seconds. Rinse with water, blue, cover slip with aqueous mounting media.
Results:
Fat   brilliant red
Nuclei   blue.

Nile blue sulfate method distinguishes between the acid lipids from neutral lipids because the stain solution contains two components, firstly blue-oxazine (Nile blue) which is the main component that stains fatty acid and phospholipids by ionic bonding between the lipid carboxyl groups and dye basic groups.

Secondly red-oxazone (Nile red) which produced by the Nile blue oxidation and stains neutral lipids by the general mechanism of fat stains.

$(CH_3)_2N—$ ... $=O$

Oxazone (Nile red)

Nile blue sulfate method for acidic and neutral lipids (research)
(after Cain 1947, Dunnigan 1968)

Fixation and sections:
Cryostat sections post-fixed for 1 hour in formal-calcium; short fixed frozen sections.
Preparation of stain:
Add 10 ml of 1% H_2SO_4 to 200 ml 1% Nile blue sulfate in water. Boil under reflux for 2 hours. This solution should be at pH 2 so that non-lipid reaction is minimal.
Method:
1. Dry sections onto slides.
2. Stain in the Nile blue sulfate solution at 60°C for 30 minutes.
3. Differentiate sections in 1% acetic acid for 1-2 minutes.
4. Wash well and counterstain nuclei with 1% chloroform-washed methyl green for 5 minutes.
5. Wash well and mount in glycerin jelly.
Results:
Unsaturated hydrophobic lipids   pink
Free fatty acids   pink to blue
Phospholipids   blue.

- **Birefringence of lipids**

Lison (1936) divided lipids into three groups according to physical state, crystallisation and birefringence type:

Lipids without birefringence:
Most lipids in liquid state are never birefringence (isotopic) except cholesterol ester, sphingolipids and glycolipids can be but are not always so.

Lipids birefringence without Maltese cross:
All lipids show a birefringence of the crystalline type without Maltese cross and with four extinction position (360°) in the solid state.

Lipids show Maltese cross birefringence:
It is only for cholesterol ester, sphingolipids and glycolipids which existing as spherocrystals and show black cross (Maltese cross).

Nature of lipids birefringence:
Lipids become birefringence when exist in special state known as liquid crystal or mesomorphic state, which is intermediate between solid and liquid state. This state classified into lyotropic and thermotropic, the latter subdivided into enantiotropic and monotropic. The enantiotropic is only one concern us here, is formed by heating the crystalline state or by cooling the isotropic liquid.
Liquid crystalline exist in three distinct mesophases, firstly the smectic in which the molecules are arranged in parallel and in distinct layers, secondly the nematic in which the molecules parallel but not arranged in layers and thirdly the cholesteric in which the molecules like nematic but twisted.

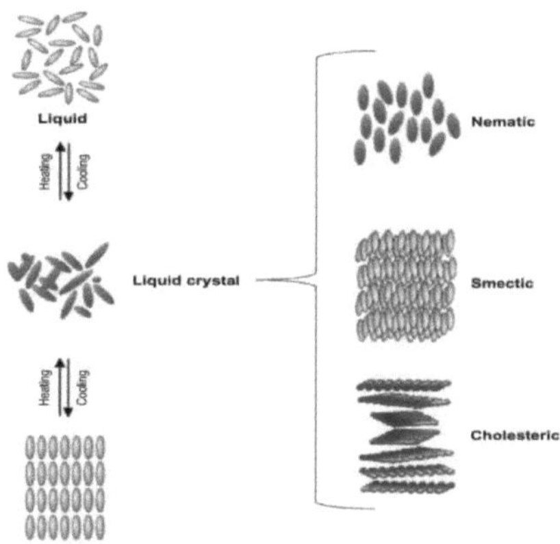

Maltese cross birefringence

As it known, this type of birefringence concerns with some types of lipids especially the cholesterol and other like sphingo-lipids and glycol-lipids.

The cholesterol is the most important one of these groups and belong to cholesteric phase which the latter subdivided according to the degree of twisting into fan-shape and conic-shape which are both known as Maltese cross shape.

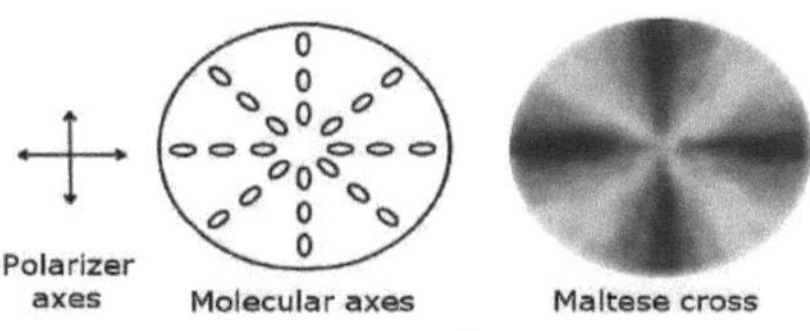

When polarized light passes through the cholesterol texture, it gives a special type of birefringence know as uniaxial indicatrix which is a subtype of interference figure birefringence and Maltese cross belong to it.

Histochemical methods

It includes eleven types of lipids.

- **Free-fatty acids**

Holczinger (1959) method is the most sensitive and specific variant of a group of copper-soap procedures. The copper acetate reacts with free fatty acids to forms soap, then the latter reacts with rubeanic acid to produces dark green color complex.

Copper Rubeanic acid method for free fatty acids (research) (Holczinger 1959)

Fixation:
Cryostat sections post-fixed in formal-calcium; fixed frozen sections.

Method:
1. Mount duplicate sections onto slides and air dry.
2. Treat with 1 M HCl for 1 hour at room temperature to desaponify calcium soaps.
3. Wash well in distilled water and dry in air.
4. Extract free fatty acids from one section with acetone at 4°C for 20 minutes and rapidly dry in air.
5. Immerse both sections in 0.005% cupric acetate for 3 hours.
6. Wash twice for 10 seconds with 0.1% EDTA adjusted to pH 7.0 with NaOH.
7. Wash thoroughly in distilled water.
8. Treat sections for 10 minutes with 0.1 % rubeanic acid (dithiooxamide) in 70% ethanol, **or** treat sections for 18 hours with 0.025% p-dimethyl aminobenzylidine rhodanine in 70% ethanol.
9. Rinse in 70% ethanol.
10. Counterstain nuclei with Kernechtrot (for rubeanic acid) or Carazzi's hematoxylin (for p-dimethylaminobenzylidine rhodanine).
11. Wash in water and mount in glycerin jelly.

Results:
Free fatty acids—dark green (rubeanic acid), or red (p-dimelthylaminobenzylidine rhodanine).

- **Sphingomyelin**

Most sphingomyelin methods base on the principle that metal salts act as mordant to increase affinity of sphingomyelin for hematoxylin. Baker (1946) devised a dichromate-acid hematin (DAH) method for frozen sections in which the chrome ion reacts with fatty acid unsaturated bonds (-c=c-) of sphingomyelin to forms chromium lipid complex, then the complex reacts with acid-hematin to gives dark blue complex (Lillie1969).

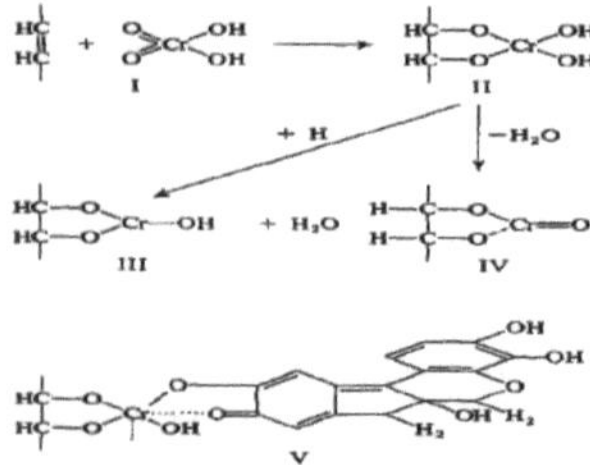

Dichromate-acid hematein (DAH) method for choline-containing phospholipids (routine/research) (after Baker 1946)

Fixation and sections:
Unfixed cryostat sections are recommended; short-fixed frozen sections can be used.

Preparation of stain:
0.1% hematoxylin   50 ml
1 % sodium periodate 1ml
Heat to boiling, cool, and add 1 ml glacial acetic acid. Use on day of preparation.

Method:
1. Treat sections with 5% potassium dichromate containing 1% calcium chloride for 18 hours at room temperature, followed by a further 2 hours at 37°C.

2. Wash thoroughly in distilled water for 30 minutes.
3. Stain with acid hematein solution for 2 hours at 37°C.
4. Wash well and differentiate in an aqueous solution containing 0.25% sodium tetraborate and 0.25% potassium ferricyanide, for 1 hour at 37°C.
5. Counterstain nuclei with 1% methyl green (optional).
6. Wash well and mount in glycerin jelly.

Results:
Lecithins and sphingomyelin   blue-black.

Phospholipids divide into glycerophospholipids and sphingophospholipids according to type of alcohol that forming it which in the first is glycerol and in the other sphingosine. The glycerophospholipids include all types of phospholipids except sphingomyelin while sphingophsophlipids joins phingomyelin only.

Adams and Bayliss (1963) introduced a stage of alkaline hydrolysis by sodium hydroxide before dichromate acid hematin to increase selectivity for sphingomyelin because the sodium hydroxide disrupts glycerophospholipids while sphingophospholidpids are not affected because the glycerophospholipids have ether bonds while the sphingophospholipids have amide bonds which the latter not hydrolysis by sodium hydroxide.

Sodium hydroxide-ferric hematoxylin/DAH method for sphingomyelin

Fixation and sections:
As above, preferably mounted on chrome-gelatin subbed slides.

Method:
1. Treat sections with 2 M sodium hydroxide for 1 hour at room temperature.
2. Wash gently but thoroughly in a large volume of water.
3. Rinse in 1% acetic acid for 5 seconds.

4. If section has become detached from the slide, remount it and proceed with the ferric hematoxylin method described above.

Results:

Sphingomyelin   blue.

Other method by Elleder and Lojda (1973) which they used pre-treatment by chloroform: methanol (2:1) to extract all lipids except phospholipids then mordation by formal calcium to links with ferric hematoxylin.

Ferric hematoxylin (FeH) method for phospholipids (Elleder & Lojda 1973)

Fixation and sections:

Ideally unfixed cryostat sections; otherwise, short fixed frozen sections.

Preparation of reagent:

Solution a.

Distilled water   298 ml

Concentrated HCI 2 ml

$FeCI_3.6H_2O$ 2.5 g

$FeSO_4.7_H2O$ 4.5 g

This solution can be stored.

Solution b.

Distilled water 10 ml

Hematoxylin   0.1 g

Dissolve by gentle heat. This solution must be fresh.

Working solution:

Mix three parts of (a) with one part of (b) and use within the hour.

Method:

1. Treat duplicate sections as follows:

a. Extract one section in chloroform: methanol (2:1) for 1 hour at room temperature.

b. Extract the other with dry acetone at 4°C for 15 minutes.

2. Fix both sections in formal-calcium for 30 minutes.

3. Rinse in distilled water.

4. Stain in the ferric-hematoxylin solution for 7 minutes.

5. Wash in distilled water.

6. Dip several times in 0.2% HCI.

7. Wash in tap water.

8. Dehydrate in acetone, clear in xylene and mount in DPX.

Results:

Phospholipids   blue

Nuclei   blue.

▪ Unsaturated lipids

The reaction of unsaturated lipids depends on ethylene groups (double bonds) which can reduce osmium tetroxide.

Osmium tetroxide method for unsaturated lipids (research)

Fixation and sections

Preferably unfixed cryostat sections; otherwise use short fixed frozen sections.

Method:

1. Immerse sections in 1% aqueous OsO_4 for1 hour at room temperature.

2. Wash well in distilled water and mount in glycerin jelly.

Results:

Unsaturated lipids are stained brown to black.

Saturated lipids and free cholesterol do not react.

Belt and Hayes (1956) also observed that unsaturated lipids give positive Schiff reaction after oxidation to aldehyde groups by ultraviolet (UV) light.

Ultraviolet-Schiff method for unsaturated lipids (research) (Belt & Hayes 1956)

Fixation and sections:
Preferably unfixed cryostat sections; otherwise use short-fixed frozen sections.

Method:
1. Mount sections onto slides and expose to a source of ultraviolet light for 2 hours.
2. Treat with Schiff's reagent (page 88) for 15 minutes, together with a non-irradiated control section to exclude non-lipid aldehydes.
3. Rinse in distilled water and wash well in tap water.
4. Mount sections in glycerine jelly.

Result
Unsaturated lipids   magenta.

- **Triglycerides**

Adams (1966) devised an enzymatic calcium lipase method for triglycerides in which lipase enzyme hydrolyse the triglycerides to their constituent fatty acids then, in the present of calcium salts these fatty acids precipitated as calcium soaps. The calcium is then base-exchanged with lead to covert calcium soaps to lead soaps, which the later brown color by ammonium sulphide.

Calcium lipase method for triglycerides (research) (Adams et al. 1966)

Fixation and sections:
Cryostat sections post-fixed in formal-calcium; formal-calcium fixed frozen sections.

Preparation of incubating medium:
Tris buffer at pH 8.0   15 ml
2% calcium chloride   10 ml
Distilled water lipase   25 ml
Porcine pancreatic lipase 50 mg
Warm solution to 37°C and filter before use.

Method:
1. Incubate free-floating frozen or slide-mounted cryostat sections in the lipase medium at 37 CC for 3 hours.

2. Wash sections well and mount onto slides.
3. Treat with 1% lead nitrate for 15 minutes.
4. Wash very thoroughly in several changes of distilled water.
5. Immerse for 10 seconds in dilute ammonium sulfide (3 drops to a Coplin jar of water).
6. Wash well, counterstain with Carazzi's hematoxylin **or** Mayer's hematoxylin for 3 minutes.
7. Wash in tap water, followed by a rinse in distilled water.
8. Mount sections in glycerin jelly.
For control sections, start at step 3.
Results:
Triglycerides   brown.

- **Phosphoglycerides**

Adams (1963) devised a gold-hydroxamic acid method for phosphoglycerides by depends on hydrolysis of the ester bond of phosphoglycerides with alkaline hydroxylamine to form hydroxamic acid.

The aldehyde groups in the later acid, able to reduce silver to metallic and finally to purple color by gold chloride toning.

Gold hydroxamic acid method for phosphoglycerides (research) (Adams et al. 1963)

Fixation and sections:
Cryostat sections post-fixed for 1 hour in formal-calcium; short fixed frozen sections.

Preparation of reagents:
a. Hydroxylamine solution
Hydroxylamine hydrochloride   2.5 g
Sodium hydroxide   6 g
Distilled water   100 ml
b. Silver solution
Silver nitrate   0.1 g
Ammonium nitrate 0.2 g
Distilled water   100 ml
Adjust pH to 7.8 with dilute sodium hydroxide.

Method:
1. Treat free-floating frozen sections or slide mounted cryostat section in the hydroxylamine solution for 20 minutes.
2. Wash the sections thoroughly in three changes of distilled water, 5 minutes each change.
3. Immerse in the silver solution for 2 hours at room temperature.
4. Wash well, rinse in 1% acetic acid and again in distilled water.
5. 'Tone' the sections for 10 minutes with 0.2% yellow gold chloride.
6. Rinse in water.
7. Remove any unreduced silver by immersing in 5% sodium thiosulfate for 5 minutes.
8. Wash well, and mount sections onto slides.
9. Counterstain nuclei with 1% methyl green for 5 minutes.
10. Mount in glycerin jelly or dehydrate, clear and mount sections in Canada balsam or synthetic resin.

Results:
Phosphoglycerides (lecithins and cephalins) purple.

▪ Plasmalogen

Feulgen and Voit (1924) used mercuric chloride to hydrolyse the plasmalogen unsaturated ether bond to aldehyde groups, which is visualized with Schiff reagent.

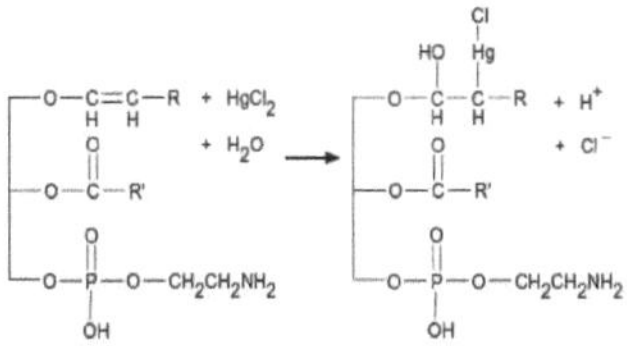

Plasmal reaction for plasmalogen phospho lipids (research) after (Hayes 1949)

Fixation and sections:
Unfixed cryostat sections, stained as soon as possible after cutting.

Method:
1. Air dry duplicate sections onto separate slides
2. Hydrolyse one section in 2% mercuric chloride for 10 minutes.
3. Wash thoroughly in distilled water, three changes.
4. Stain both sections with Schiff's reagent for 10 minutes.
5. Rinse in distilled water and wash in running tap water for 10 minutes to develop the color.
6. Counterstain nuclei with Mayer's hematoxylin for 3 minutes.
7. Wash again in tap water, rinse in distilled water and mount sections in glycerin jelly.

Results
Plasmalogen phospholipids (mainly phosphatidyl ethanolamine)   magenta.

▪ Cholesterol

A perchloric acid naphthoquinone (PAN) method, devised by Adams (1961). Perchloric acid is believed to condense cholesterol to cholesta-3, 5-dene, which is then converted by 1,2-naphthoguinone to a blue pigment.

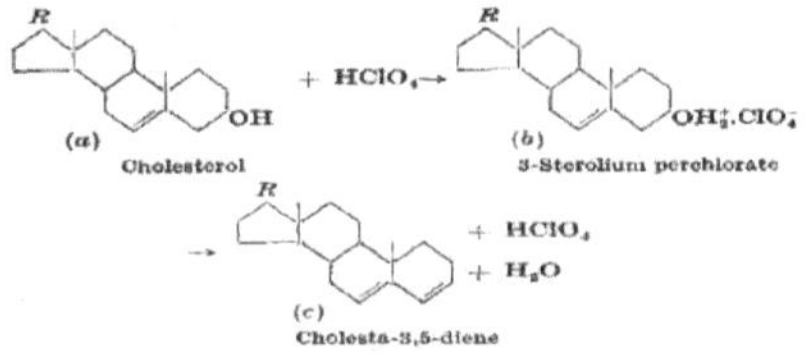

Percholoric acid naphthoquinone (PAN) method for cholesterol (research) (Adams, 1961)

Fixation and sections:
Formal-calcium fixed frozen section; cryostat sections post-fixed in formal calcium.

Preparation of reagent;
1:2 naphthoquinone-4-sulfonic acids   40 mg
Ethanol   20 ml
60% perchloric acid   10 ml
40% formaldehyde   1 ml

Distilled water   9 ml

Mix and use within 24 hours.

Method:

1. Air dry sections onto slides.

2. Treat with 1% ferric chloride for 4 hours.

3. Wash well in distilled water.

4. Carefully paint the sections sparingly with the reagent using a soft camel-hair brush. (Note: wash the brush thoroughly with water after each use, and dry.) Heat them on a surface at 70°C for 1 or 2 minutes, until the color develops. The sections are kept moist by gently replenishing the reagent from time to time.

5. Place a drop of perchloric acid on a cover-glass and lower section into position.

Results:

Cholesterol and related steroids   blue.

Digitonin-PAN is another method for cholesterol, but it is more specific for non-esterified (free cholesterol) in section. Digitonin, a naturally occurring glucoside, is a precipitating agent forms crystalline complexes with non-esterified cholesterol.

Digitonin-PAN method for free cholesterol (research) (Adams & Bayliss 1974, after Schnabel 1964)

Fixation:

As for previous method.

Method;

1. Dry sections onto slides.

2. Precipitate free cholesterol with 0.5% digitonin in 40% ethanol for two hours at room temperature.

3. Extract cholesterol esters with acetone for 1 hour at room temperature.

4. Proceed as for the PAN technique, described above.

Results:

Free cholesterol   blue.

A more recent method for non-esterified (free) cholesterol uses filipin a mixture of three similar antifungals and classified as macrolide polyenes (Kiernan 2015).

The mechanism of staining is hydrophobic interactions between hydrocarbon parts of the molecules are reinforced by hydrogen bonding of cholesterol only OH to an OH at one end of the filipin molecule (Kiernan 2015).

Filipin method for free cholesterol (routine and research) (Kruth & Vaughan 1980)

Fixation and sections:

Cryostat sections, post-fixed; frozen sections of fixed tissue.

Preparation of reagent:

Stock solution

2.5 mg filipin in 1 ml dimethyl formamide

Staining solution

Filipin stock solution   0.2 ml

Phosphate buffered saline   10 ml

Method:

1. Wash sections in PBS.

2. Stain for 30 minutes in filipin solution.

3. Wash in PBS (x2).

4. Mount in PBS or glycerin jelly.

5. Examine by fluorescence microscopy (excitation BG12 with 515 am barrier filter).

Results:

Free cholesterol shows strong silvery fluorescence.

- **Cerebrosides**

The cerebroside and related lipids can be demonstrated by reactions specific for their hexose molecule. The PAS is one of methods that stain cerebroside by oxidation of the 1,2-glycol group in the hexose molecule to aldehyde, then the later give Schiff positive reaction. Adams and Bayliss (1963) used the chloramine T to coverts all amino groups to carbonyl groups and performic acid to oxidize ethylene bonds to aldehydes and then blocked by dinitrophenyl hydrazine.

Modified PAS reaction for cerebroside (Adams & Bayliss 1963)

Fixation and section:
Cryostat sections post-fixed in formal calcium; fixed frozen sections.

Preparation of reagent:

Performic acid

98% formic acid	45 ml
100 vol hydrogen peroxide	4.5 ml
Concentrated H_2SO_4	0.5 ml

Prepare an hour before use and stir occasionally with a glass rod, inside a fume hood, to release bubbles of gas from the solution.

Method:
1. Mount duplicate sections onto separate slides and extract one of these with chloroform methanol (2:1 v/v) for 1 hour at room temperature.
2. Deaminate both sections in 10% aqueous chloramine T for 1 hour at 37°C.
3. Wash slides vigorously and as rapidly as possible, one at a time, in a large volume of water before transferring them immediately to performic acid for 10 minutes. The washing must be swift yet thorough, to avoid swelling and detachment of sections from slides.
4. Wash well in distilled water.
5. Treat with a filtered saturated solution of 2:4 dinitrophenyl hydrazine in M HCl at 4°C for 2 hours.
6. Wash well in water.
7. Treat with 0.5% periodic acid for 10 minutes.
8. Wash in distilled water.
9. Stain in Schiff's reagent for 15 minutes.
10. Rinse in distilled water and wash in tap water for 15 minutes to develop colour.
11. Counterstain nuclei with Mayer's hematoxylin or Carazzi's hematoxylin if wished.
12. Wash in tap water, distilled water and finally mount sections in glycerine jelly.

Results:
Cerebroside   magenta
Indicated by the difference in staining intensity between the two sections.

▪ Sulfatides

These sulphuric acid esters of cerebrosides and the only lipids that are sufficiently acidic to induce a metachromatic shift in a variety of basic aniline dyes like toluidine blue (Bodian and Lake 1963).

Toluidine blue-acetone method for sulfatide (routine) (Bodian & Lake 1963)

Fixation and sections:
Post-fixed cryostat sections; formal calcium fixed frozen sections.

Reagents:
0.01% toluidine blue in phosphate-citrate buffer at pH 4.7.

Buffer solution

0.2 M Na_2HPO_4	96 ml
0.1 M citric acid	104 ml

Method:
1. Mount sections onto slides.
2. Stain for 16-18 hours in buffered toluidine blue.
3. Wash in water.
4. Dehydrate with acetone for 5 minutes.
5. Mount in DPX.

Result:
Sulfatide deposits appear metachromatic red-brown or yellow.

Acriflavine-DMAB method (Hollander 1963) used cationic fluorochrome dye (acriflavine) to combine with negative groups of sulfatides then the complex converted to red color product by the p-dimethylaminobenzaldehyde (DMAB).

Acriflavine-DMAB method for sulfatide (Hollander 1963)

Fixation and sections:
Post-fixed cryostat sections; formal calcium fixed frozen sections.

Preparation of reagents:

a. Acriflavine stock solution

Acriflavine	100 mg
Distilled water at 80°C	20 ml

Store in the dark at 4°C.

b. Acriflavine working solution

0.1 M citrate-HCI buffer pH 2.5	99 ml
Stock acriflavine solution	1 ml

c. DMAB solution

p-dimethylaminobenzaldehyde	0.6 g
20% hydrochloric acid	30 ml
Isopropanol	70 ml

Method:
1. Mount sections onto slides.
2. Stain for 6 minutes in acriflavine solution.
3. Differentiate for 1 minute in two changes of 70% isopropanol.
4. Treat with DMAB reagent for 30-45 seconds.
5. Rinse in distilled water for 2-3 minutes.
6. Counterstain nuclei in Mayer's or Carazzi's hematoxylin.
7. Blue in tap water, rinse in distilled water and mount sections in glycerin jelly.

Results:

Sulfatide	red.

- **Gangliosides**

Gangliosides are a type of glycolipids distinguish by their constituent neuraminic acid and its acyl derivatives (sialic acid) so can be detected by PAS method.

Roberts (1977) devised amodification of the PAS method for gangliosides by reducing the concentration of the oxidizing agent (periodate) from 1% to 0.01% due to rapid oxidation of sialo groups.

Also, the destroying any existing aldehyde groups by reduction with sodium borohydride (BH).

$$4RCHO + NaBH_4 \longrightarrow 4RCH_2OH + B(OH)_3 + Na^+ + OH^-$$

Borohydride Periodate Schiff (BHPS) method

Fixation and sections:
Cryostat sections post-fixed in formal calcium; frozen sections of fixed tissue.

Method;
1. Destroy existing aldehyde groups (endogenous or from formalin or glutaraldehyde fixation) by reduction with 0.1 M (0.38%) sodium borohydride in 1% disodium hydrogen phosphate for 1 hour at room temperature.
2. Wash thoroughly in distilled water.
3. Oxidize with 1.2 mM (0.03%) sodium periodate for 30 minutes at room temperature.
4. Wash twice for 5 minutes each time in distilled water.
5. Stain with Schiff's reagent for 10 minutes.
6. Rinse in distilled water and wash well in tap water.
7. Counterstain with Mayer's hematoxylin or Carazzi's hematoxylin.

8. Blue in tap water, rinse in distilled, then mount sections in glycerin jelly.

Results:

Gangliosides (in Tay-Sachs' disease and GMl gangliosidosis)   red.

Nuclei   blue.

▪ Lipofuscins

Lipofuscins are auto-fluorescent compound (i.e. produce fluorescent without addition of any fluorochrome dye). The most derivative responsible from this property are Schiff bases and 1,4-dihydropyridines, which are produced during lipid peroxidation.

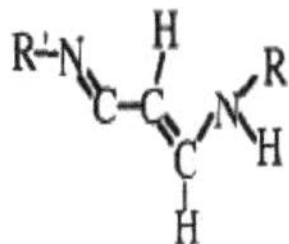 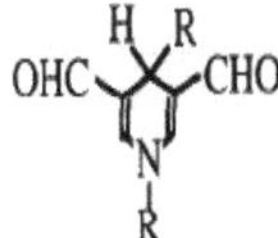

Shiff Bases   **1,4-Dihydropyridines**

UV method for lipofuscins

Fixation and sections:

Cryostat sections (5-10 um) air-dried; frozen sections of fixed tissue; paraffin sections.

Method:

1. Bring sections to xylene and mount in DPX
2. Examine by fluorescence microscopy (dark ground transmission) or epi-illumination. Excitation filter 300-370 nm (UG5) with barrier filter at 410 nm.

Results:

Lipofuscin (wear and tear pigment) has orange-yellow fluorescence.

· Further reading:

· Adams, C.W.M. (1961) A perchloric acid-utiphtho-quinone method for the histochemical localization of cholesterol, Nature (London), 193: 331.

· Adams, C.W.M., Abdulla, Y.H., Bayliss, O.B. & Weller, R.O. (1966) Histochemical detection of triglyceride esters with specific lipases and a calcium lead sulphide technique. Journal of Histochemistry and Cytochemistry. 14:385.

· Adams, C.W.M. & Bayliss, O.B. (1963) Histochemical observations on the localization and origin of sphingomyelin, cerebroside and cholesterol in normal and atherosclerotic human artery. Journal of Pathology and Bacteriology, 85:113.

· Adams, C.VV.M. & Bayliss, O.B. (1963) Histochemical observations on the localization and origin of sphingomyelin, cerebroside and cholesterol in normal and atherosclerotic human artery. Journal of Pathology and Bacteriology, 85: II3.

· Adams, C.W.M. & Bayliss. O.B. (1974) Lipid histochemistry. In: Click. D. & Rosenbaum, R.M. (eds). Techniques of Biochemical and Biophysical Morphology, vol. 2. New York: Wiley-In jour science, 99-156.

· Baker, J.R. (1946) The histochemical recognition of lipine. Quarterly journal of Microscopical Science, 87:441.

· Bayliss, O.B. & Adams, C.W.M. (1972) Bromine Sudan Black (BSB). A general stain for tissue lipids including free cholesterol. Histochemical journal, 4: 505.

· Bayliss High, O.B. (1981) The histochemical versatility ofSudan Black B. Acta Histochemica, Suppl.-Band. XXIV,5: 247.

· Belt, VV.D. & Hayes, E.R. (1956) An Ultraviolent-Schiff reaction tor unsaturated lipids. Stain Technology. 31:117.

· Bodian, M. & Lake, B.D. (1963) The rectal approach to neuropathology. British journal of Surgery, SO: 702.

· Cain, A. (1947) Use of Nile Blue in the examination of lipoids. Quarterly journal of Microscopical Science. 88:383.

- Churukian, C. J. (2005). Manual of the special stains laboratory (8th ed.). Rochester University of Rochester.
- Dapson RW (2005) Dye-tissue interactions: Mechanisms, quantification and bonding parameters for dyes used inbiological staining. Biotech. & Histochem. 80: 49-72.
- Dunnigan. M.G. (1968) The use of Nile blue sulphate in the histochemical identification of phospholipids. Stain Technology. 43: 249.
- Elleder, M. & Lojda, Z. (1973) New, rapid, simple and selective method for the demonstration of phospholipids. Histochemie, J6: 149.
- Feulgen, R. & Voit, K. (1924) Ueber einen Weitverbreiteten lesten Aldehyd seine lintstehung aus einer Varstufe, sein mikrochemischer Nachweis und die Wege zu seiner proparativen. Darstellung. Pfliigers Archiv fur die gesamte Physiologic des Menschen und der Tiere. 206: 389.
- Hayes, B.R. (1949) A rigorous re-definition of the plasma reaction. Stain Technology. 24: 19.
- Holczinger, L. (1959) Histochemischer Nachweis freier Fattsiiuren. Acta Histochemica, 8: 167.
- Hollander, H. (196 3) A staining method for cerebroside-sulphuric-esters in brain tissue. Journal of Histochemistry and Cytochemistry, 11: 118.
- Horobin, R.W. (]982) Histochemistry: An Explanatory Outline of Histochemistry and Biophysical Staining. Stuttgart: Fischer, and London: Butterworths.
- Kiernan, J.A. (2015) Histological and Histochemical Methods: Theory and Practice. 5th edition, Scion Publishing.
- Kruth, H.S. & Vaughan, M. (1980). Quantification of low density lipoprotein binding and cholesterol accumulation by single human fibroblasts using fluorescence microscopy. Journal of Lipid Research. 21:123-1 30.
- Lillie, R.D.: Mechanisms of chromation hematoxylin stains. Histochemie 20:338, 1969.
- Lison, L. (1936) In: Histochemie Animale. Paris: Gauthier-Villars.
- Pearse A.G.E. (1985) Histochemistry, Theoretical and Applied, Vol. 2, 4th edn. Edinburgh: Churchill Livingstone.
- Prento P (2001) A contribution to the theory of biological staining based on the principles for structural organization of biological macromolecules. Biotech. & Histochem.76: 137- 161.
- Pfuller, U., Franz, H., Glockner, R.: Histochemische Darstellung von sauren Mucopolysacchariden mit nichtkationischen Farbstoffen. 71. Vers. d. Anatom. Ges., Rostock 1976. Anat. Anz.
- Roberts, G.P. (1977) Histochemical detection of sialic acid residues using periodate oxidation. Histochemical Journal, 9: 97.
- Schnabel, R. (1964) Eine topochemischc Method zur Differenzierung des freien und veresterten Cholesterins. Acta Histochimica, 18: 161.

All amino acids have a common structure of amine ($-NH_2$) and carboxyl ($-COOH$) functional groups, along with a side chain (R group) specific to each amino acid. There are about 300 amino acids occurring in nature, but only 20 of them occur in proteins. The staining reaction of proteins and protein containing compounds will depend on the amino-acid composition and the pH of the staining solution. The precise histochemical reactions of proteins are due to their reactive groups, and these are not peculiar to one amino-acid or one type of protein.

Fixation:

The type of fixative used will depend on the reactive groups involved in the method to be employed; but Freeze-dried sections which yield good results may be preferred and recommended as it appropriates for each technique.

Tyrosine

Tyrosine amino acid contains the hydroxy phenyl group and can be give red or pink color by million reactions. Firstly, tissue treated with nitrous acid, which reacts with phenolic ring to causing C-nitrosation (Kiernan 2015).

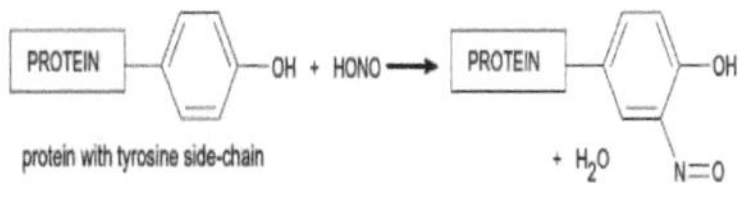

Then this nitroso compound forms red stable chelate with mercuric ions (Kiernan 2015).

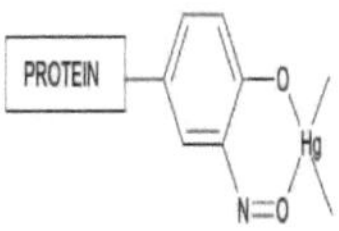

Millon reaction for tyrosine (Baker 1956)

Fixation:

Neutral buffered formalin; formaldehyde vapor (for freeze-dried tissue).

Control section:

Paraffin, fixed cryostat, freeze-dried or celloidin.

Solution a:

10 g of mercuric sulphate is added to a mixture of 90 ml distilled water and 10 ml of concentrated sulfuric acid, and dissolved by heating. After cooling to room temperature 100 ml of distilled water is added.

Solution b:

250 mg of sodium nitrite is dissolved in 10 ml of distilled water.

Staining solution:

5 ml of solution b is added to 50 ml of solution a.

Method:

1. Take sections to water.
2. Immerse sections in staining solution in a small beaker and gently bring to boil; simmer for 2 min.
3. Allow to cool to room temperature.
4. Wash in three changes of distilled water, 2 min each.
5. Dehydrate through alcohols, clear in xylene, and mount in DPX.

Result:

Tyrosine-containing proteins   red or pink.

Tryptophan

Amino acids like tryptophan contain indole groups. The most reliable method for demonstration of tryptophan is DMAB-nitrate method.

Section firstly treated with P-dimethyl amino-benzaldehyde (DMAB) which reacts with indole ring leading to formation of β-carboline (Kiernan 2015).

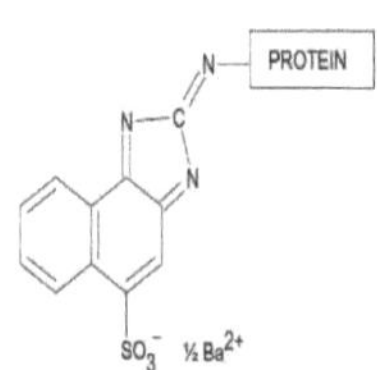

The later (β-carboline) oxidized by the nitrite solution to produce a deep blue pigment (Kiernan 2015).

DMAB-nitrite method for tryptophan (Adams, 1957)

Fixation:
Neutral buffered formalin; formaldehyde vapor (for freeze-dried tissue).
Control section:
Paraffin, freeze-dried, cryostat.
Solutions:
DMAB solution:
5 g of p-dimethylaminobenzaldehyde is dissolved in 100 ml of concentrated hydrochloric acid.
Nitrite solution:
1 g of sodium nitrite is dissolved in 100 ml of concentrated hydrochloric acid.
Method:
1. Take sections to alcohol.
2. Celloidinize in 0.5 per cent celloidin.
3. Place sections in DMAB solution for 1 min.
4. Transfer sections to nitrite solution for 1-2 min.
5. Wash gently in tap water for 30 sec.
6. Rinse in acid alcohol for 15 sec.
7. Wash in water and optionally counterstain in1 percent aqueous neutral red for 5 min.
8. Dehydrate through alcohols, clear in xylene and mount in DPX.

Results:

Tryptophan   dark blue.
Nuclei   red.

Arginine

The only amino acid which has guanidyl group is arginine. Arginine can be demonstrated in tissues by a histochemical method based on the sakaguchi reaction. Sections are treated with a solution containing sodium hypochloride and α-naphthol in which the sodium hybochloride oxidizes the α-naphthol to 1,2-naphthoquinone 4-sulphoric acid (Lillie et al. 1971).

The Guanidyl groups react with 1,2-naphtho quinone 4-sulphoic acid to produce an orange-red product (Lillie *et al.*1971)

The modified Sakaguchi reaction for arginine (Baker, 1947)

Fixation:
Neutral buffered formalin; formaldehyde vapor (for freeze-dried tissue). Formaldehyde mixtures.
Sections:
Paraffin, freeze-dried, fixed cryostat.
Incubating solution:
1 % sodium hydroxide 2 ml
1 % α-naphthol in 70 % alcohol 2 drops alcohol
1 % Milton 4 drops in distilled water

Pyridine—chloroform solution:

Pyridine	30 ml
Chloroform	10 ml

Method:
1. Celloidinize sections (optional).
2. Take sections to water.
3. Rinse in 70 per cent alcohol.
4. Flood slide with incubating solution for 15 min
5. Drain and gently blot dry.
6. Immerse in pyridine-chloroform solution, 2 min.
7. Mount in fresh pyridine-chloroform solution and ring coverslip.

Result:

Arginine	orange-red.

Cystine and Cysteine

Adam and Sloper (1955) developed a method for disulphide groups of cystine. The method depends on oxidation of disulphide by performic acid to anionic cystic acid.

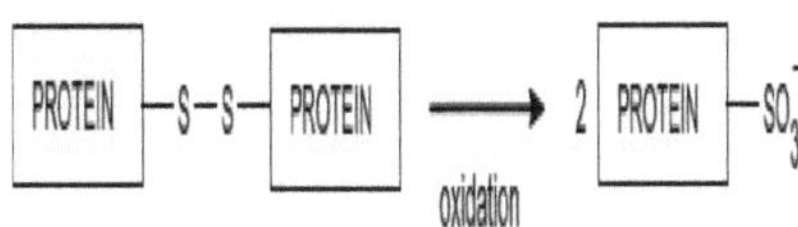

Then later links with cationic alcian blue to give blue color.

Performic acid-Alcian blue method (Adams & Sloper 1955)

Fixation:
Neutral buffered formalin; formaldehyde vapor (for freeze-dried tissue).

Sections:
Paraffin, freeze-dried, cryostat.

Performic acid:

98 % formic acid	40 ml
100 vol. hydrogen peroxide	4 ml
Concentrated sulfuric acid	0.5 ml

Alcian blue:

Alcian blue	1 g
98 per cent sulfuric acid	2.7 ml
Distilled water	47.2 ml

Method:
1. Take sections to water; blot to remove surplus water.
2. Stand sections in performic acid solution, 5 min.
3. Wash well in tap water,10 min.
4. Dry in 60°C oven until just dry.
5. Rinse in tap water.
6. Stain in Alcian blue solution at room temperature, 1 hour.
7. Wash in running tap water.
8. Counterstain (e.g., neutral red) if required.
9. Wash in tap water.
10. Dehydrate through alcohols, clear in Xylene and mount in DPX

Result:

Disulfides	blue.

The DDD reaction also have been used for cysteine demonstration. The reagent (dihydroxy-dinaphyl-disulphide) combines with sulfhydryl groups of cysteine to forms a naphthyl disulphide compound and free naphthols which the latter removed by washing in alcohol and ether; while the naphthyl-disulphide reacts with fast blue to give colored product.

Dihydroxy- dinaphthyl- disulphide (DDD) technique (Barnett and Seligman 1954)

Fixation:

Use Carnoy, formalin and so on.

Reagents:

DDD (Dihydroxy-dinaphthyl-disulphide):

DDD   25 mg

Absolute alcohol   15 ml

Dissolve DDD in alcohol, and add to 35 ml of 0.1 M veronal-acetate buffer (pH 8.5).

Fast blue B salt solution

Fast blue B salt   50 mg

0.1 M Phosphate buffer (pH 7.4)   50 ml

It must be freshly prepared.

Method:

1. Bring sections to water.
2. Incubate in DDD reagent for 1 hour at 50^0C.
3. Cool to room temperature, and rinse in distilled water.
4. Wash for 10 minutes in two changes of distilled water acidified to pH 4 with acetic acid.
5. Remove the free naphthols by washing in 70, 80, 95 and 100% alcohol, followed by two washes in absolute ether for 5 minutes each.
6. Rinse in distilled water.
7. Immerse for two minutes (at room teperature) in fast blue B salt solution.
8. Wash in running tap-water.
9. Dehydrate, clear and mount.

Result:

Blue staining indicates a high concentration of SH groups; red staining indicates areas of lower concentration.

Further reading:

- Adams, C.W.M. & Sloper, J.C. (1955) Technique for demonstrating neurosecretory material in the human hypothalamus, lancet, i: 651.
- Adams, C.W.M. (1957) A p-dimethyl aminobenzaldehy-denitrite method for the histochemical demonstration of tryptophane and related compounds, journal of Clinical Pathology. 10: 56.
- Baker, J. R. (1947) The histochemical recognition of certain guanidine derivatives. Quarterly Journal of Microscopical Science, 88: 115.
- Baker, J.R. (1956) The histochemical recognition of phenols, especially tyrosine. Quarterly journal of Microscopical Science. 97: 161.
- Barnett, R. j. and Seligman, A.M. (1958). Histochemical demonstration of protein bound alpha-acyl amido carboxyl groups. J. Biophys. Biochem. Cytol., 4, 169-176.
- Drury R A B and Wallington E A. Carleton Histological Techniques, fifth edition, Oxoford University press, London 1980; pp 121.
- Kiernan, J.A. (2015) Histological and Histochemical Methods: Theory and Practice. 5th edition, Scion Publishing.
- Lillie, R.D., Pizzolato, P., Dessauer, H.C. and Donaldson, P.T. (1971). Histochemical reactions at tissue arginine sites with alkaline solutions of a-naphthoquinone -4- sodium sulfonate and other o-quinones and oxidized o-diphenols. Journal of Histochemistry and Cytochemistry 19: 487–497.

The term nucleic acid is the overall name for deoxyribonucleic acid (DNA) which is mainly found in the nucleus and ribonucleic acid (RNA) which is located in the cytoplasm of cells, mainly in the ribosomes.

The basic structural units of the nucleic acids are called nucleotides which are made of three components, a 5-carbon sugar (deoxyribose in DNA and ribose in RNA) a phosphate group and a nitrogenous base (adenine, cytosine, guanine and thymine in DNA and adenine, cytosine, guanine and uracil in RNA).

When nucleotides link each other to form poly-nucleotides polymer which is single strand in RNA and double strand in DNA.

Most demonstrating methods depend upon the Presence of phosphoric acids which gives an electronegative character to nucleic acids and presence of pentose permits certain methods to be used for sugar detection.

Nucleic acid demonstration

Fixation:

Good fixatives are alcoholic and acidic fixatives like carnoys fluid, which contain both alcohol and glacial acetic acid. Formalin to use as neutral formalin at 4^0 C.

Decalcification:

If decalcification is needed, must be applicable by using weak acids for short period of time.

Feulgen reaction

Most reliable and specific method for DNA, which occurs in two stages:

Aldehydes liberation:

In this stage, aldehyde groups liberate from DNA by breaking its purine-deoxyribose bonds and hydrochloric acid considered one of common hydrolyser agent (Kiernan2015).

Schiff's reaction:

This stage subdivided into two steps:

Firstly, preparation of Schiff reagent by decolourisation of the coloured fuchsin solution (due to visible wavelength absorbance of its central quinoid structure) to colourless fuchsin (due to delocalization of pi-electron system and resonance in the parent molecule) by sulphurous acid.

$$H_2O + SO_2 \rightleftharpoons H_2SO_3 \rightleftharpoons H^+ + HSO_3^- \rightleftharpoons 2H^+ + SO_3^{2-}$$

Secondly, the reaction of aldehyde groups with leuco Schiff reagent to convert it to coloured Schiff as below simplified chart (Horobin and Kiernan, 2002).

Feulgen nucleal reaction for DNA (Feulgen & Rossenbeck 1924)

Fixation:

Not critical but avoid the bouin's fluid.

Preparation of solutions:

a. 1 M hydrochloric acid:

Hydrochloric acid (conc)	8.5 ml
Distilled water	91.5 ml

b. Schiff's reagent: (see page 88)

c. Bisulfite solution:

10 % potassium metabisulfite	5 ml
1 M hydrochloric acid	5 ml
Distilled water	90 ml

Method:

1. Bring all sections to water.
2. Rinse sections in 1 M HCI at room temperature.
3. Place sections in 1 M HCI at 60°C
4. Rinse in 1 M HCI at room temperature, 1 min.
5. Transfer sections to Schiff's reagent, 45 min.
6. Rinse sections in bisulfite solution, 2 min.
7. Repeat wash in bisulfite solution, 2 min.
8. Repeat wash in bisulfite solution, 2 min.
9. Rinse well in distilled water.
10. Counterstain if required in 1 per cent light green, 2 min.
11. Wash in water.
12. Dehydrate through alcohols to xylene and mount.

Results

DNA	red-purple
Cytoplasm	green.

Feulgen reaction control:

Naphthoic acid hydrazine (NAH) method is a control method for the standard Feulgen reaction. According to (Nohammer1989) the liberated aldehyde groups are reacting with 3-hydroxy-2-naphthoic acid hydrazide to form 3-hydroxy-2-naphthoic acid hydrazine then the latter coupled to the fast blue B to form coupled azo dye.

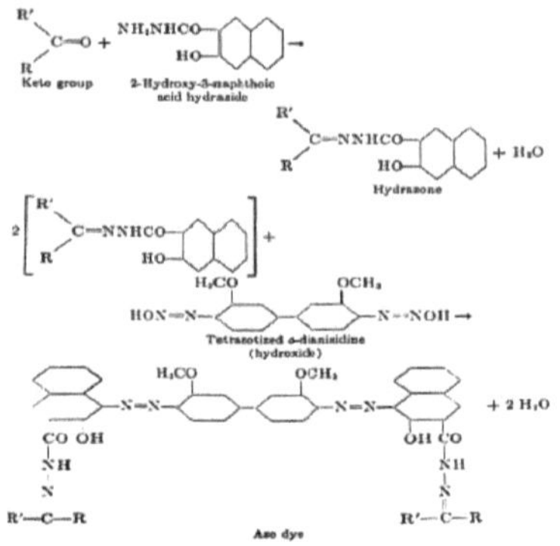

Naphthoic acid Hydrazine-Feulgen method for DNA (Pearse 1951)

Fixation:

Not critical.

Preparation of solutions:

a. I M hydrochloric acid

Hydrochloric acid	8.5 ml
Distilled water	91.5 ml

b. NAH solution

2-hydroxy-3-naphthoic acid	50 mg
Absolute alcohol	47 ml
Acetic acid (cone.)	3 ml

c. Fast blue B solution

Fast blue B	50 mg
Veronal acetate buffer, pH 7.4	50 ml

This solution must be freshly prepared.

Method

1. Bring all sections to water.
2. Rinse briefly in 1 M HCI.
3. Place sections in 1 M HCI at 60°C
4. Rinse sections in 1 M HCI at room temperature, 1 min.
5. Rinse sections in distilled water, 1 min.
6. Rinse sections in 50 % alcohol, 1 min.
7. Place sections in NAH solution at room temperature, 3-6 hours.
8. Rinse sections in 50 % alcohol, 10 min.
9. Rinse sections in 50 % alcohol, 10 min.
10. Rinse sections in 50 % alcohol, 10 min.
11. Rinse sections in distilled water, 1 min.

12. Place sections in fresh fast blue B solution, 3 min.
13. Dehydrate through alcohols to xylene and mount in DPX.

Result:

DNA   blue to bluish-purple
Protein material   purplish-red.

Methyl green-pyronin

It is a mixture of two cationic dyes, methyl green and pyronin Y.

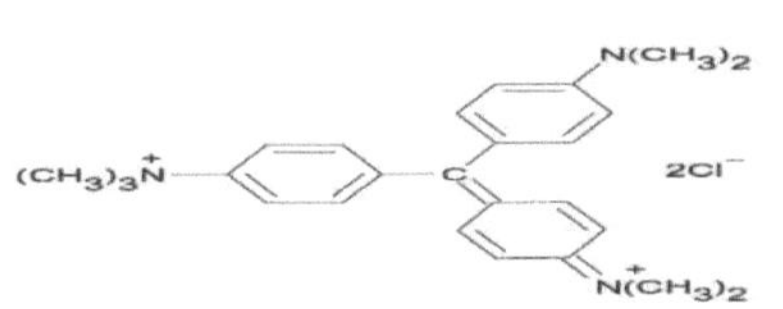

Methyl green

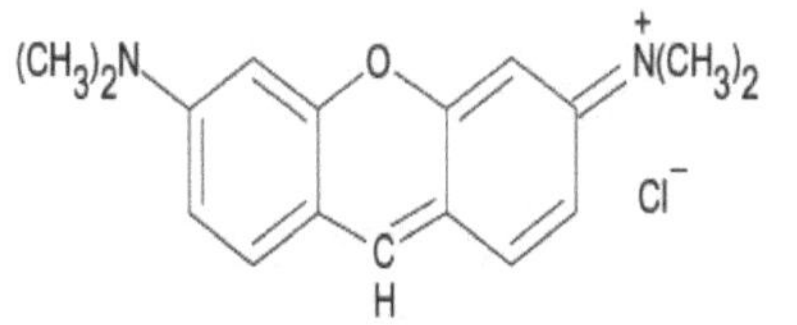

Pyronin Y

The methyl green contains two cationic groups and links with DNA to gives it green color, while pyronin contains one cationic group and stains RNA to acquires it red color. The phosphate groups are the most anionic groups in nucleic acid link with these dyes.

In spite of both dyes are cationic dyes, they produce differences in their staining of tissue and that explained by many theories. Kurnick (1950) suggested that the degree of polymerization of DNA and RNA accounted for differences in staining, and if DNA is depolymerized it loses its methyl green staining.

Vercauteren (1950) claimed that the stereochemical factor in the nucleic acid molecule which accounted for its high affinity for methyl green was the presence of negatively charged phosphate residues at a distance corresponding to that between two possible sites for positive charges on the methyl green molecule. The solution pH also effects in this differentiation because if pH was (1.5) the pyronine staining predominates and when pH (9.0) methyl green predominates therefore pH (4.8) is suitable for both dyes.

Methyl green-pyronin method (Pappenheim 1899; Unna 1902)

Fixation:
Carnoy preferred, but formalin acceptable.

Staining solution:

2 % methyl green	9 ml
2 % pyronin Y	4 ml
Acetate buffer pH 4.8	23 ml
Glycerol	14 ml

Mix well before use.

Method:
1. Take sections down to water.
2. Rinse in acetate buffer pH 4.8.
3. Place in staining solution for 25 min.
4. Rinse in buffer.
5. Blot dry.
6. Rinse in 93% alcohol, then in absolute alcohols.
7. Rinse in xylene and mount in DPX.

Results

DNA   green-blue
RNA   red.

Gallocyanin chrome alum

Gallocyanin is an oxazine dye which acts in aqueous solution as a weakly acid stain.

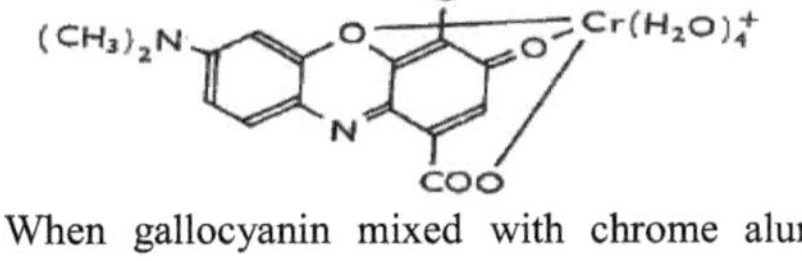

When gallocyanin mixed with chrome alum formed three lakes which are lake-cation, lake hydroxide and lake sulphate (Einarson 1951).

Einarson (1951) postulated that lake-cation responsible for nucleic acid staining and other lakes for background.

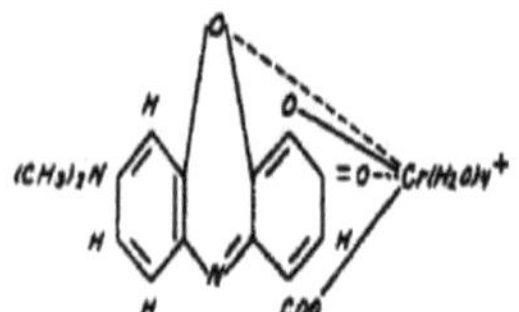

Horobin (1968) disagreed with Einarson (1951) in that cationic-lake and considered it unsuitable for staining and not specific for nucleic acid, so he postulated 2:1 Gallocyanin chromium (G_2Cr) which the latter contains cationic groups that combine with phosphate groups of nucleic acid therefore it behaves like basic dyes.

Gallocyanin-chrome alum method for RNA and DNA (Einarson 1932. 1951)

Solution:

Chrome alum   5 g
Distilled water   100 ml
Gallocyanin   150 mg

The chrome alum is dissolved in the distilled water, the gallocyanin added and the solution slowly heated until it boils. It is allowed to boil for 5 min. When the solution has cooled to room temperature, the volume is adjusted to 100 ml. The solution is filtered before use.

Method:

1. Bring sections down to water.
2. Stain in gallocyanin chrome alum solution 18-48 hours.
3. Wash in tap water.
4. Dehydrate through alcohols and mount in DPX.

Results:

RNA, DNA   blue.

Nucleic acids extraction

Enzymatic extraction of nucleic acids

Both deoxyribonuclease and ribonuclease have been used to nucleic acids extraction.

Enzyme extraction of DNA (Brachet 1940):
Principle:
The deoxyribonuclease (DNase) acts on the phosphate group attached to position 5 of those deoxyribose units of DNA.

Fixation:
Potassium dichromate will inhibit digestion, and should be avoided.

Extraction solution:

Deoxyribonuclease   10 mg
0.2 M Tris buffer, pH 7.6   10 ml
Distilled water   50 ml

Method:

1. Bring both test and control sections to water.
2. Place test section in extraction solution, control in Tris buffer, pH 7.6 both at 37°C, for 4 hours.
3. Wash in running tap water.
4. Stain both sections by the Feulgen method.

Result

Test section   DNA negative
Control section   DNA red.

Enzyme extraction of RNA (Brachet 1940):
Principle:
The ribonuclease (RNase) acts on the phosphate group attached to position 3 of those ribose units of RNA (Kiernan 2015).

Fixation:
Potassium dichromate and mercuric chloride should be avoided, as digestion is inhibited.

Preparation of solution:

Ribonuclease   8 mg
Distilled water   10 ml

Method:
1. Bring both test and control slides to water.
2. Place test slide in ribonuclease solution, and control slide in distilled water, at 37°C for 1 hour.
3. Wash in distilled water.
4. Apply methyl green-pyronin method.

Results

Test slide   RNA negative, DNA green
Control slide   RNA red, DNA green.

Chemical extraction of nucleic acids

Many acids like perchloric acid, trichloroacetic acid and hydrochloric acid are used for nucleic acids extraction because it is cheaper than enzymes. These acids hydrolyse the bonds between the sugars and the bases and between sugars and phosphoric acid (Kiernan 2015).

Extraction with perchloric acid:

Preparation of solutions:

Solution a:
Perchloric acid   2.5 ml
Distilled water   47.5 ml
Solution b:
Perchloric acid   5 ml
Distilled water   45 ml
Solution c:
Sodium carbonate   1 g
Distilled water   100 ml

Method:

To remove RNA only
1. Bring sections down to water.
2. Place sections in 10% perchloric acid (solution b) at 4°C overnight.
3. Briefly rinse in distilled water.
4. Transfer to the sodium carbonate (solution c), 5 min.
5. Wash in tap water.
6. Employ nucleic acid method.

To remove both RNA and DNA

place sections in 5 % perchloric acid (solution a) at 60°C for 30 min at stage 2, then continue method.

Extraction with Trichloroacetic acid:

Bring sections to water and treat with 4 per cent trichloroacetic acid at exactly 90°C for 15 min. Wash and stain with toluidine blue. Both types of nucleic acid are extracted by this procedure.

Extraction with Hydrochloric acid:

Bring sections to water and treat with 1 M HCI for 3 hours at 37°C. Wash and stain with dilute methylene blue at pH 5.7 for 12-24 hours, or with any other suitable basic dye for shorter periods. This method removes both types of nucleic acid.

Further reading:

- Kiernan, J.A. (2015) Histological and Histochemical Methods: Theory and Practice. 5th edition, Scion Publishing.
- Kruth, H.S. & Vaughan, M. (1980). Quantification of low density lipoprotein binding and cholesterol accumulation by single human fibroblasts using fluorescence microscopy. Journal of Lipid Research. 21:123-130.

- Lillie, R.D.: Mechanisms of chromation hematoxylin stains. Histochemie 20:338, 1969.
- Lison, L. (1936) In: Histochemie Animale. Paris: Gauthier-Villars.
- Pearse A.G.E. (1985) Histochemistry, Theoretical and Applied, Vol. 2, 4th edn. Edinburgh: Churchill Livingstone.
- Prento P (2001) A contribution to the theory of biological staining based on the principles for structural organization of biological macromolecules. Biotech. & Histochem.76: 137- 161.

Definition:

It is an extracellular, proteinaceous fibrillar deposit exhibiting β-sheet secondary structure and identified by apple-green birefringence when stained with congo red under polarized light.

Composition:

About 85% of the amyloid material consists of fibril proteins, and the remaining 15% consists of amyloid P component (AP).

Structure:

Amyloid formed of long unbranched fibrils which generally composed of several protofilaments that interact laterally as flat ribbons. Each protofilament possesses the typical cross-β structure and may be formed by several β-sheets stacked on each other.

Formation:

Amyloid is formed through the polymerization of hundreds to thousands of monomeric peptides or proteins into long fibers. Amyloid formation involves three phases:

Nucleation phase:
In which unfolded or partially unfolded polypeptide chains (monomers) converted into nucleus.

Elongation phase:
In which fibrils grow subsequently from nuclei throw the addition of monomers, dimers, oligomers and protofibrils.

Saturation phase:
It is the final phase in which protofibrils are extend and aggregate to form mature amyloid fibrils.

Classification:

Primary amyloid occurs spontaneously in the absence of apparent predisposing illness and often affects tissue of mesodermal origin such as muscle, heart, skin and tongue. Often with localized deposits.

Secondary amyloid occurs in association with a wide range of predisposing or coexistent pathology. In the past these were often chronic infective diseases such as syphilis or tuberculosis, but nowadays inflammatory conditions such as rheumatoid arthritis are the more common cause.

Myeloma-associated amyloid is found in aproportion of patients with plasma cell diseases such as multiple myeloma.

Demonstration of amyloid:

Most amyloid useful fixatives are alcohol and mercuric chloride. The cryostat and free-floating frozen sections are best for amyloid demonstration.

Congo red

It is an acidic diazo dye comprises two identical halves each composed of a phenyl ring bounded to a naphthalene moiety by a diazo group. The two phenyl groups are bound together by a diphenyl bond linked so as to give a linear molecule that is largely hydrophobic (Turnell & Finch, 1992).

From the above structure, there are three sets of potential bonding sites according to Dapson 2019:

Paired sulfonic acids of the upper edge for ionic bonding.

Paired amines on the lower edge for hydrogen bonding.

Large conjugated system for Van der Waal forces.

According to Yakupova *et al.* 2019 there are three main hypothetical models of binding of congo red to amyloids:

Hydrogen bonding between primary hydroxyl groups of the peptide chains of amyloid protein and the amino groups of congo red (Punchtler 1962).

Ionic bonding between positively charged amino acid residues along amyloid peptide chains and the sulfonic groups of congo red (Klunk *et al.* 1989).

Van Der Waal forces between large conjugated system of congo red and amyloid protein (Reinke and Gestwicki 2011).

Due to staining of many tissue components beside amyloid, some modifications and pretreatment are very important to increasing to specify of amyloid staining (Llewellyn, 2012). Modifications include:

Polarity of the solution:
As it known that using a less polar solution reduces ionisation and tends to lessen the intensity of staining. So it is that background staining can be paler with congo red if ethanol is used as the solvent, while amyloid to be seen more easily.

The pH:
Usually, acid is added to acid dyes to increase the amount which will attach to basic tissue components, and alkalis added to basic dyes to increase attachment to anionic tissue components. The reverse may also be done, that is, an alkali may be added to acid dye solutions to inhibit ionisation and decrease ionic staining. Since amyloid hydrogen bonding is not affected by altering pH, this becomes an effective means of suppressing attachment of the dyes to basic tissue components. Usually, a pH in the neighbourhood of 10 is sufficient.

Presence of salts:
When a salt such as sodium chloride dissolved, it ionises to positively charged cations and negatively charged anions. Since like repels like and opposites attract, it is to be expected that the positively charged sodium ion will be attracted to negatively charged groups in the tissue, effectively annulling their charge, so they can no longer repel negatively charged dye molecules. Due to the elimination of these repulsive forces, the dye can closely approach tissue components with either a like charge or an opposite charge, resulting in increased likelihood of amyloid hydrogen bond formation should it be possible.

Highman's Congo red technique (Highman 1946)

Fixation:
Not critical; formal saline gives satisfactory results.
Solutions:
0.5% Congo red in 50% alcohol
0.2% potassium hydroxide in 80% alcohol
Method:
1. Take sections to water, removing pigment where necessary.

2. Stain in Congo red solution 5 minutes.
3. Differentiate with the alcoholic potassium hydroxide solution, 3-10 seconds.
4. Wash in water, stain nuclei in alum hematoxylin, differentiate and blue.
5. Dehydrate, clear and mount.

Results:

Amyloid, elastic fibers, eosinophil granules red
Nuclei blue.

Alkaline Congo red technique (Puchtler *et al.* 1962)

Fixation:
Not critical.

Stock solutions:

Stock solution A
Saturated sodium chloride in 80% ethanol

Stock solution B
Saturated Congo red in 80% ethanol saturated with sodium chloride.

1% aqueous sodium hydroxide

Working solutions
To 100 ml of stock solution A add 1 ml 1% aqueous sodium hydroxide and filter.
To 100 ml of stock solution B add 1 ml 1% aqueous sodium hydroxide and filter.

Method:
1. Sections to water, removing pigment where necessary.
2. Stain nuclei in alum hematoxylin, differentiate and blue.
3. Immerse in alkaline sodium chloride solution for 20 minutes.
4. Transfer directly to the alkaline Congo red solution for 20 minutes.
5. Rinse briefly in alcohol, clear and mount.

Results:

Amyloid, elastic fibers, eosinophil granules red
Nuclei blue.

High pH Congo red technique (Eastwood and Cole, 1971)

Fixation:
Not critical.

Preparation of solutions:
Glycine buffer, pH 10.0
0.1 M glycine 30 ml
0.1 M sodium chloride 30 ml
0.1 M sodium hydroxide 40 ml
Staining solution
0.5% Congo red in equal parts pH 10.0 glycine buffer and ethanol.

Method:
1. Sections to water, removing pigment where necessary.
2. Stain nuclei in alum hematoxylin, differentiate and blue.
3. Stain in staining solution, 10-20 minutes.
4. Rinse in 70% alcohol until background is clear, few seconds.
5. Dehydrate, clear and mount.

Results:

Amyloid, elastic tissue, eosinophil granules red
Nuclei blue.

Congo red apple green birefringence

Congo red gives a colored birefringence with amyloid under polarized microscope due to a phenomenon known as anomalous dispersion of refractive index. In which the refractive index is not constant at every wave length, but changes dramatically around an absorption peak (i.e., the index sinks to a minimum on the short-wave side, and jump to a maximum on the long wave side). (Howie 2009).

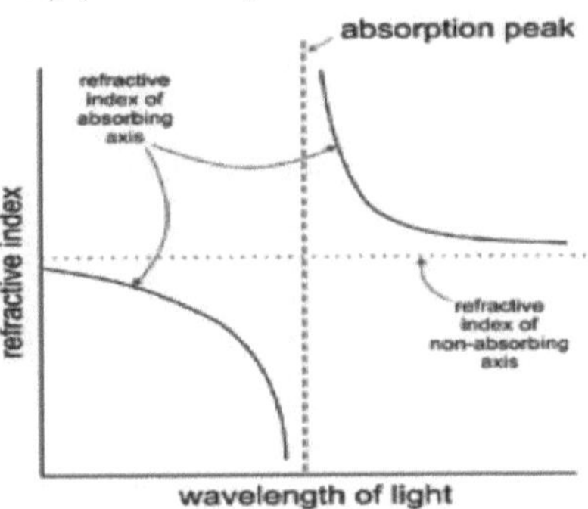

By this phenomenon, amyloid absorbs in both ends of the spectrum (i.e., the violet and red). Absorption of the violet alone gives yellow color and absorption of red gives blue color, so the green color is a mixture of blue and yellow.

Congo red dichroism

At the molecular level, light is only absorbed when it is polarized parallel to a light-absorbing atomic bond, so if amyloid is oriented (i.e., all its bonds are parallel) an appropriate wave length will be maximally absorbed from white light which is polarized parallel to the bonds and will give red color. In other hand, when polarized perpendicularly to the bonds of amyloid not red color and amyloid appears colorless (Howie *et al.* 2009).

This property is called dichroism, which means that either a material has different planes (i.e., from colored to colorless) depend on the plane of polarization.

The material orientated on the specimen stage of a microscope fitted with a polarizer or an analyser but not both, and either the stage or the polarizing filter is rotated to change the appearance from color to colorless (Howie *et al.* 2008).

Crystal violet

It is a mixture of tetra, penta and hexamethyl pararosaniline.

N(CH3)2
(CH3)2N
C
Cl⁻
N(CH3)2

The staining of amyloid is probably selective affinity for one of these derivatives (i.e., amyloid takes the color of less methylated derivatives

while the background takes the crystal violet color).

Crystal violet method (Hucker and Conn, 1928)

Preparation of solution:
Dissolve 2 g crystal violet in 20 ml of 95% alcohol. Add 80 ml of 1% aqueous ammonium oxalate. Dissolve using the minimum of heat. Cool and filter.

Method:
1. Take sections to water, removing pigment where necessary.
2. Stain in crystal violet solution, 5 min.
3. Wash and differentiate in weak (c. 0.2%aqueous) acetic acid, controlling the differentiation microscopically, arresting differentiation in water, and repeating until good contrast is obtained between amyloid and the background.
4. Wash and mount in modified Apathy's medium.

Results:

Amyloid, mucin, renal hyaline	red purple
Background	blue.

Thioflavine T:

It is a benzothiazole salt which is used principally as cationic fluorochrome dye.

It has a hydrophobic end with a dimethyl amino group attached to a phenyl group, linked to a more polar benzothiazole group containing the polar N and S.

H3C
S
N⁺
CH3
CH3
N
CH3
Cl⁻

Likewise, it binds to amyloid beta-sheet by hydrogen bonds along amyloid axis like congo red and displays enhanced fluorescence. Thioflavine T prior to binding to amyloid fibril emits weakly around 527 nm, but when excited by immobilized; the two rotational planes of the two rings of Thioflavine T (i.e., benzylamine and benzathiole ring that are connected through a carbon-carbon bond and rotate freely when thioflavine T in staining solution) produce a strong fluorescence signal at approximately 482 nm (Biancalana 2010).

Khurana *et al.* 2005 suggested thioflavine T exists as micelles and these micelles cause fluorescence when linked by amyloid (involving both ionic and hydrophobic bonds).

Thioflavine T method (Vassar and Culling, 1959)

Fixation:
Not critical.

Preparation of solution:
1% aqueous thioflavine T.

Method:
1. Sections to water, removing pigment where necessary.
2. Treat with alum hematoxylin solution, 2 minutes.
3. Wash in water and stain in thioflavineT solution, 3 minutes.
4. Rinse in water and differentiate excess fluorochrome from background in 1% acetic acid, 20 minutes.
5. Wash well in water, dehydrate, clear and mount in a nonfluorescent mountant.

Results:
Using UV light source (mercury vapor lamp), UG1 exciter filter, BG38 red suppression filter, and K430 barrier filter.
Amyloid, elastic tissue etc.—silver-blue fluorescence.
Using blue light fluorescence quartz-iodine or mercury vapor lamp with BG12 exciter filter and K530 barrier filter.
Amyloid, elastic tissue etc.— yellow fluorescence.

Further reading:

- Biancalana M, Koide S (2010). Molecular mechanism of Thioflavin-T binding to amyloid fibrils. *Biochimica et Biophysica Acta.* 1804 (7): 1405–12.
- Dapson, RW. Amyloid from a histochemical perspective. A review of the structure, properties and types of amyloid, and a proposed staining mechanism for Congo red staining. Biotech Histochem. 2018;93(8):543-556.
- Eastwood, H. and Cole. K.R. (1971) Staining of amyloid by buffered Congo red in 50 per cent ethanol. Stain Technology. 46(4): 208-209.
- Elmira I. Yakupova, Liya G. Bobyleva, Ivan M. Vikhlyantsev, et al. Congo Red and amyloids: history and relationship. Bioscience Reports. 2019, Vol.39, No. 1.
- Highman, B. (1946) Improved methods for demonstrating amyloid in paraffin sections. Archives of Pathology, 41: 559.
- Howie A.J.; Brewer D.B. (2009) Optical properties of amyloid stained by Congo red: history and mechanisms. Micron. 40: 285-301.
- Hucker, G.J. and Conn, ll. J. (1928) Gram stain. 1. A quick method for staining Gram-positive organisms in the tissues. Archives of Pathology. 5: 828.
- Khurana, R., Coleman, C., Ionescu-Zanetti, C., Carter, S., Krishna, V., Grover, R. & Singh, S., (2005) Mechanism of thioflavin T binding to amyloid fibrils., Journal of structural biology. 151: 229-238.
- Klunk, W.E., Pettegrew, J.W. and Abraham, D.J. (1989) Quantitative evaluation of congo red binding to amyloid-like proteins with a beta pleated sheet conformation. J. Histochem. Cytochem. 37, 1273–1281.
- Llewellyn, B.D., (2012) Direct dyes for amyloid (Stainfile Site)

- Puchtler, H., Sweat, F., et al. (1962) On the binding of Congo red by amyloid. Journal of Histochemistry and Cytochemistry. 10: 355.
- Reinke, A.A. and Gestwick, J.E. (2011) Insight into amyloid structure using chemical probes. Chem. Biol. Drug Des. 77, 399–411.
- Turnell, VV.G. and Finch, J.T. (1992) Binding of the dye congo red to the amyloid protein pig insulin reveals a novel homology amongest amyloid-forming peptide sequences, journal of Molecular Biology. 227(4): 1205-I223.
- Vassar. PS. and Culling, F.A. (1959) Fluorescent stains with special reference to amyloid and connective tissue. Archives of Pathology. 68: 487.

Connective tissue

The term connective tissue was traditionally applied to describe a basic type of tissue of mesodermal origin that provides structural and metabolic support. It consists of 3 different components: cells, fibers, and amorphous ground substance. Connective tissue cells include fibroblasts, mast cells, histiocytes, adipose tissue, reticular cells, osteoblasts, osteocytes, chondroblasts, chondrocytes and blood forming cells, etc. The ground substance is usually composed of amorphous (non-sulfated and sulfated mucopolysaccharides). Connective tissue fibers are three types; collagen fibers, elastic fibers and reticular fibers. These components vary in amount between four types of connective tissue, which are connective tissue proper, cartilage, bone and blood (B.young and Heath, j.w., 2000).

Collagen Fibers

Collagen fibers are the most abundant type of connective tissue fibers which are straight or wavy bundles. Collagen fibers are formed of a protein known as collagen which the later itself consists of three alpha polypeptide chains, with each chain formed of 1050 amino acids with of about 300 nm in length and 1.5 nm in diameter. Collagen contains 33% glycine, 10% proline, 10% hydroxyproline and 1% hydroxylysine. The synthesis of collagen involves the initial uniting of two α_1 chains and one of chain α_2 to form procollagen. Then this latter is transformed to tropocollagen when its non-helical domains are cleaved by peptidase. The tropocollagen self-aggregates in a staggered array to form a collagen fibril and finally many such fibrils cross-link side-by-side to form a collagen fiber.

Types of collagen fibers:

Type I:It formed by fibroblasts, osteoblasts and odontoblasts and formed of thick fibrils assembled in parallel bundles. This is the principal collagen of loose connective tissue, white fibrocartilage, bone, fascia and tendons.

Type II: It formed by chondroblasts and present in hyaline and elastic cartilage.

Type III:It formed by fibroblasts and smooth muscle cells, occurs in skin, muscle, lung, reticular fibers and other internal organs.

Type IV:It formed by fibroblasts and endothelial cells. This is the principal collagen of all basement membranes.

Type V:It formed by fibroblasts and present in placenta.

Collagen Staining

Acid dye mixtures are one of the oldest methods for collagen demonstration. These anionic mixtures divided into two major groups:

- ***Two-anionic dye mixtures:***
This type is a mixture of two anionic dyes imparts one color to collagen and another to cytoplasm, including that of muscle fibres and erythrocytes. Van Gieson method and its variants are the most common methods of this type all of them contain picric acid and other stains like acid fuchsin, Sirius red, aniline blue, indigo carmine and methylene blue (Kiernan2015). There are many theories to explain action of these mixtures which include:

Physical theory(Mann 1902, Baker 1958, Horobin and Flemming1988):

This theory depends on two concepts, firstly dye size and molecular weight (i.e., picric acid is small dye with low molecular weight while acid fuchsin and other similar dyes are medium to large dye with high molecular weight), secondly tissue density and permeable (i.e., the collagen fiber less dense and more permeable while other cytoplasmic structures denser and less permeable). According to these concepts, the small picric acid penetrates all of the tissues rapidly, but are only firmly retained in the close textures like RBCS and muscle while the large fuchsin displaces picric acid from collagen because collagen has large pores and allow larger molecules to enter.

Chemical theory (Lillie 1964, Puchtler and Sweat 1964):

This theory explains the staining of collagen by acid fuchsin. Firstly, Lillie1964 postulated two mechanisms depends on pre-treatment with nitrous acid and mixture of acetic anhydride, acetic acid and sulphuric acid which are ionic-bonding between sulphonate groups of dye and arginine side chains and hydrogen bonding between dye nitrogen atoms and hydroxy groups of serine, threonine and the hydroxylysine. Secondly, Puchtler and Sweat 1964 considered acid fuchsine like other direct cotton dyes that react with hydrogen bond.

Van Gieson technique (van Gieson 1889)

Sections:
paraffin. Celloidin sections are washed in distilled water after van Gieson solution.

Solution:

Saturated picric acid solution	50 ml
1% aqueous acid fuchsin	9.0 ml
Distilled water	50 ml

Method:
1. Deparaffinize sections and bring to water.
2. Stain nuclei by the celestine blue-hematoxylin sequence.
3. Wash in tap water.
4. Differentiate in acid alcohol.
5. Wash well in tap water.
6. Stain in van Gieson solution for 3 minutes.
7. Blot and dehydrate through alcohols.
8. Clear in xylene and mount in permanent mounting medium.

Results:

Nuclei	blue/black
Collagen	red
Other tissues	yellow.

- ***Heteropolyacid mixtures***

This type is a mixture of phosphotungestic acid or phosphomolybdic acid with two, three or rarely four anionic dyes. Most famous types of it are Masson trichrome and Mallory trichrome. There are three theories to explain their action which are described by (Kiernan 2015):

First theory (Mann 1902, Baker 1958, Horobin and Flemming1988): it is similar to physical theory of van Gieson, but here the tissue firstly stained by a small or medium dye which penetrates most tissue components, but links tightly with more dense structures like RBCS, then addition of polyacid competes small and medium dye in the combination in all tissue parts except fine textures like RBCS because polyacid can't able to reach it, finally section stained by large dye (collagen stain) which replaces and competes polyacid from linkage with collagen fiber and that needs time control because any time increase make collagen stain covers all section by its colour.

The second theory (Puchtler and Lsler 1958): this theory considered collagen stains as amphoteric dyes and can link directly by its negative charged groups to protonated amino and guanidino groups of collagens electrovalently or by its cationic charged groups and free negatively charged groups of the collagen-bound ions of polyacid.

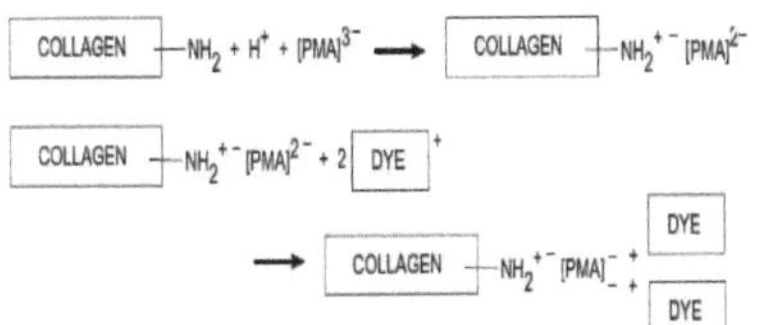

Third theory (Everett and Miller 1974) this theory postulates two modes of polyacids binding, firstly ionic binding with cytoplasmic proteins and secondly non-ionic binding (may be hydrogen bond) with collagen only.

Masson trichrome technique (Masson 1929)

Fixation:
Formal sublimate or formal saline.
Sections:
All types.
Solutions
Solution a:

Acid fuchsin	0.5 g
Glacial acetic acid	0.5 ml
Distilled water	100 ml

Solution b:

Phosphomolybdic acid	1.0 g
Distilled water	100 ml

Solution c:

Methyl blue	2.0 g
Glacial acetic acid	2.5 ml
Distilled water	100 ml

Method:
1. Deparaffinize sections and bring to water.
2. Remove mercury pigment by iodine, sodium thiosulfate sequence.
3. Wash in tap water.
4. Stain nuclei by the celestin blue-hematoxylin method.
5. Differentiate with 1 % acid alcohol.
6. Wash well in tap water.
7. Stain in acid fuchsin (solution a) for 5 minutes.
8. Rinse in distilled water.
9. Treat with phosphomolybdic acid (solution b), 5 minutes.
10. Drain.
11. Stain with methyl blue solution c for 2-5 minutes.
12. Rinse in distilled water.
13. Treat with 1% acetic acid 2 minutes.
14. Dehydrate through alcohols.
15. Clear in xylene, mount in permanent mounting medium.

Result:

Nuclei	blue-black
Cytoplasm, muscle and erythrocytes	red
Collagen	blue.

Elastic fibers:

Elastic fibers re thinner fiber than collagen (0.1 – 0.2) nm, run singly (not in bundles), branch and anastomoses with other fibers.

Elastic fibers are composed mainly of protein called elastin (which rich in proline and glycine with unusual amino acids like desmosine) and microfibril (which is very fine fibril consisting of glycoproteins).

Elastic fibers are formed via a process known as elastogenesis. In this process tropoelastin (monomeric precursor of elastic protein) produced by elastogenic cells and chaperoned to the cell surface, then a number of them link up by (Lox and Fibulin-4) to make elastin and this process called coacervation.

Also, elastogenic cells produce fibrillin-1 (monomeric precursor of microfibril) which a number of them link up by (MFAP-4) to make microfibril. When elastin links with microfibril, the elastic fibers will be formed.

There are other fibers related to elastic fibers. Thus, oxytalan fibers are bundles of microfibrils, 10-12 nm in diameter, which do not contain elastin. Elaunin fibers are filaments that cross discontinuous aggregates of elastin.

Resorcin-fuchsin method (Weigert, 1898)

Principle:
It is a mixture of di and polynuclear products derived from pararosaniline by oxidative coupling under the influence of ferric ions (Pearse1980).

According to Puchtler (1961) staining mechanism occurs by hydrogen bond between phenolic hydroxyl groups of dyes and the carbonyl oxygen of elastic acid polysaccharide ester groups. Horobin and Flemming (1980) postulated the role of van der Waals forces in staining mechanism.

Preparation of Weigert resorcin fuchsin:
To 100 ml of distilled water, add 1 g of basic fuchsin and 2 g of resorcin. Boil. Add 12.5 ml of freshly prepared 30% ferric chloride solution. Continue boiling for 5 minutes. Cool and filter, discarding the filtrate. Dissolve the whole of the precipitate in 100 ml of 95% ethanol, using a hot plate or waterbath for controlled heating and add 2 mL of concentrated hydrochloric acid. As an improved solvent, the precipitate may be dissolved in:

2 methoxyethanol	50 ml
Distilled water	50 ml
Concentrated hydrochloric acid	2 ml

Staining time is reduced with this solvent.

Method:
1. Deparaffinize sections and bring to alcohol.
2. Place in staining solution in a Coplin jar, 1-3 hours at room temperature or 1 hour at 56°C.
3. Rinse in tap water.
4. Remove background staining by treating with 1% acid alcohol.
5. Rinse in tap water.
6. Counterstain as desired
7. Dehydrate through alcohols.
8. Clear in xylene and mount in permanent mounting medium.

Results:

Elastic tissue fibers   brown to purple.

Verhoeff's method for elastic fibers (Verhöeff, 1908)

Principle:
Horobin and Flemming (1980) speculated that this was a 2:1 hematein-iron coordination complex, such as the one down below.

The four phenolic hydroxyl groups of hematin are able to form hydrogen bond with elastic fibers (Arshid 1956). Horobin and flemming (1980) suggested the dye link to elastin occur by van der Waals forces. The role of ferric and iodine in staining mechanism, unknown exactly.

Verhoeff's method for elastic fibers (Verhöeff, 1908)

Preparation of stain:

Solution a:

Hematoxylin	5 g
Absolute alcohol	100 ml

Solution b:

Ferric chloride	10 g
Distilled water	100 ml

Solution c: (Lugol's iodine solution)

Iodine	1 g
Potassium iodide	2 g
Distilled water	100 ml

Solution d: (working solution)

Solution (a)	20 ml
Solution (b)	8 ml
Solution (c)	8 ml

Add in the above order, mixing between additions.

Method:

1. Deparaffinize sections and bring to water.
2. Verhoeff's solution 15-30 minutes.
3. Rinse in water.
4. Differentiate in 2% aqueous ferric chloride until elastic tissue fibers appear black on a gray background.
5. Rinse in water
6. Rinse in 95% alcohol to remove any staining due to iodine alone.
7. Counterstain as desired
8. Blot to remove excess stain.
9. Dehydrate rapidly through alcohols.
10. Clear in xylene and mount in permanent mounting medium.

Results:

Elastic tissue fibers	black

Other tissues according to counterstain.

Aldehyde fuchsin method for elastic fibers

Principle:

There are several aldehyde fuchsine components, three being mono-, di- and tri Schiff base derivatives of pararosaniline (Horobin and Kiernan 2002).

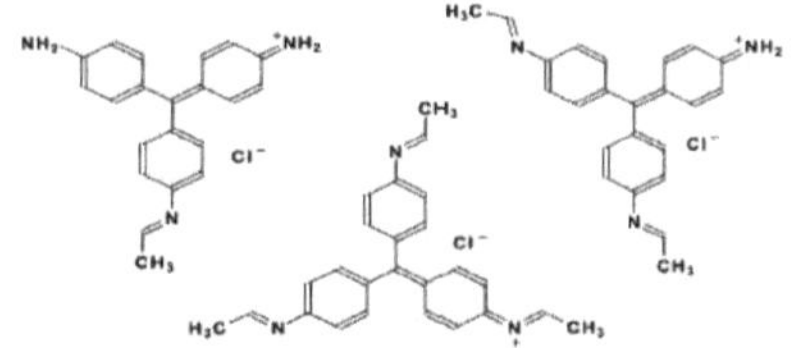

According to Pearse (1980) the staining mechanism fall into three main categories. Firstly, ionic-bond with polyanions specially when these are sulphated, secondly covalent bond with sulphonic acid, carboxyl and tautomeric enamine and thirdly non-ionic such as hydrogen bond.

Horobin and Flemming (1980) postulated aldehyde fuchsine bonds to elastin by van der Waals forces.

Aldehyde fuchsin method for elastic fibers

Preparation of staining solution:

Dissolve 1 g of basic fuchsine in 100 ml of 70% ethanol; heat may be used to speed the process. After cooling and filtering add 1 ml of concentrated hydrochloric acid and 2 ml of paraldehyde. Stand at room temperature for 2 days to complete the ripening process, which is indicated by a conversion from red to purple. Ripening time may be reduced by increased temperature at 50-60°C. The ripened solution should be refrigerated for storage. Batches of basic fuchsin suitable for the production of Schiff's reagent are usually satisfactory for the preparation of aldehyde fuchsin. Paraldehyde may lose some potency upon storage but this may be partially compensated by the addition of an extra 0.5 ml of this solution. The staining potential of aldehyde fuchsin is greatest at between 2 and 4 days after preparation, but may be adequate for the demonstration of elastic tissue fibers for several weeks if stored at 4°C.

Method:

1. Deparaffinize sections and bring to water.

2. Oxidize in 1% potassium permanganate, 5 minutes.
3. Rinse in tap water.
4. Remove permanganate staining by treatment with 1% oxalic acid.
5. Rinse in tap water.
6. Rinse in 70% ethanol.
7. Place in sealed container of aldehyde fuchsin for 15 minutes.
8. Rinse well in 70% ethanol.
9. Rinse in tap water.
10. Counterstain as desired
11. Dehydrate through alcohols.
12. Clear in xylene and mount in permanent mounting medium.

Results:

Elastic tissue fibers   blue-purple
Other tissues according to counterstain.

Horobin and Flemming general theory of elastic fiber staining, based on structure-staining correlations:

Horobin and Flemming (1980) argued that since dyes which stained elastic fibers all had large conjugated systems, the major factor which favoured staining of elastic fibers was van der Waals binding, with a contribution from hydrophobic bonding in some cases. They argued in this after adopting a structure-staining correlation approach, and used the number of conjugated bonds in a dye to assess whether it was likely to stain elastic fibers.

Reticular Fibers:

Reticular fibers are long, very thin, and extracellular fibers with 100 - 150 nm diameter. They crosslink to form a fine network (reticular) for supporting soft tissue such as liver, bone marrow and lymphatic tissues.

They are composed of type III collagen but differ from collagen (especially collagen type I) by they are many fibers, have uneven thickness, do not form bundles and contain carbohydrates (6% - 12%).

Silver impregnation:

There are many variations of silver methods for reticular fibers, but most of them are similar in major steps of mechanism:

- Oxidation of the adjacent glycol groups of the hexose sugars of Reticular Fibers glycoprotein to aldehydes by oxidizer agent as phosphomolybdic acid, potassium permanganate or periodic acid.

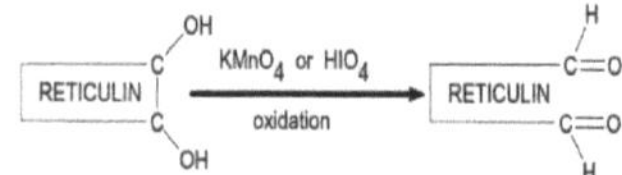

- Bleaching only required following oxidization with potassium permanganate by oxalic acid to remove manganese dioxide by converting it into soluble reduced manganese, carbon dioxide and water.

- Sensitization usually by iron alum (ferric ammonium sulfate) or with another sensitizer like uranyl nitrate and dilute solution of silver nitrate. The exact chemical reaction is not known, but some explanations have been given like that ferric ion combines with binding sites freed up by the permanganate oxidation and attaches to reticular fibers predominantly, with much lower amount attaching to other components or by formation of metal-organic compound with tissue with metals or by partial blocking or deblocking of active groups, oxidation, reduction and pH induced changes.

- Treatment by an ammoniacal or diamine complex to reduce a few of silver ions or to metallic silver (i.e., formation of silver nuclei at Reticular Fibers reducing groups) while other silver ions form ionic bonds by ionized groups in tissue.

$$\text{RETICULIN} \begin{cases} \overset{\displaystyle H}{\underset{}{\overset{|}{C}}}=O \\ \overset{}{C}=O \\ \overset{\displaystyle |}{H} \end{cases} + 2[Ag(NH_3)_2]^+ + 2H_2O + 3OH^-$$

$$\longrightarrow \text{RETICULIN} \begin{cases} \overset{OH}{\underset{}{\overset{|}{C}}}=O \\ \overset{}{C}=O \\ \overset{\displaystyle |}{OH} \end{cases} + 4Ag(s) + 8NH_4OH$$

- Reduction of tissue attached unreduced silver by formalin near original sites of reduction and how it is possible to visualize under microscope.

$$2[Ag(NH_3)_2]^+ + HCHO + 2OH^- \rightarrow$$
$$2Ag + 4NH_3 + HCOOH + H_2O$$

- Toning by gold chloride to replace metallic silver precipitate by gold and the deposit changes from brown-black to purple black.

$$3Ag + (AuCl_4)^- \rightarrow Au + 3AgCl + Cl^-$$

- Fixing by sodium thiosulfate treatment to removes un-reduced silver or gold complex formation.

$$Ag^+ + 2\,Na_2S_2O_3 \rightarrow Na^+ + Na_3Ag(S_2O_3)_2$$

- Counterstaining according to what other components are to be demonstrated.

Gordon & Sweets' method for reticular fibers (Gordon & Sweets, 1936)

Preparation of silver solution

To 5 mL of 10% aqueous silver nitrate solution add concentrated ammonia, drop by drop, until the precipitate first formed dissolves, taking care to avoid any excess of ammonia. Add 5 mL of 3% sodium hydroxide solution. Re-dissolve the precipitate by the addition of concentrated ammonia, drop by drop, until the solution retains a trace of opalescence. If at this stage any excess of ammonia is present, indicated by the absence of opalescence, add a few drops of 10% silver nitrate solution, to produce a light precipitate. Make up the volume to 50 mL with distilled water. Filter before use. Store in a dark bottle.

Method:
1. Deparaffinize sections and bring to water.
2. Treat with 1% potassium permanganate solution, 5 minutes.
3. Rinse in tap water.
4. Bleach in 1% oxalic acid solution.
5. Rinse in tap water.
6. Treat with 2.5% iron alum solution for at least 15 minutes.
7. Wash well in several changes of distilled water.
8. Plate in a Coplin jar of silver solution, 2 minutes.
9. Rinse in several changes of distilled water.
10. Reduce in 10% aqueous formalin solution, 2 minutes.
11. Rinse in tap water.
12. Tone in 0.2% gold chloride solution, 3 minutes.
13. Rinse in tap water.
14. Treat with 5% sodium thiosulfate solution, 3 minutes.
15. Rinse in tap water.
16. Counterstain as desired.
17. Dehydrate through alcohols.
18. Clear in xylene and mount in permanent mounting medium.

Results

Reticular fibers	black
Nuclei	black or unstained

Other elements according to counterstain.

Gomori's method for reticular fibers (Gomori 1937)

Preparation of silver solution:
To 10 ml of 10% potassium hydroxide solution add 40 ml of 10% silver nitrate solution. Allow the precipitate to settle and decant the supernatant. Wash the precipitate several times with distilled water. Add ammonia drop by drop until the precipitate has just dissolved. Add further 10% silver nitrate solution until a little precipitate remains. Dilute to 100 ml and filter. Store in a dark bottle.

Method:

1. Deparaffinize sections and bring to water.
2. Treat with 1% potassium permanganate solution, 2 minutes.
3. Rinse in tap water.
4. Bleach in 2% potassium metabisulfate solution.
5. Rinse in tap water.
6. Treat with 2% iron alum, 2 minutes.
7. Wash in several changes of distilled water.
8. Place in Coplin jar of silver solution, 1 minute.
9. Wash in several changes of distilled water.
10. Reduce in 4% aqueous formalin solution, 3 minutes.
11. Rinse in tap water.
12. Tone in 0.2% gold chloride solution, 10 minutes.
13. Rinse in tap water.
14. Treat with 2% potassium metabisulfite solution, 1 minute.
15. Rinse in tap water.
16. Treat with 2% sodium thiosulfate solution,1 minute.
17. Rinse in tap water.
18. Counterstain as desired.
19. Dehydrate through alcohols.
20. Clear in xylene and mount in permanent mounting medium.

Results:

Reticular fibers	black
Nuclei	gray

Other tissues according to counterstain.

Fibrin and Fibrinoid

Fibrin is an insoluble fibrillar protein material derived from fibrinogen one of the plasma proteins by polymerization. Its primary function is to stop bleeding. Fibrin is an important constituent of the acute inflammatory exudate thus it may be found wherever there is recent tissue damage. Although fibrin is not tissues, but the stains used for the demonstration of connective tissues are also used for its identification. It is acidophilic, often can be seen in H &E as distinctly pink but less brilliant than erythroctes. In paraffin sections, fibrin is strongly eosinophilic and stains blue black with Mallory's Phosphotungstic Acid Hematoxylin (PTAH) stain, but old fibrin tends to stain red (as collagen). It is yellow after Van Gieson stain and weekly to moderately PAS positive (Bancroft and et al. 2008). Lendrum et al. (1962) recommended Lendrum's Martius, Scarlet and Blue (MSB) which is a popular trichrome staining method to demonstrate fibrin and to distinguish between fibrin of varying ages. MSB is a modification of Masson's trichrome stain, it can demonstrate older fibrin. Early fibrin deposits may also be stained, although phosphotungstic acid blocks muscle staining, Collagen and most connective tissue fibers.

The ending -oid means "like", so fibrinoid means like fibrin. Fibrinoid is a hyaline eosinophilic material seen in some diseases, often auto immune, which has identical staining reactions to fibrin but occurs in tissues in different situations and disorders. Now it is generally accepted that fibrinoid is fibrin that is mixed with or which has trapped other materials which alter its staining reactions. It is a mixture of exudates and altered cytoplasmic constituents, forming a homogenous eosinophilic material which gives the same staining reaction as fibrin.

Techniques for the selective demonstration of fibrin are of three types: Gram-Weigert, Phosphotungstic acid-hematoxylin and Trichrome methods.

MSB technique for fibrin (Lendrum *et al.*, 1962)

The standard MSB technique employs Martius yellow (acid yellow 24) CI 10315, brilliant crystal scarlet (acid red 44) CI 16250, and soluble or methyl blue (acid blue 93) CI 42780.

Preparation of solutions
Martius yellow solution

Martius yellow	0.5 g
PTA	2 g
95% alcohol	100 ml

Martius yellow is dissolved in alcohol before adding the phosphotungstic acid.

A satisfactory substitute for Martius yellow is the larger molecule dye, lissamine fast yellow, which has the advantage of being less easily removed by the subsequent red dye.

Brilliant crystal scarlet solution

Brilliant crystal scarlet	1 g
Glacial acetic acid	2 ml
Distilled water	100 ml

A number of medium sized molecule anionic red dyes may be substituted for the brilliant crystal scarlet, e.g. Ponceau de xylidine and azofuchsin.

PTA solution

PTA	1 g
Distilled water	100 ml

Methyl blue solution

Methyl blue	0.5 g
Glacial acetic acid	1 ml
Distilled water	100 ml

Many large molecule blue or green dyes may be substituted for the methyl blue e.g. durazol blue, pontamine sky blue, fast green FCF or naphthalene black 10B. The replacement of methyl blue by pontamine sky blue reduces the tendency of fibrin coloring by the blue dye due to the larger molecular size.

1% acetic acid

Glacial acetic acid	1 ml
Distilled water	100 ml

Method
1. Deparaffinize sections and take to water.
2. Remove mercury pigment with iodine, sodium thiosulfate treatment.
3. Stain nuclei by the celestine blue-hematoxylin sequence.
4. Differentiate in 1% acid alcohol.
5. Wash well in tap water.
6. Rinse in 95% alcohol.
7. Stain in Martius yellow solution for 2 minutes.
8. Rinse in distilled water.
9. Stain in brilliant crystal scarlet solution for 10 minutes.
10. Rinse in distilled water.
11. Treat with PTA solution until no red remains in the collagen.
12. Rinse in distilled water.
13. Stain in methyl blue solution until collagen is sufficiently stained.
14. Rinse in 1% acetic acid.
15. Dehydrate through ascending grades of alcohol.
16. Clear in xylene and mount in permanent mounting medium.

Results

Nuclei	blue
Erythrocytes	yellow
Muscles	red
Collagen	blue

Fibrin red (early fibrin may stain yellow and old fibrin, blue).

Muscular tissue

Muscles provide power and movement to the body by contractile properties of the myofibrils and subcellular components. Muscles provide power and movement by contracting their cells, shortening their overall length, and thus pulling the points where the muscle is attached closer together. Many cells in the body share this ability to contract and change shape and this is due to the presence of three proteins and the interaction between them: α-Actin, Actin and Myosin. Muscular tissue is divided into three basic types, all types have similar constituents and their mode of providing power and movement is also similar.

- *Voluntary striated muscle*

Widely distributed over all parts of the skeleton, thus it called skeletal muscle. Skeletal muscle movement can be voluntarily controlled, it composed of large elongated eosinophilic myofibers, and have striations or stripes which cross the fibers at right angle to their long axes. Myofiber is made up of thinner myofibrils separated by a well-developed system of mitochondria and sarcoplasmic reticulum. Skeletal muscle contains abundant of glycogen storage that provides immediate source of energy.

- *Involuntary smooth muscle*

Derived from mesenchymal tissue, composed of smaller tapered myofibers with eosinophilic cytoplasm containing glycogen. Like skeletal muscle, the myofiber contains bundles or myofilament or myofibrils. Smooth muscles comprise the wall of the gastrointestinal tract, urogenital tract and blood vessels, whose contractions cannot be controlled at will.

- *Striated cardiac muscle.*

Only found in the heart, known as the myocardium. Its cytoplasm contains myofibrils and sarcoplasm. It is striated, but the striations are less distinct as myofibrils are not arranged regularly like the voluntary skeletal muscle.

Demonstration of muscle striations

All types of muscle, whether voluntary, involuntary or cardiac, contain considerable amount of connective tissue or collagenous fibers that surround and divide muscle fibers into bundles.

Many staining techniques for demonstration of connective tissue are therefore also applicable to muscle tissue. H&E and trichrome methods demonstrate muscle striations, but better definition is seen using Heidenhain's iron hematoxylin and Mallory's PTA hematoxylin.

Further reading:

- Arshid, F.M., Connelly, R.F., Desai, J.N., Fulton, R.G., Giles, C.H. & Kefalis, J.C. (1954) A study of certain natural dyes. Part 2. The structure of the metallic lakes of Brazilwood and Logwood colouring matters. 3. *SOC. Dyers. Colour.* 70, 402.
- Baker, J.R. (1958). *Principles of Biological Microtechnique.* London: Methuen.
- Everett, M.M. and Miller, W.A. (1974). The role of phosphotungstic and phosphomolybdic acids in connective tissue staining. *Histochemical Journal* 6: 25–34.
- Gordon. H. & Sweets, H.H. (1936) A simple method for the silver impregnation of reticulum. American journal of Pathology. 12: 545.
- Gomori, G. (1950) Aldehyde-fuchsin, a new stain for elastic tissue. American Journal of Clinical
- Horobin, R.W. and Flemming, L. (1988). One-bath trichrome staining: investigation of a general mechanism based on a structure–staining correlation analysis. *Histochemical Journal* 20: 23–34.
- Horobin, R.W. and Flemming, L. (1980). Structure–staining relationships in histochemistry and biological staining. II. Mechanistic and practical aspects of the staining of elastic fibres. *Journal of Microscopy* 119: 357–372.
- Horobin R W & Kiernan J A, (2002). Conn's Biological Stains, 10th ed. BIOS Scientific Publishers, Oxford, UK
- Kiernan, J.A. (2015) Histological and Histochemical Methods: Theory and Practice. 5th edition, Scion Publishing.

- Lillie, R.D. (1964). Histochemical acylation of hydroxyl and amino groups. Effect on the periodic acid–Schiff reaction, anionic and cationic dye and van Gieson collagen stains. *Journal of Histochemistry and Cytochemistry* 12: 821–841.
- Mann, G. (1902). Physiological Histology. Methods and Theory. Oxford: Clarendon Press.
- Masson, P. (1929) Some histological methods. trichrome stainings and their preliminary technique. Bulletin of the Jntcrnational Association of Medicine. 12: 75
- Prento, P. (1993). Van Gieson's picrofuchsin: the staining mechanisms for collagen and cytoplasm, and an examination of the dye diffusion rate model of differential staining. *Histochemistry* 99: 163–174.
- Pearse, A.G.E. and Stoward, P.J. (1980,1985,1991). *Histochemistry, Theoretical and Applied,* 4th edn, Vols 1–3. Edinburgh: Churchill-Livingstone.
- Puchtler, H., Sweat. F., Bates, R. & Brown, J.H. (1961) On the mechanism of resorcin-fuchsinstaining. *3. Histochem. Cyrochem.* 9, 553.Pathology. 20: 665.
- Puchtler, H. and Sweat, F. (1964). Histochemical specificity of staining methods for connective tissue fibers: resorcin–fuchsin and van Gieson's picro-fuchsin. *Histochemie* 4: 24–34.
- Puchtler, H. and Isler, H. (1958). The effect of phosphomolybdic acid on the stainability of connective tissues by various dyes. *Journal of Histochemistry and Cytochemistry* 6: 265–270.
- van Gieson, I. (1889) Laboratory notes of technical methods for the nervous system. York medical Journal, 50: 57
- Verhiieff, F.H. (1908) Some new staining methods of wide applicability, including a rapid differential stain for elastic tissue. Journal of American Medical Association. 50: 876.
- Weigert, C. (1898) Liber eine Methode zue Farbung elastischer Fasern. Zentralblatt fur Allgcmeine Pathologic und Pathologische Anatomic, 9: 289.
- Young. B. and heath. j.w. (2000). functional histology, fourth edition, ISSN 04430-56129.

The term *pigment* refers to any of the various coloring agents, frequently deposited as cytoplasmic inclusions or granules, in cells and tissues and absorb visible light (electromagnetic energy within narrow range (400 – 800) nm). It is not necessary to stain pigments with biologic dyes because they are colored (yellow, brown or black), however, special stains may be necessary in differentiation of similarly colored pigments. Various pigment may greatly differ in origin, chemical composition and biological significance. They can be either organic or in organic compound that are insoluble in most solvent.

Pigments have an important role in the diagnosis of diseases such as gout, kidney and gallstones, jaundice, melanomas, albinism, hemorrhage and tuberculosis (Irons RD, *et al.* 1977).

Pigments can be classified in three categories.
1. Endogenous Pigments:
These pigments are produced either within tissues and serve a physiological function, or may be products of normal metabolic processes. They are further subdivide into:

hematogenous (blood-derived) pigments (hemosiderin, hemoglobin, bile pigment and porphyrins), ***non-hematogenous*** (such as melanin, lipofuscin and chromaffin), and ***endogenous minerals*** (such as iron, calcium and copper). Endogenous pigments become pathologic when they are deposited in excessive quantity or found in abnormal locations.
2. Exogenous Pigments:
These pigments consist of foreign materials, usually have no physiological function. They enter the body accidentally through a variety of methods. Entry into the body may occur either by inhalation into the lungs or by implantation into the skin. Most exogenous pigments are

minerals, few of which are actively pigment. Exogenous pigments include carbon, silica, asbestos, lead, sliver and tattoo pigments.
3. Artifact Pigments:
These are pigments usually lie on top of tissue instead of within the cells. They are produced due to the interactions between certain tissue components and some chemicals during the course of histological techniques and most commonly result from fixation. Artifact pigments include formalin, malaria, schistosome, mercury, chromic oxide and starch.

Endogenous pigments

Hematogenous endogenous pigments

It contains the following blood-derived pigments: hemosiderin, hemoglobin, bile pigment and porphyrins

Hemosiderin

It is an iron-storage complex that is composed of partially digested ferritin and lysosomes and result from the breakdown of heme or the abnormal metabolic pathway of ferritin. Hemosiderin is most commonly found in macrophages and is especially abundant in situations following haemorrhage, suggesting that its formation may be related to phagocytosis of red blood cells and hemoglobin. Hemosiderin deposits are small and commonly in apparent without special stains like perls Prussian blue. The deposition of larger amounts of hemosiderin due iron over load in tissues known as hemochromatosis.

Perls' Prussian blue reaction for ferric iron (Perls, 1867)

Principle:
The hydrochloric acid liberates ferric ions from tissue to react with potassium ferrocyanide, lead

to formation of ferric ferrocyanide (Prussian blue).

$$4Fe^{3+} + 3[Fe(CN)_6]^{4-} \longrightarrow Fe_4[Fe(CN)_6]_3(s)$$

Fixation:
Avoid the use of acid fixatives. Chromates will also interfere with the preservation of iron.
Sections:
Works well on all types of sections including resin.
Ferrocyanide solution:
1% aqueous potassium Ferrocyanide 20 ml

2% aqueous hydrochloric acid   20 ml
Preferably freshly prepared just before use.
Method:
1. Take a test and control section to water
2. Treat sections with the freshly prepared acid ferrocyanide solution for 10-30 minutes
3. Wash well in distilled water.
4. Lightly stain the nuclei with 0.5% aqueous neutral red or 0.1% nuclear fast red.
5. Wash rapidly in distilled water.
6. Dehydrate, clear and mount in synthetic resin.
Results:

Ferric iron	blue
Nuclei	red.

Hukill& Putt's method for ferrous and ferric iron (Hukill & Putt, 1962)

Principle:
Both ferrous and ferric ions form red complex chelate with bathophenanthroline.

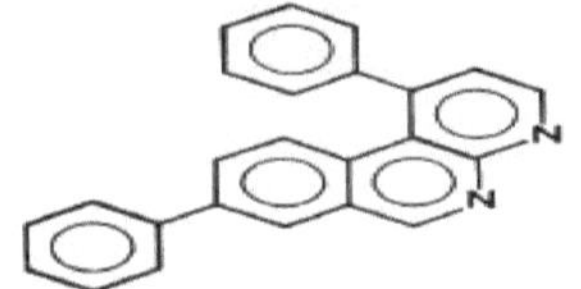

Fixation:
Not critical but avoid prolonged exposure to acidic fixatives.
Sections:
All types of tissue sections may be used including resin.
Solution:
Bathophenanthroline
(4,7-diphenyl-1,10-phenanthroline)   100 mg
3% aqueous acetic acid   100 ml
Place in oven at 60°C for 24 hours, agitating at regular intervals. Cool to room temperature and filter. This solution is stable for about 4 weeks. Before use add thioglycolic acid to a concentration of 0.5% (this should be replenished each time before use as it rapidly undergoes oxidation on exposure to air).
Method:
1. Take test and control sections to distilled water.
2. Stain sections in bathophenanthroline solution for 2 hours at room temperature.
3. Rinse well in distilled water.
4. Counterstain in 0.5% aqueous methylene blue for 2 minutes.
5. Rinse well in distilled water.
6. Stand slides on end until completely dry.
7. Dip slides in xylene and mount in synthetic resin.
Results:

Ferrous iron	red
Nuclei	blue.

Hemoglobin

It is the iron-containing oxygen-transport metalloprotein mainly in the red blood cells or in the A9 dopaminergic neurons in the substantia nigra, macrophages, alveolar cells, lungs, retinal pigment epithelium, hepatocytes, mesangial cells in the kidney, endometrial cells, cervical cells and vaginal epithelial cells.
It consists of a protein part called globin (a protein with four peptide chains joined together by

non-covalent bonds) that is tightly bound to 4 heme molecules (non-protein part).

Several kinds of haemoglobin are HbA, HbA_1, HbA_2 and HbF. Production of Hb continues in the cell throughout its early development from the proerythroblast to the reticulocyte in the bone marrow when the heme part is synthesized in a series of steps in the mitochondria and the cytosol of immature red blood cells, and the globin protein parts are synthesized by ribosomes in the cytosol link together.

Leuco Patent Blue V method for hemoglobin (Dunn & Thompson, 1946)

Principle:
In the presence of hydrogen peroxide, the colorless leuco patent blue V converted to colored leuco patent blue V by peroxidase enzyme.

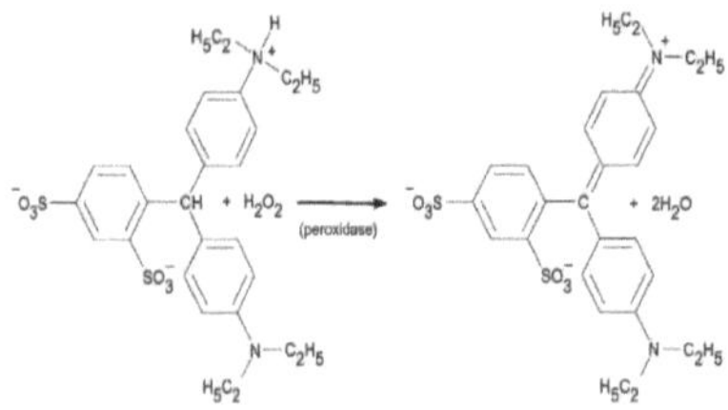

Fixation:
Formalin or formal mercury.

Preparation of solutions:

Stock solution:

1 % aqueous patent blue V (CI 42045)	100 ml
Powdered zinc	10 g
Glacial acetic acid	2 ml

Boil in a 500 ml flask, until colorless (usually takes 10 minutes). Cool, filter and store in the refrigerator in an airtight bottle. The solution is stable for about one week.

Staining solution:

Stock solution	10 ml
Glacial acetic acid	2 ml
3% hydrogen peroxide	1 ml

Prepare immediately before use.

Method:
1. Take test and control sections to distilled water
2. Stain in Patent blue solution for 5 minutes at room temperature.
3. Rinse in distilled water
4. Lightly counterstain in 0.5% aqueous neutral red or 0.1% aqueous nuclear fast red for 1 minute.
5. Rinse in distilled water.
6. Dehydrate, clear and mount in synthetic resin.

Results

Hemoglobin peroxidase (red blood cells and neutrophils)	dark blue
Nuclei	red.

Bile pigments

Bile pigments are biological pigments of linear arrangements of four pyrrole rings (tetrapyrroles) formed as a metabolic product of certain porphyrins.

At the end of the red cells life span (120 days), they are removed from circulation by the cells of reticuloendothelial (RE) system mostly present in liver, spleen and bone marrow, where they are lysed and hemoglobin comes out, giving globin molecule (which hydrolyzes into free amino acids) and heme ring (which gives biliverdin and bilirubin).

Modified Fouchet's technique for liver bile pigments (Hall 1960)

Principle:
The bilirubin oxidizes by ferric chloride to biliverdin in the presence of trichloroacetic acid.

Fixation:
Any fixative appears suitable.

Sections:
Any sections.

Solutions:

Fouchet's solution

25% aqueous trichloracetic acid	36 ml
10% aqueous ferric chloride	4 ml

Freshly prepared before use.

Van Gieson stain

Dissolve 100 mg of acid fuchsin (CI 42685) in 100 ml of saturated aqueous picric acid.

Method:

1. Take test and control sections to distilled water
2. Treat with the freshly prepared Fouchet's solution for 10 minutes.
3. Wash well in running tap water for 1 minute.
4. Rinse in distilled water.
5. Counterstain with van Gieson solution for 2 minutes.
6. Dehydrate, clear and mount in synthetic resin.

Results:

Bile pigments	emerald to blue green
Muscle	yellow
Collagen	red.

Gmelin technique (Tiedermann & Gmelin 1826)

Principle:

When bile pigments react with nitric acid its color change according to the sequence yellow, green, blue, violet or red.

The Gmelin reaction depends on the dehydrogenation of bilirubin to the greenish- blue bilatriene (verdin), and the green stage of the reaction is due to mixtures of bilatriene and unoxidized bilirubin. Similarly, the blue stage is also due to a mixture, this time of bilatriene with violet pigments (purpurins) produced by its further oxidation to biladienedol. Finally, the blue and violet compounds are oxidized to yellow choletelins (pearse 1980).

Sections:

Paraffin.

Method:

1. Sections to distilled water and mount in distilled water.

2. Place mounted section under the microscope using an objective with reasonable working distance.
3. Place 2-3 drops concentrated nitric acid to one side of the cover glass and draw under the cover glass by means of a piece of blotting paper on the opposite side.
4. Remove excess solution and observe pigment for color changes.

Results:

Bile pigments will gradually produce the following spectrum of color change: yellow-green-blue-purple-red.

Porphyrins

Porphyrins are normal pigment present in haemoglobin, myoglobin and cytochrome. The porphyrias are rare pathological conditions due to inherited and acquired deficiencies in the heme biosynthesis pathway resulting in genetic deficiency of one of the enzymes required for the synthesis of haem, leading to excessive accumulation of porphyrins. The site of abnormal heme metabolism and porphyrin accumulation classifies porphyria as *hepatic* (more common and have a normal erythroid precursor, but have a defect in synthesis of haem in the liver) or *erythropoietic* (defective synthesis of haem in the red cell precursors in the bone marrow). In erythropoietic protoporphyria, the pigment is seen as focal dark-brown pigment and under polarized light shows a bright red color with a centrally located dark Maltese cross on liver sections, while on frozen section, exhibit brilliant red fluorescence that rapidly fades with exposure to UV light.

Non-hematogenous endogenous pigments

Contains the following:

- Melanins
- Lipofuscins
- Chromaffin

- Pseudomelanosis (melanosis coli)
- Dubin-Johnson pigment
- Ceroid-type lipofuscin
- Hamazaki-Weisenberg bodies

Melanin

It is a broad term for a group of natural pigments found mainly in the skin and several internal sites, notably the eye, the cochlea and some neurons in the brain stem. There are five basic types of melanin: eumelanin, pheomelanin, neuromelanin, allomelanin and pyomelanin but the common type is eumelanin, of which there are two subtypes brown eumelanin and black eumelanin.

Melanin is produced through a multistages chemical process known as melanogenesis, where the oxidation of the amino acid tyrosine to dihydrophenylalanine (DOPA) and then to melanin by polymerization.

A number of methods can be used for the identifcation of melanin:

- **Reducing method for Melanin:**

Melanin is a strong reducing agent, so it used by three ways:

- The reduction of ammoniacal silver solution to metallic silver without the aid of reducing agent is known as the argentaffin reaction. Masson method is widely used for routine purposes.
- Melanin reduces ferricyanide to ferrocyanid then Prussian blue in the presence of ferric salts. The schmorl reaction is an example of it.
- Lillie ferrous-ion uptake method in which melanin forms ferrous melanin complexes when reacts with ferrous sulfate, then ferrous melanin complexes react with the ferricyanide to produce ferrous ferricyanide (Turbull blue).

Masson-Fontana method for melanin (Fontana 1912, Masson 1914)

Fixation:
Formalin is best; chromate and mercuric chloride should be avoided.

Sections:
Works on all types of sections, although some adjustment may be necessary for resin sections.

Silver solution preparation (after Fontana)
Place 20 ml of a 10% aqueous silver nitrate solution in a glass flask. Using a fine-pointed dropper pipette, add concentrated ammonia drop by drop, constantly agitating the flask until the formed precipitate almost dissolves. This titration is critical if the method is to work consistently well. The end point of the titration is seen when a faint opalescence is present, and is best viewed using reflected light against a black background. If too much ammonia is inadvertently added, then the addition of a few drops of 10% silver nitrate will restore the opalescence. To this correctly titrated solution add 20 ml triple distilled water and then filter into a dark bottle. Store the solution in the refrigerator and use within 4 weeks. Ammoniacal silver solutions are potentially explosive if stored incorrectly.

Method:
1. Take test and control sections to distilled water
2. Treat with the ammoniacal silver solution in a Coplin jar, which has been covered with aluminium fail, for 30-40 minutes at 56°C or overnight at room temperature.
3. Wash well in several changes of distilled water.
4. Treat sections with 5% aqueous sodium thiosulfate (hypo) for 1 minute.
5. Wash well in running tap water for 2-3 minutes.
6. Lightly counterstain in 0.5% aqueous neutral red or 0.1% aqueous nuclear fast red for 5 minutes.
7. Rinse in distilled water.

8. Dehydrate, clear and mount in a synthetic resin.

Results:

Melanin, argentaffin, chromaffin and some lipofuscins   black
Nuclei   red.

Schmorl's reaction (taken from Lillie, 1954)

preparation of solutions:

Freshly prepared 0.4% aqueous potassium ferricyanide   4 ml
Freshly prepared 1% aqueous ferric chloride (or
1% ferric sulfate)   30 ml
Use this solution soon after mixing.

Method:

1. Take test and control sections to distilled water.
2. Treat sections with the ferric-ferricyanide
solution for 5-10 minutes.
3. Wash well in running tap water for several
minutes to ensure that all residual ferricyanide
is completely removed from the section.
4. Lightly counterstain with 0.5% aqueous neutral red or 0.1% aqueous nuclear fast red for 5
minutes.
5. Dehydrate, clear and mount in synthetic resin.

Results:

Melanin, argentaffin cells, chromaffin, some
lipofuscins, thyroid colloid and bile:
                                        dark blue
Nuclei   red.

- **Enzymetic method**

Cells containing tyrosinase are able to oxidase
dihydroxyphenylalanine (DOPA) to dihydroxyphenylalanine quinone (DOPA quinone) after
which the synthesis continues spontaneously to
melanin.

DOPA oxidase (tyrosinase) method for tissue sections (Bloch. 1917. Laidlaw &Blackberg 1952)

Sections:

Fresh frozen or frozen sections cut from tissue
fixed in buffered formalin for no longer than 2-
3 hours.

Preparation of solutions:

pH buffer 7.4

Dissolve 42.8 g sodium cacodylate and 9.6 ml
M hydrochloric acid in 1 litter distilled water.

Primary fixative

10% formalin in the pH 7.4 buffer to which is
added 0.44 M sucrose.

Incubating medium

0.1% DOPA in the pH 7.4 buffer.

Method:

1. Place sections in distilled water for a few
seconds.
2. Place the test section in the DOPA solution
for 30 minutes at 37°C. Place the control section in buffer only for the same time and temperature as the test section.
3. Replace with fresh solutions and then examine microscopically every 30 minutes or so
to observe the developing reaction. The color of
the solution will change from a reddish color to
light brown in 2-4 hours. By this stage the reaction should be completed.
4. Wash sections well in several changes of distilled water.
5. Stain in Mayer's hematoxylin for 2 minutes.

6. Wash well to 'blue' the section, dehydrate, clear and mount in synthetic resin.

Results:

DOPA oxidase   brown

Nuclei   blue.

- **Formalin-induced fluorescence (FIF)**

Melanin precursors, especially Dopamine (DA) is the one of important catecholamine that give a yellow primary fluorescence when exposed to formaldehyde. These amines firstly converted to tetrahydroisoquinoline by formaldehyde, then dehydrogenated (-2H) to give dihydroisoquinoline which the later exist in a pH-dependant equilibrium with its tautomeric quinoidal form.

Dopamine: R' = H, Noradrenaline: R' = OH, Formaldehyde: R'' = H

Formaldehyde-induced fluorescence method for melanin-precursor cells (Franko 1955)

Fixation:

Formaldehyde only.

Sections:

Cryostat, or 5 um paraffin sections.

Method:

1. Deparaffinize sections in xylene. Fix frozen sections in 10% buffered formalin for 5 minutes, dehydrate and place in xylene.
2. Rinse in fresh xylene.
3. Mount in a media that is fluorescent-free.
4. Examine using a fluorescence microscope with BG38, UG1 and a barrier filter.

Results:

Melanin precursor cells weak yellow fluorescence.

- **Solubility and bleaching methods:**

Melanin is tightly bonded with its protein component; so it is insoluble in most organic solvents or in anything that will significantly destroy the tissue that contains them. Using strong oxidizing agents, such as permanganate, chlorate, chromic acid, peroxide and peracetic acid, will bleach melanin, although the process is slow, usually taking 16 hours.

The method of choice is peracetic acid, but treatment with 0.25% potassium permanganate followed by 2% oxalic acid also works well.

Bleaching melanin pigment using hydrogen peroxide (H_2O_2) (Orchard, 2007)

Fixation

10% neutral buffered formalin.

Solution

40% H_2O_2 5 ml

Phosphate buffered saline (pH 7.6)   45 ml

(Dissolve PBS tablets according to instructions in 200 ml of distilled water per tablet.). Make the solution fresh and place in a 50 ml Coplin jar.

Method:

1. Take test and control sections to distilled water.
2. Prepare the incubating solution fresh and place in a water bath or oven at 60°C for 10 minutes.
3. Place slides into the incubating solution and ensure the Coplin jar lid is securely placed over the jar.
4. Incubate in the jar for 1 hour.
5. Remove slides and wash in running tap water for 3 minutes.
6. Continue with immune-histochemical procedures (heat-mediated or enzyme digestion antigen retrieval techniques).

Lipofuscin

Commonly referred to as "wear and tear" pigments. Lipofuscin is fine yellow-brown pigment granules formed within lysosomes by covalent combination of proteins with oxidation products of unsaturated fatty acids in addition to sugars and metals like aluminium, iron, copper and zinc.

It found in the liver, kidney, heart muscle, retina, adrenals, nerve cells, and ganglion cells. Some staining methods for lipofuscin are:

Fat stains: The lipofuscin derivate from lipids. (hydrophobic character)

Acidophilia: Due to cationic nitrogenous that found in lipofuscin peptide.

Basophilia: Prevented by methylation and restored due to carboxyl groups by saponification.

PAS: Due to its carbohydrate content and free aldehydes in addition to aldehydes from unsaturated lipids oxidation.

Bleaching: By 10% H_2O_2 for 48 h at room temperature.

Schmorl reaction: No certain groups detected.

Masson-Fontana: Due to aldehyde groups result from unsaturated lipids oxidation.

Aldehyde-Fuchsin: By strong oxidation of unsaturated fatty acids to carboxyl groups by potassium permanganate, then link with fuchsine.

Long Ziehl-Neelsen: The cationic carbol fuchsin reacts with carboxyl groups of lipofuscin but that need over-right instead of 10 minutes, so the name is long ziehlneelsen. The phenol acts as pH adjuster.

Long Ziehl-Neelsen method (Pearse 1953)

Fixation:
Any fixative.

Sections:
Works well on all types of tissue sections.

Method:
1. Slides to distilled water.
2. Stain in a Coplin jar with filtered carbol fuchsin using a 60°C water bath for 3 hours.
3. Wash well in running tap water.
4. Differentiate in 1% acid alcohol until the background staining is removed
5. Wash well in running tap water.

6. Counterstain nuclei with 0.25% aqueous methylene blue in 1% aqueous acetic acid for 1 minute.
7. Dehydrate, clear and mount in synthetic resin.

Results:

Lipofuscin	magenta
Nuclei	blue
Background	pale magenta to pale blue.

Sudan black B technique

Method:
1. Take paraffin sections to 70% ethyl alcohol.
2. In a Coplin jar, stain overnight in filtered saturated Sudan black B in 70% ethyl alcohol at room temperature.
3. Rinse well in 70% ethyl alcohol to differentiate excess dye in the background.
4. Wash in water and mount in an aqueous mountant (e.g. Apathy's mounting media).

Results:

Lipofuscin pigment and red blood cells	black
Background	pale gray.

Aldehyde fuchsin technique (Gomori 1950)

Solutions:

Acidified potassium permanganate solution
(0.25% aqueous potassium permanganate in 0.1% sulfuric acid)

2% aqueous oxalic acid
Aldehyde fuchsin:
Dissolve 1 g pararosanilin (CI 42500) in 100 ml aqueous 70% ethanol. Add 1 ml concentrated hydrochloric acid and 2 ml paraldehyde, shaking the mixture thoroughly. Stand for 2-3 days at room temperature or preferably longer, near natural light, to allow the solution to blue. Store solution at 4°C. The solution will remain viable for approximately 2 months. Any increase in the background staining will indicate deterioration of the staining solution.

Method:
1. Sections to distilled water.

2. Treat with acidified potassium permanganate solution for 5 mins.
3. Wash well in distilled water and treat 2 mins with oxalic acid solution to bleach section.
4. Wash well in distilled water.
5. Rinse in 70% ethyl alcohol.
6. Stain section in aldehyde fuchsin for 5 minutes. Longer staining times will be needed as the solution ages.
7. Rinse in 70% ethyl alcohol followed by a rinse in three changes of distilled water.
8. Counterstain with 0.1% aqueous tartrazine (CI 19140) in 0.2% acetic acid for 1 minute.
9. Rinse well in distilled water.
10. Dehydrate, clear and mount in synthetic resin.

Results:

Lipofuscin	purple
Background	yellow.

Chromaffin:

This pigment is seen as dark brown granular material in the cells of adrenal medulla in physiological and pathological conditions. This pigment gives chromaffin reaction, which is development of a brown color following treatment of fresh tissue by chromate salt or chromic acid (other oxidant agent such as aldehyde can be used). Chromate oxidation rapidly produce the brown pigment in adrenalin and noradrenalin, but iodate oxidizes noradrenalin more quickly than adrenalin, and this can be used as a way of distinguishing between the two compounds. Fixation in formalin is not recommended and fixatives containing alcohol, mercuric chloride or acetic acid should be avoided. Dichromate fixative is recommended. Chromaffin can be demonstrated by Schmorl's reaction, Nile Blue, Masson-Fontan, PAS techniques and Giemsa staining after dichromate fixation.

Pseudomelanosis pigment (melanosis coli).

Sometimes seen in the macrophage in the lamina propria of the large intestine and appendix. It is endogenous pigment similar to Ceroid type of lipofuchsin.

Dubin- Johnson pigment:

Found in the liver of patient with Dubin-Johnson syndrome due to defective canalicular transport of bilirubin. It is characterized by brownish black colour, granular, intracellular pigment located in the centrilobular hepatocyte. Histochemically it is similar to the lipofuchsin, but there are ultrastructural differences.

Ceroid –type lipofuchsin:

It differs from lipofuchsin because it fails to stain with ferric ferrocynide reaction.

Hamazaki- weisenberg:

Small yellow brown spindle shaped structures found in the sinuses of lymphonodes, either lying free or as cytoplasmic inclusion (sarcoidosis). Also, their presence associated with melanosis coli. Histochemically is similar to the lipofuchsin. Under electron microscope (EM) appear as lysosomal residual bodies.

Endogenous minerals:

Calcium

Calcium are distributed throughout all the tissues and body fluids, such compounds are in a state of solution and cannot be demonstrated histologically. The deposition of calcium is normally restricted to bone in as the form of bone salts, mainly crystalline hydroxy apatite (hydrated calcium phosphate, with traces of carbonate, citrate and other ions).

In certain disorders of calcium metabolism, excessive calcium is deposited in insoluble form in tissues which normally do not contain calcium, and the deposition of calcium is common in many degenerative and chronic inflammatory diseases (e.g. atherosclerosis and tuberculosis).

Methods to demonstrate calcium are widely applied to sections of undecalcified bone in the diagnosis of some types of bone disease, particularly in distinguishing between the two bone diseases, osteoporosis and osteomalacia.

Calcium can be demonstrated by various dyes which act by forming chelate complex. These dyes include; alizarine red S, purpurin, naphthochrome green B and nuclear fast red. In general, these dyes demonstrate medium to large amount of calcium better than particulate deposits which stains weekly & the exception being alizarin red S that tends to give reliable results with small deposits. None of these methods is specific for calcium.

Alizarin red S method for calcium (Dahl 1952, McGee-Russell 1958. Luna 1968)

Principle:
It forms chelates in which a quinone oxygen and a phenolic oxygen link with calcium (Kiernan 2015).

Fixation:
Buffered neutral formalin, formal alcohol and alcohol.

Sections:
Paraffin or frozen.

Solution:
1% aqueous alizarin red S (CI 58005) adjusted to pH 4.2 or 6.3-6.4 with 10% ammonium hydroxide.

Method:
1. Sections to 95% alcohol.
2. Stand slides an end and thoroughly air dry.
3. Place sections in a Coplin jar filled with the alizarin solution for 1-5 minutes. This stage must be controlled microscopically.
4. Rinse quickly in distilled water.
5. Blot and rinse in acetone for 30 seconds
6. Treat with equal parts acetone-xylene for 15 seconds.
7. Rinse in xylene and mount in synthetic resin.

Results:
Calcium deposits   orange-red.

Copper

Copper is present in many tissues in concentrations too small to be detectable by histochemical means. In the disease called Wilson's disease (hepato-lenticular degeneration) there is a disorder of copper metabolism leading to excessive deposition of copper in the liver and in the basal ganglia region of the brain. The methods of choice are the rubeanic Acid and rhodanine-technique.

Rubeanic acid method for copper (Okamoto &Utamura 1938, Uzman 1956)

Principle:
Rubeanice acid (dithiooxamide) forms an insoluble dark-green chelate with cupric ions in presence of ethanol and acetate in alkaline solution (Kiernan 2015).

Solution:

0.1% rubeanic acid (dithiooxamide) in absolute

ethyl alcohol   5 ml

10% aqueous sodium acetate   100 ml

Prepare fresh before use.

Method:

1. Take the test section, together with a known positive control section, to distilled water.
2. Place sections in a Coplin jar filled with rubeanic acetate solution for at least 16 hours at 37°C. Times may need to be extended and the method is best carried out in a water bath.
3. Wash in 70% ethyl alcohol.
4. Rinse briefly in distilled water.
5. Drain section and blot dry.
6. Lightly counterstain with 0.5% aqueous neutral red or 0.1 % aqueous nuclear fast red for 1 minute.
7. Rinse in distilled water.
8. Dehydrate, clear and mount in synthetic resin.

Results:

Copper   greenish black

Nuclei   pale red.

Modified rhodanine technique (Lindquist 1969)

Principle:

The p-dimethyl-aminobenzylidene rhodanine forms a red complex with cuprous ions. Copper probably replace the hydrogen attached to the nitrogen atom in the five membered ring (Kiernan 2015)

Solutions:

Rhodanine stock solution

5-p-Dimethylaminobenzylidine rhodanine

                                       0.05 g

Absolute ethanol   25 ml

Prepare fresh and filter prior to use.

Working solution:

Take 5 ml of the stock rhodanine solution and add to 45 ml of 2% sodium acetate trihydrate.

Borax solution:

Disodium tetraborate   0.5 g

Distilled water   100 ml

Method:

1. Take test and control sections to water.
2. Incubate in the rhodanine working solution at 56°C for 3 hours or overnight in a 37°C oven
3. Rinse in several changes of distilled water for 3 minutes.
4. Stain in acidified Lillie-Mayer or other alum hematoxylin for 10 seconds.
5. Briefly rinse in distilled water and place immediately in borax solution for 10 seconds.
6. Rinse well in distilled water.
7. Mount with Apathy's mounting media.

Results:

Copper and copper associated protein

                           red to orange-red

Nuclei   blue

Bile   green.

Uric acid & Uurates:

Uric acid is the breakdown product of the body's purine (nucleic acids) metabolism, but a small proportion is obtained from diet. Most but not all uric acid is secreted by the kidneys.

Uric acid circulating in the blood in the form of monosodium urate (acidic) which is high in patient with gout forming a super saturated solution which may results in urate deposition causing:

- Subcutaneous nodular deposit of urate crystals (tophi).
- Synovitis & arthritis.
- Renal disease and renal calculi.

Pseudogout or chondrocalcinosis is a pyrophosphate arthropathy result in calcium pyrophosphate being deposited in joints; the cause of deposition is unknown and is more commonly in elderly, affecting mainly large joints.

The crystals of urates are birefringant, argentaffin and slightly soluble in dilute alkalis but insoluble in saturated ammonia and alcohol.

Lithium carbonate extraction-hexamine silver technique (Gomori 1936, 1951; Grocott 1955)

Principle
The urate deposits reduce the hexamine silver solution due to their argentaffin properties. It distinguished from phosphate and carbonates deposits by their solubility in dilute solutions of lithium carbonate.

Fixation
Urate crystals are water soluble, therefore fixation in alcohol will give a more specific reaction.

Sections
Paraffin, frozen, or celloidin.

Solutions
Grocott's hexamine silver solution
Saturated aqueous lithium carbonate solution
2% aqueous sodium thiosulfate (hypo)
0.2% aqueous light green solution in 0.2% acetic acid.

Method
1. Take two test sections and two control sections to 70% ethyl alcohol.
2. Place one section from each pair in saturated aqueous lithium carbonate solution for 30 minutes.
3. Rinse all sections in distilled water.
4. Place all sections in a Coplin jar filled with hexamine silver solution for 1 hour at 45°C.
5. Wash sections in distilled water.
6. Treat sections with hypo for 30 seconds.
7. Counterstain with light green solution for 1 minute.
8. Wash in water, dehydrate, clear, and mount in synthetic resin.

Results
Extracted sections:
urates only are extracted.
Unextracted sections:
urates and possibly pyrophosphates are blackened.
Background   green.

Although often listed as being exogenous pigments, the majority of them are, in fact, colorless in reactive while others can be visualized by histochemical method.

Tattoo pigment:
Associated with skin and adjacent lymph area. If viewed using reflected light, the various colour used to create the tattoo can be seen.

Amalgam tattoo is brown to black areas in the mouth which may result from traumatic introduction of mercury and silver during dental procedures.

Histologically brown granules may deposit in collagen, basement membrane, nerve sheet, blood vessels wall and elastic fibers. The pattern of distribution is similar to that in the skin in argyria.

Carbon:
Commonly found in the lung and lymphoid tissues of human and other animals living in a dusty atmosphere. Inhaled carbon particles generally are trapped by the thin film of mucus in the nose, pharynx, trachea and bronchi, but a small amount will find its way into the alveoli of the lung.

Lung anthracosis is a black pigmentation of the lung as a result of massive accumulation of carbon in coal workers.

It is not reactive and cannot be demonstrated by all staining method, so the site and nature of carbon make identification easy. It may be confused with melanin but treatment with bleaching agent will show carbon unaffected where melanin will be dissolved.

Silica:

Found in the same sites as carbon. It causes fibrosis of the lung and may be recognized by the birefringant and their resistance to microincineration (anisotropic).

Asbestos:

A special form of silica has been used as fire resistant, there are several types of asbestos and the fibers that cause pulmonary disease in man are amphiboles. The most dangerous type is corcidolite (cape blue asbestos).

Asbestos found in the body as long beaded rods which are birefringant and resistant to microincineration. They become coated with protein and haemosidrin to develop yellow colour and loss their birefringant appearance.

Lead

Lead poisoning is now uncommon but used to lead paints, Lead pipes that carried much of the domestic water lead in paint, batteries, gasoline and working in industries involving lead. The rhodizonate method is Probably more specific.

Rhodizonate method for lead salts (Lillie, 1954)

Principle:

The sodium rhodizonate forms black chelates with lead salt.

Fixation:

Avoid the use of mercury-containing fixatives. Bones containing lead salts can be decalcified in 5-10% sulfuric acid containing 5-10% sodium sulfate. This procedure should convert lead deposits into insoluble lead sulfate.

Sections:

Paraffin.

Preparation of solution:

Sodium rhodizonate	200 mg
Distilled water	99 ml
Glacial acetic acid	1 ml

Method:

1. Sections to distilled water.
2. Place in rhodizonate solution for 1 hour.
3. Rinse well in distilled water.
4. Counterstain in 0.1% aqueous light green in 0.2% acetic acid for 2 minutes.
5. Rinse briefly in distilled water.
6. Mount in glycerin jelly.

Results:

Lead salts	red
Background	green.

Aluminium and beryllium

Aluminium and Beryllium usually gains entry to the body by inhalation of particles into the lung in industrial exposure or by traumatization of skin. Several methods are available for demonstration of aluminium and beryllium, which are usually by the same methods as solochrome azurine.

Solochrome azurine method for beryllium and aluminum (Pearse 1957)

Principle:

Aluminium and beryllium form deep blue chelates with solochrome azurine.

Fixation:

Not critical.

Sections:
Paraffin or frozen.
Preparation of solutions:
a. 0.2% solochrome azurine (syn Pure Blue B)
b. 0.2% solochrome azurine in normal sodium hydroxide.
Method:
1. Take two test sections to distilled water.
2. Stain one section in solution a and one in solution b for 20 mins.
3. Wash in distilled water.
4. Lightly counterstain in 0.5% aqueous neutral red or 0.1% aqueous nuclear fast red for 5 mins.
5. Wash in distilled water and mount in synthetic resin.

Results:

Solution A: aluminum and beryllium	blue
Solution B: beryllium only	blue-black
Nuclei	red.

Silver

This metal may be found in the skin, alimentary tract and other organs in silver workers; it gives the skin a peculiar slate-grey appearance (argyria) and now more commonly seen as a localized change in the mouth (amalgam tattoo) or in association with silver ear rings in ineptly pierced lobes. In sections, the particles appear as dark brown to black granules.

Silver can be demonstrated in tissues by the Dimethylaminobenzylidene Rhodanine method.

Rhodanine method for silver (Okamoto &Utamura 1958)

Principle:
The p-dimethylaminobenzylidene rhodanine forms reddish brown chelates with silver deposits.

Fixation:
Not critical but avoid the use of mercury-containing fixatives.

Sections:
Paraffin; frozen.

Incubating solution:

p-Dimethylaminobenzylidene rhodanine (saturated solution in 90 % alcohol)	3.5 ml
M nitric acid	3 ml
Distilled water	93.5 ml

Method:
1. Paraffin sections to distilled water.
2. Incubate sections in rhodanine solution at 37°C for 24 hours.
3. Wash well in distilled water.
4. Mount in glycerine jelly.

Results:

Silver deposits	reddish-brown.

Iron

The iron stored in the body is found in loose combination with protein in the form of a golden brown pigment called hemosiderin. Another storage form of iron is ferritin, in which iron is bound to a protein called apoferritin. The iron can be separated from the protein by reducing agents such as hydrosulphite. Other iron in the tissues is much more strongly bound to protein (e.g. in haemoglobin, myoglobin) and the iron is not available for demonstration; treatment for a short time by 100 of hydrogen peroxide may release sufficient iron for demonstration by the Perls' reaction. Iron demonstrated histochemically like hemosiderin.

Artifact Pigments

Formalin pigment:

It is dark brown, birefringant often with no relationship to the tissue (i.e., the precipitate appears adjacent to tissues or within interstices or vessels), especially in postmortem and blood-containing tissues fixed with acid formaldehyde. As these solutions age, formic acid develops from the formaldehyde content and lowers the pH. This in turn causes crystals of formalin pigment, or acid formaldehyde hematin, to be deposited throughout the tissues. Formalin pigment may be easily stopped from forming by using 10% neutral buffered formalin (NBF) as the fixative. Since its formation is dependent on an acidic pH, buffering to pH7 effectively stops it. However, it may still form if tissues are stored in NBF for much extended periods without changing the solution. The NBF should be changed every six months at a minimum.

Formalin pigment can be removed from sections prior to staining by 1% alcoholic solution of sodium hydroxide (NaOH) or by saturated alcoholic picric acid.

Removing formalin pigment (Suvarna 2013, Kiernan 1999)

Method 1
1. Bring sections to water via xylene and ethanol.
2. Place into 1.8% picric acid in absolute alcohol for 1 hour.
3. Optionally, treat with saturated aqueous lithium carbonate to remove Picric acid discoloration.
4. Wash well with water.
5. Continue with the staining method.

Method 2
Solution:
Alcohol-Ammonia Solution

95 % alcohol   50 ml
Concentrated ammonia   15 ml
Mix before use.

Method:
1. De-paraffinize and hydrate to distilled water.
2. Place in Alcohol-ammonia solution for 1 (one) hour.
3. Wash in water.
4. Stain using H&E or other technique.

Method 3
Solution:

Ammonia Water 28%   2 ml

Alcohol 70%   100 ml
Method:
1. Place in solution for 30-60 minutes.
2. Rinse and place in 1% aqueous acetic acid.
3. Wash thoroughly in tap water and stain as desired.

Method 4
Solution:

Hydrogen Peroxide 3%   50 ml
Acetone   50 ml
Ammonium Hydroxide 28%   1 ml
Method:
1. Place in solution for 5-10 minutes.
2. Wash thoroughly in running tap water and stain as desired.

Removing Formalin Pigment (Garvey' s Technique):

Solutions:
Alkylphenol ethoxylate(APE)
Phenol   5 ml
HCl   5 ml
Absolute ethanol   90 ml
Method:
1. Place sections in alkylphenol ethoxylate (APE) for 5 minutes.
2. Wash in water for 5 minutes.
3. Treat with 5% potassium permanganate for 2 minutes.
4. Wash in water for 2 minutes.
5. Decolorize in 5% oxalic acid, 2 minutes.

Malaria pigment:
Morphologically similar to formalin pigment, and occasionally identical. It is soluble in alcoholic picric acid and birefringant, it is intracellular and this may be sufficient to separate it from formalin which is extracellular. Malarial pigment, can be removed from tissue sections with saturated alcoholic picric acid, but usually requires 12–24 hours' treatment for complete removal. Much less time is required to remove the pigment so 10% ammonium hydroxide can be used.

Extraction method for formalin and malarial pigment

Solutions

10% ammonium hydroxide in 70% ethyl alcohol.

Method

1. Sections to 70% ethyl alcohol.
2. Place sections in a Coplin jar containing ammonium hydroxide alcohol for 5–15 minutes.
3. Wash well in distilled water.
4. Apply staining method desired.

Mercury deposit:

Dark brown to black granular deposit, distributed uniformaly throughout the tissue, these deposits occur in all tissues fixed in liquids containing mercuric chloride, including B5, Heidenhain's Susa, Helly's and Zenker 's fluid. Addition of a few drops of saturated alcoholic iodine solution during dehydration will remove the pigment. The pigment is converted by iodine to mercuric iodide which is alcohol soluble, but this will tend to make tissues brittle. Hence, final removal of the mercurial deposit by subsequent bleaching with a weak sodium thiosulfate (hypo) after sectioning and before staining is recommended.

Method

Solutions:

Lugol's Iodine

Iodine	1.0 g
Potassium iodide	2.0 g
Distilled water	100 ml

5 % Aqueous Sodium Thiosulfate

Method:

1. Bring sections to water.
2. Place in Lugol's iodine for 15 minutes.
3. Wash in water.
4. Place in thiosulphate for 3 minutes.
5. Wash in water.
6. Stain with H&E or other technique.

Osmium Tetroxide Deposits(Ellis, 1979)

Osmic acid appears as black deposits on tissues which have not been properly washed out. To remove by bleaching, the following procedures may be used:

Method

1. Sections to 70% alcohol.
2. Place the tissue in solution containing 2 ml of Hydrogen Peroxide and 70% Alcohol (48 ml.)
3. Expose to sunlight for 15-30 minutes to bleach.
4. Take down to water and wash thoroughly.

Chrome deposition:

Occur as fine brown or black granules after dichromate fixation (zinker). It can be removed from the tissue by washing in running tap water and from section by acid alcohol.

Starch:

This pigment is introduced by talcum powder from the gloves. It is positive PAS and maltes cross configuration.

Stains may cause precipitate due to faulty technique. They are highly coloured, usually amorphus and granular. Stain precipitates may be a problem in automatic staining machines.

Further reading:

Bloch, B. (1917) Des Problem Pigment bildung in der Haul. Archives Dermato-syphili graphiques. 124: 129.

Dunn, R.C. & Thompson, E.C. (1946) A simplified stain for hemoglobin in tissue and smears using patent blue. Stain Technology. 21; 65.

Fontana, A. (1912) Verfahrenzur intensiven und raschen Farbung des Treponema pallidum und anderer Spirochaten. DermatologischeWochenshrift, 55: 1003.

Eranko, O. (1955) Distribution of adrenalin and noradrenalin in the adrenal medulla. Nature, 175: 88.

Gomori, G. (1950) Aldehyde fuchsin: a new stain for elastic tissues. American Journal of Clinical Pathology, 20: 665.

Hall, M.J. (1960) A staining reaction for bilirubin in tissue sections. American Journal of Clinical Pathology,34: 313.

Hukill, P.B. & Putt, LA. (1962) A specific stain for iron using 4-7 diphenyl-1-10 phenanthrotine. Journal of Histochemistry, 10: 490.

Laidlaw, G.F. &Blackberg, S.N. (1932) Melanoma studies: DOPA reaction in normal histology. American journal of Pathology. 8: 491.

Lillie, R.D. (1954) Histopathologic Technic and Practical Histochemistry. New York: Blakiston.

Masson, P. (1914) La glande endocrine de I'intesune chez rhomme. Comptes Rendus Hehdamadmres des Seances de I, Academic des Sciences, 158: 59.

Pearse, A.G.E. (1953) Histochemistry. Theoretical and Applied. London: Churchill.

Perls, M. (1867) Nachweis von Eisenoxyd in geweissen Pigmentation. Virchows Archiv fur Pathologische Anatomic und Physiologic und fur Klinische Medizin. 39:42.

Tiedermann, F. & Gmelin, L. (1826) Die Verdauungnach Versuchen. Heidelberg: K. Gross, vol. 1, 89.

Microorganisms are organisms seen only by microscope. Medically important microorganisms include five main groups: Bacteria, Fungi, Viruses, Protozoa and Helminths.

Bacteria

Bacteria are tiny, single-celled organism with genetic material and cell wall. The bacterial shape provides a basis for classification, therefor are classified as cocci when it spherical-shaped or bacilli when it is rod-shaped or spirochetes when it spiral-shaped. Many pathogenic bacteria identification methods like culturing, staining and biochemical testing are used in the microbiology lab, however in the histopathology lab depends on the shape and staining characteristics of bacteria when present in large numbers in tissue especially in abscess or in vegetation.

The gram stain is the most common differential method that allows bacteria to be classified into gram-positive and gram-negative bacteria.

Gram method for paraffin section

Principle:
Bacteria have a cell wall composed of peptidoglycan which take the colour of crystal violet iodine then the section decolorized by alcohol or acetone to removes crystal violet in the first step, but it found that the color removes from gram-negative not from gram-positive bacteria and that due to the large crystal violet iodine molecular complex cannot easily wash out of the intact peptidoglycan layer of gram-positive bacteria while this complex easily removes from gram-negative bacteria which the alcohol disrupts its outer lipopolysaccharide layer so the remaining thin peptidoglycan cell wall cannot retain the complex.

Finally, a counter stain is applied to color the gram-negative bacteria.

Sections:
Formalin-fixed, paraffin embedded.

Solutions:
Crystal violet solution
0.5% crystal violet in 25% alcohol
Gram's and Lugol's iodine

Iodine	1.0 g
Potassium iodide	2.0 g
Distilled water	10 ml

Shake together distilled water and potassium iodide until dissolved; add iodine. Make up to 300 ml with distilled water for Gram's iodine, or 100 ml for Lugol's.
1% aqueous neutral red.

Method:
1. Deparaffinize and rehydrate through graded alcohols to distilled water.
2. Stain with filtered crystal violet solution, 2 min.
3. Rinse in tap water and drain.
4. Iodine solution, 2 min.
5. Rinse in tap water, blot and flood with acetone, 1-2 seconds.
6. Wash in tap water.
7. Counterstain in neutral red, 3 min
8. Blot, dehydrate rapidly, clear and mount.

Results:
Gram-positive organisms, fibin, some fungi, Paneth cells granules, keratohyalin, and keratin blue
Gram-negative organisms red.

Mycobacteria
Mycobactria are rod-shaped bacteria that contain large amounts of lipid in their cell wall, exhibit filamentous growth and cause tuberculosis.

It resists decolorization with dilute mineral acid, so it called acid-fast bacteria and this property due to long-chain fatty acid known as mycolic acid in their capsule. Also, mycobacteria contain carbohydrates in their cell walls, so it can give PAS positive.

Ziehl-Neelsen (ZN) stain for Mycobacterium bacillus

Principle:
The lipid capsule of mycobacteria takes up carbol-fuchsin and stains red. This step enhanced by the phenol and alcohol which present in carbol-fuchsin in addition to heating which forces this dye into the mycobacteria. Secondly is decolorization by acid alcohol which removes carbol-fuchsin from almost other structure except mycobacteria and that due to that mycobacteria have a waxy capsule consists of mycolic acid.

Sections:
Formalin or fixative other than Carnoy's, paraffin.

Solutions:
Carbol-fuchsin
1 g basic fuchsin dissolved in 10 ml of absolute alcohol; add 100 ml of 5% aqueous phenol. Mix well and filter before use.

Acidified methylene blue
0.25% methylene blue in 1% acetic alcohol.

Method:
1. Deparaffinize and rehydrate through graded alcohols to distilled water.
2. Flood sections with freshly filtered carbol-fuchsin and heat to steaming with intermittent flaming, 15 minutes, or stain in Coplin jar at 56°-60°C, 30 min.
3. Wash well in tap water.
4. Differentiate in 1% acid alcohol, 10 min.
5. Wash well in tap water.
6. Counterstain in methylene blue solution, 30 seconds.
7. Blot and differentiate by alternate dehydrationand rehydration until the background is a delicate pale blue.
8. Dehydrate, clear and mount.

Results:
Mycobacteria, hair shafts, Russell bodies, Splendore-Hoeppli immunoglobulins around actinomycetes and some fungal organisms   red
Background   pale blue.

Fluorescent method for Mycobacterium bacilli (Kuper & May 1960)

Principle:
The staining solution is a mixture of two cationic fluorochrome dyes which are Rhodamine B and Auramine O, these two dyes in staining solution together make one cationic complex which links with negative groups of mycolic acid.

Auramine O

Rhodamine B

Sections:
Formalin-fixed, paraffin.

Solution:

Auramine O	1.5 g
Rhodamine B	0.75 g
Glycerol	75 ml
Phenol crystals (liquefied at 50°C)	10 ml
Distilled water	50 ml

Method:
1. Deparaffinize (1-part groundnut oil, and 2 parts xylene for M. leprae).
2. Pour on pre-heated (60°C), filtered staining solution, 10 min.
3. Wash in tap water.
4. Differentiate in 0.5% hydrochloric acid in alcohol for M. tuberculosis, or 0.5% aqueous hydrochloric acid for *M. leprae.*
5. Wash in tap water, 2 min.
6. Eliminate background fluorescence in 0 5% potassium permanganate, 2 min.
7. Wash in tap water and blot dry.
8. Dehydrate (not for *M. leprae*), clear and mount in a fluorescence-free mountant.

Results:
Mycobacteria   golden yellow (using blue light fluorescence below 530 nm)
Background   dark green.

Mycobacteria leprae

M. Leprae is a type of mycobacteria that attack and destroy nerves; especially in the skin and cause leprosy. It is weak acid-fast mycobacteria because it is more easily decolorization by acid or alcohol than other mycobacteria, so the differentiation must be very carefully controlled and fite-modification method for standard Zhiel-Neelsen method is good.

Wade-Fite technique for leprosy bacilli
(Wade, 1957)

Principle:
The *Mycobacterium leprae* takes carbol-fuchsin then the decolorization by sulphuric acid instead of alcohol because the later remove weak waxy capsule layer of *Mycobacterium leprae*. Also, the peanut oil added to xylene in deparaffination step.

Sections:
Formalin-fixed, paraffin.
Solutions:
Same as for ZN technique.

Method:
1. Warm sections and deparaffinize using 1-part groundnut or peanut oil or clove oil and 2 parts xylene to remove paraffin, 10 minutes.
2. Repeat blotting and washing in water until-section is uniformly wet.
3. Stain in filtered carbol-fuchsin at room temperature, 30 min.
4. Wash in tap water and blot dry.
5. Decolorize in 5% sulfuric acid.
6. Wash in tap water.
7. Counterstain in 0.2% methylene blue, 5-10 seconds, OR an alum hematoxylin followed by bluing in tap water.
8. Blot dry and complete drying in an oven at 60°C.
9. Clear and mount.

Results:
Leprosy and other *Mycobacteria, Nocardia*
                red
Background   blue
Nuclei   blue-black (if hematoxylin is used).

Helicobacter bacteria

Helicobacter are spiral vibrio bacteria that are adherent to the luminal surface of the epithelial cells of gastric glands and cause chromic gastritis, which are frequently seen in endoscopic biopsies.

Some cationic dyes like carbol-fuchsin, cresyl violet and toluidine blue stain helicobacter by combination with negative groups of bacteria ribosomes (contain RNA).

Cresyl violet acetate method for *Helicobacter* sp.

Sections:
Formalin-fixed, paraffin.
Method:
1. Deparaffinize and rehydrate through graded alcohols to distilled water.

2. Filter 0.1% cresyl violet acetate onto slide or into Coplin jar, 5 min.
3. Rinse in distilled water.
4. Blot, dehydrate rapidly in alcohol, clear and mount.

Results:

Helicobacter and nuclei	blue-violet
Background	shades of blue-violet.

Gimenez method for *Helicobacter pylori* (Gimenez 1964, McMullen *et al*. 1987)

Sections:
Formalin-fixed, paraffin.

Solutions:

Buffer solution (phosphate buffer at pH 7.5, or 0.1 M)
0.1M sodium dihydrogen orthophosphate 3.5 ml
0.1Mdisodium hydrogen orthophosphate 15.5 ml.

Stock carbol-fuchsin

Commercial cold acid-fast bacilli stain OR Basic fuchsin	1.0 g
Absolute alcohol	10 ml
5% aqueous phenol	10 ml

Working carbol-fuchsin

Phosphate buffer	10 ml
Stock carbol-fuchsin	4 ml

Filter before use.

Malachite green

Malachite green	0.8 g
Distilled water	100 ml

Method:
1. Deparaffinize and rehydrate through graded alcohols to distilled water.
2. Stain in working carbol-fuchsin solution, 2 min.
3. Wash well in tap water.
4. Stain in malachite green, 15-20 seconds.

5. Wash thoroughly in distilled water.
6. Repeat steps 4 and 5 until section is blue-green to the naked eye.
7. Blot sections dry, and complete drying in air.
8. Clear and mount.

Results:

Helicobacter	red-magenta
Background	blue-green.

Toluidine blue in Sorenson's buffer for Helicobacter

Sections:
Formalin-fixed, paraffin.

Solutions:
Toluidine blue in pH 6.8 phosphate buffer

Sorenson's phosphate buffer pH 6.8	50 ml.
1% aqueous toluidine blue	1.0 ml.

Method:
1. Deparaffinize and rehydrate through graded alcohols to distilled water.
2. Stain in buffered toluidine blue, 20 min.
3. Wash well in distilled water.
4. Dehydrate, clear and mount.

Results:
Helicobacter dark blue against a variably blue background.

Spirochetes bacteria
The treponema pallidum is a very important bacterium in this group because this bacterium is causatives bacteria of syphilis. Most demonstrating methods of spirochetes depend on sliver reduction method like warthin-starry method and Steiner and Steiner method.

The silver methods of spirochetes are similar in mechanism which that firstly tissue stained by silver and a large number of silver ions from coordinate bond to protein molecules especially the imidazole side chain of the histidine, but unfortunately small numbers of silver atoms at certain specific sites in bacteria, in the second stage these nuclei of silver ion atoms in bacteria catalyse local reduction of more silver ion by a reducing agent until enough colloidal metal has been deposited to display the organism as black objects of characteristic form. The reducing agent (developer) may be pyrogallic acid in levaditi method or hydroquinone in Warthin-Starry and Steiner and Steiner method.

Warthin-Starry method for Spirochetes (Warthin & Starry, 1920)

Sections:
Formalin-fixed, paraffin.

Solutions:
Acetate buffer, pH 3.6
Sodium acetate   4.1 g
Acetic acid   6.25 ml
Distilled water   500 ml
1% silver nitrate in pH 3.6 acetate buffer.

Developer
Dissolve 3 g of hydroquinone in 10 ml pH 3.6 buffer, and mix 1 ml of this solution and 15 ml of wormed 5% Scotch glue or gelatin; keep at 40°C. Take 3 ml of 2% silver nitrate in pH 3.6 buffer solution and keep at 55 CC. Mix these two solutions immediately before use.

Method:
1. Deparaffinize and rehydrate through graded alcohols to distilled water.
2. Celloidinize in 0.5% celloidin, drain and harden in distilled water, 1 min.
3. Impregnate in preheated 55-60°C silver solution (b), 90-105 minutes.
4. Prepare and preheat developer in a water bath.
5. Treat with developer (solution c) for 3 minutes and 30 secs at 55°C. Sections should be golden-brown at this point.
6. Remove from developer and rinse in tap water for several minutes at 55-60°C, then buffer at room temperature.
7. Tone in 0.2% gold chloride.
8. Dehydrate, clear and mount.

Results:
Spirochetes   black
Background   golden yellow.

Modified Steiner for filamentous and non-filamentous bacteria (modified Swisher, 1987)

Sections:
Formalin-fixed, paraffin.
Solutions:
1.0% uranyl nitrate
Uranyl nitrate   1 g
Distilled water   100 ml

1.0% silver nitrate
Silver nitrate   1 g
Distilled water   100 ml
Make fresh each time and filter with #1 or #2 filter paper before use.

0.04% silver nitrate
Silver nitrate   0.04 g
Distilled water   100 ml
Refrigerate and use for only one month.

2.5% gum mastic
Gum mastic   2.5 g
Absolute alcohol   100 ml
Allow to dissolve for 24 h then filter until clear yellow before use. Refrigerate unused portion.

2% hydroquinone
Hydroquinone   1 g
Distilled water   25 ml
Make fresh solution each use.

Reducing solution:
Mix 10 ml of 2.5% gum mastic, 25 ml of 2.0% hydroquinone, and 5 ml absolute alcohol. Make just prior to use and filter with #4 filter paper; add 2.5 ml of 0.04% silver nitrate. Do not filter this solution. When gum mastic is added, solution will have a milky appearance.

Method:

1. Deparaffinize and rehydrate through graded alcohols to distilled water.
2. Sensitize sections in room temp. 1% aqueous uranyl nitrate, and place in microwave oven until solution is just at boiling point, approx. 20-30 seconds; do not boil. Alternatively, place in preheated 1% uranyl nitrate at 60°C in a water bath for 15 min., or in microwave oven and bring to boiling point do not boil; 2% zinc sulfate in 3.7% formalin may be substituted.
3. Rinse in room temp, distilled water until uranyl nitrate residue is eliminated.
4. Place in room temp. 1% silver nitrate and microwave just until boiling point is reached. Do not boil. Remove from oven, loosely cover jar and allow to stand in hot silver nitrate, 6-7 min. Alternatively, preheat silver nitrate 20-30 min. in a 60°C water bath, add slides and allow to impregnate for 1 h and 30 min.
5. Rinse in 3 changes of distilled water.
6. Dehydrate in 2 changes each of 95% alcohol and absolute alcohol.
7. Treat with 2.5% gum mastic, 5 min.
8. Allow to air dry, 5 min.
9. Rinse in 2 changes of distilled water. Slides may stand here while reducing solution is being prepared.
10. Reduce in preheated reducing solution at 45°C in a water bath for 10-25 min., or until sections have developed satisfactorily with black microorganisms against a light yellow background. Avoid intensely stained background.
11. Rinse in distilled water to stop reaction.
12. Dehydrate, clear and mount.

Results:

Spirochetes, cat-scratch organisms, Donovan-bodies, nonfilamentous bacteria of L. pneumophila   dark brown black
Background   bright yellow golden yellow.

Fungi

Fungi are unicellular or multicellular primitive plants that have a distinct membrane-bound nucleus containing genetic material. Their identification depends on culture appearance and microscopic morphology, like filamentous yeast and dimorphic fungi. Most fungi rich in polysaccharides in its cell walls, hence they can be detected with PAS or Grocott-Gomori methenamine.

Grocott methenamine (hexamine) silver for fungi (Gomori 1946, Grocott 1955)

Principle:
The first step in the procedure is the oxidation of the fungal polysaccharides to aldehyde groups by chromic acid then the tissue exposed to the alkaline silver reagent in the second step, in which the aldehyde oxidation products reduce the silver nitrate to metallic silver. The methenamine is added to the silver reagent to give alkaline properties, which are necessary for proper reaction.

Sections:
Formalin-fixed, paraffin.

Solutions:
a) *5% sodium tetraborate in distilled water*
b) *Methenamine silver:*
5% silver nitrate in distilled water   5 ml
3% methenamine in distilled water   100 ml

Add silver nitrate to methenamine silver, gently shaking until formed precipitate dissolves. Mixture will keep for 1-2 months at 4°C.

Incubating solution:

Solution a (borax)	5 ml
Distilled water	25 ml
Solution b, methenamine silver	25 ml

Ideally, the methenamine silver/water solution and the borax should be preheated at 56°C and mixed prior to use, as the silver solution starts to degenerate once borax is added.

Arzac's counterstain:

Orange G	0.25 g
Light green	1 g
Phosphotungstic acid	0.5 g
50% alcohol	100 ml
Glacial acetic acid	1 ml

This solution keeps well.

Method:

1. Deparaffinize and rehydrate through graded alcohols to distilled water.
2. Oxidize in 5% aqueous chromic acid (chromium trioxide), 1 hour.
3. Wash in tap water.
4. Rinse in 1% sodium metabisulfate.
5. Wash in tap water, 5 min.
6. Rinse in distilled water, then place in preheated (56 CC) silver incubating solution in a dark place, up to 1 hour.
7. Rinse well in distilled water.
8. Tone in 0.1% gold chloride, 4 min.
9. Rinse in distilled water.
10. Place in 3% sodium thiosulfate, 5 min.
11. Counterstain in Arzac's stain, or 1% light green in 0.1% acetic acid, 15-30 seconds, or stain with H&E.
12. Blot, dehydrate, clear and mount.

Results:

Fungi, Pneumocystis, melanin	black
Mucins and glycogen	gray-black
Red blood cells	yellow
Background	pale green.

Viruses are composed of either DNA or RNA with protein and need living cells to provide it by energy and the machinery for duplication. Most viruses detected by electron microscope, but some of it aggregate within cells to produce viral inclusion bodies which can be seen with the light microscope by using special stains like phloxine-tartrazine and orcein.

Phloxine-tartrazine technique for viral inclusions (Lendrum 1947)

Principle:
Firstly, cytoplasm stained by phloxine, secondly the phloxine staining is differentiated by tartrazine solution which removes the red color from the collagen and other constituents substitutes its own yellow color in it except viral inclusion bodies because have strong phloxinophilia constituents.

Sections:
Formalin-fixed, paraffin.

Solutions:

Phloxine

Phloxine	0.5 g
Calcium chloride	0.5 g
Distilled water	100 ml

Tartrazine

A saturated solution of tartrazine in 2-ethoxyethanol, or cellosolve.

Method:

1. Deparaffinize and rehydrate through graded alcohols to distilled water.
2. Stain nuclei in alum hematoxylin (Carazzi's or Harris's), 10 min.
3. Wash in running tap water, 5 min.
4. Stain in phloxine solution, 20 min.
5. Rinse in tap water and blot dry.
6. Controlling with the microscope, stain in tartrazine until only the viral inclusions remain strongly red, 5-10 min. average.
7. Rinse in 95% alcohol.

8. Dehydrate, clear and mount.
Results:

Viral inclusions	bright red
Red blood cells	variably orange red
Nuclei	blue gray
Background	yellow.

Shikata's orcein method for hepatitis B surface antigen (modified Shikata *et al.* 1974)

Principle:
The sulphur groups of viral protein oxidize by the potassium permanganate to sulphonates which the later react with orcein to give brown-black color.

Sections:
Formalin-fixed, paraffin.
Solutions:
Acid permanganate

0.25% potassium permanganate	95 ml
3% aqueoussulfuric acid	5 ml

Orcein

Orcein (synthetic)	1 g
70% alcohol	100 ml
Concentrated hydrochloric acid (gives a pH of 1-2)	1 ml

Saturated tartrazine in cellosolve (2-ethnxij-ethmin)
Method:
1. Deparaffinize and rehydrate through graded alcohols to distilled water.
2. Treat with acid permanganate solution, 5 min.
3. Bleach until colorless with 1.5% aqueous oxalic acid, 30 seconds.
4. Wash in distilled water, 5 min., then in 70% alcohol.
5. Stain in orcein solution at room temperature, 4 hours, or in a Caplin jar of 37°C preheated orcein, 90 min.
6. Rinse in distilled alcohol and examine microscopically to determine desired staining intensity.
7. Rinse in cellosolve, stain in tartrazine, 2 min.
8. Rinse in cellosolve, clear and mount.
Results:

Hepatitis B-affected cells, elastic and some mucins	brown-black
Background	yellow.

Protozoans

Protozoans are single-celled microorganisms that possess a nucleus and cytoplasm surrounded by a cell membrane. Some of it present in the blood (malaria and trypanosomes), or in the intestine (amoebae, Balantidium coil, giardia lamblia) and other in tissues like leishmania tropica and coccidia.

Most protozoa detected in blood or faeces specimen, but we can detect in tissue section by its morphological appearance using H&E, And by Giemsa stains.

Giemsa stain for parasites

Principle:
The Giemsa stains belong to the class of polychromatic stains which consist of a mixture of dyes of different hues which provide subtle differences in staining when methylene blue prepared at an alkaline pH, it spontaneously forms like azure A, B and C (Kiernan 2010).

The azure derivatives are cationic and link with the negatively charged phosphate groups of DNA, while the eosin is anionic and links with the positive amine groups of protein (Kiernan 2010).

Sections:
Fixative is not critical, but B5 or Zenker's is preferred; thin (3 um) paraffin sections.

Solutions:
Giemsa stock
Giemsa stain powder	4 g
Glycerol	250 ml
Methanol	250 ml

Dissolve powder in glycerol at 60 C with regular shaking. Add methanol, shake the mixture and allow to stand for 7 days. Filter before use.

Working Giemsa for parasites
Giemsa stock	4 ml
Acetate buffered D.W, pH 6.8	96 ml

Method:
1. Deparaffinize and rehydrate through graded alcohols to water.
2. Rinse in pH 6.8 buffered distilled water.
3. Stain in working Giemsa, overnight.
4. Rinse in distilled water.
5. Rinse in 0.5% aqueous acetic acid until section is pink.
6. Wash in tap water.
7. Blot until almost dry.
8. Dehydrate rapidly through alcohols, clear and mount.

Results:
Protozoans and some other microorganisms	dark blue
Background	pink-pale blue
Nuclei	blue.

Further reading:

- Gimenez, D.F. (1964) Staining rickettsia in yolk sac cultures. Stain Technology, 39: 13 5-140.
- Gomori, G. (1946) A new histoehemical test for glycogen and mucin. American Journal of Clinical Pathology,16: 177.
- Grocott, R.G. (1955) A stain for fungi in tissue sections and smears. American Journal of Clinical Pathology.25: 975.
- Kumar, G. and Kiernan, J. A. (2010) *Education Guide: Special Stains and H & E.* 2nd ed. Carpinteria, CA: Dako North America.
- Kuper, S.W.A. & May, J.R. (1960) Detection of acid-fast organisms in tissue sections by fluorescence microscopy. Journal of Pathology and Bacteriology, 79: 59.
- Lendrum, A.C. (1947) The phloxine-tartrazine method as a general histological stain for the demonstration of inclusion bodies. Journal of Pathology and Bacteriology.59: 399.
- McMullen, L. Walker, M.M. Bain, L.A., Karim, Q.V & Baron, J.H. (1987) Histological identification of Campylobacter using
- Gimenez technique in gastric antral mucosa. Journal of Clinical Pathology.464-465.
- Shikata, T., llzawa, T., Yoshiwara, N., Akatsuka, T. & Yamazaki. S. (1974) Staining methods for Australian antigen in paraffin section detection of cytoplasmic inclusion bodies. Japanese Journal of Experimental Medicine. 44: 2 5.
- Swisher, B.L. (1987) Modified Steiner procedure for microwave staining of spirochetes and non-filamentous bacteria. Journal of Histotechnology.10: 241-243.
- Wade, H.W. (1957) A modification of Fite formaldehyde tissues (Fite) method for staining acid-fast bacilli in paraffin sections. Stain Technology, 32: 287

The nervous system is divided into three main sections:

Central nervous system:
Comprising the brain and the spinal cord.

Peripheral nervous system:
Consisting of peripheral nerves.

Autonomic nervous system:
Joining autonomic nerves and glia.

The major cellular components of the nervous system are: ***neurons*** (nerve cells) and ***supporting cells*** (glial cells or neuroglia).

The demonstration of nervous system falls into three groups; firstly, stains for neuronal bodies and processes, secondly stains for glial cells and processes and thirdly stains for myelin sheath.

The neuron

It is the structural and functional unit of the nervous system and formed of a nerve cell with all its processes, which are the axon and the dendrite.

The nerve cell is a branched cell with very thin membrane, central spherical nucleus rich in nuclear fluid, and all cell organoids and inclusions but with no centrioles.

The cytoplasm of nerve cell is rich by specific basophilic bodies known as Nissl substances, which consist of masses of rough endoplasmic reticular with their attached ribosomes.

The dendrite is usually a short, highly branched process that function as major sites of information input for the neuron and does not have a myelin sheath.

Axon (nerve fiber) is a neuronal process that carries nerve impulses over long distances, terminates on the dendrites or cell body of other neurons or in an effective organ like muscle, its transport maybe antegrade and retrograde and has conical-shape area at its origin from nerve cell known as axon hillock which contains neurofibrilbut not Nissl substances.

Nissl substance staining

Nissl substance primally composed of rough endoplasmic reticulum which the later ultrastructural consist of ribonucleic acid (RNA) and protein. The basic aniline dyes such as thionine, azure A and cresyl echt violet stain this substance sharply due to RNA content.

Cresyl fast violet (Nissl) stain for paraffin sections

Fixation:
Alcohol, Carnoy's or neutral formal saline.

Sections:
Paraffin 7-10 μm or 25 μm.

Preparation of stain:
Cresyl fast violet   0.5 g
Distilled water   100 ml

Differentiation solution:
Glacial acetic acid   250 μl
Alcohol   100 ml

Method:
1. Dewax sections and bring to water.
2. Cover with filtered cresyl fast violet; stain for10-20 min.
3. Rinse in distilled water.
4. Differentiate in 0.25% acetic alcohol until most of the stain has been removed (4-8 sec).

5. Briefly pass through absolute alcohol into xylene and check microscopically.
6. Repeat steps 4 and 5 if necessary, giving it less differentiation when repeat.
7. Rinse well in xylene and mount in Canada balsam or DPX.

Results:

Nissl substance	purple-dark blue
Neurons pale	purple-blue
Cell nuclei	purple blue.

Axon staining

It is formed of acytoplasm known as axoplasm containing mitochondria, neurofibrils and neurotubules. It is surrounded with a membrane known as axolemma.The axon hillock is the conical expansion of the axon at its origin from the nerve cell. it has no Nissl granules but it is rich in neurofibrils.

Axon staining divide into three groups:

Chromate precipitation methods:

Golgi (silver chromate) and Golgi-Cox (mercury chromate) are the major group of chromate precipitation methods for axon. In both methods the tissue chromate firstly by chromate or dichromate, but in Golgi method chromate tissue treated by silver nitrate to form submicroscopical of an insoluble complex of chromate and silver with the cytoplasm of nerve cells and its process (Kiernan 2015).

$$CrO_4^{2-} + 2Ag^+ \longrightarrow Ag_2CrO_4(s)$$

$$Cr_2O_7^{2-} + 4Ag^+ + H_2O \longrightarrow 2AgCrO_4(s) + 2H^+$$

In Golgi-Cox method, the chromated tissue treated by mercury to form white precipitation from mercurous chromate (Hg_2CrO_4) after $HgNO_3$ **OR** mercuric oxide chromate ($Hg_3O_2CrO_4$) after Hg (NO_3)$_2$. Then the blacking enhances by alkali (Kiernan 2015).

$$2Hg^+ + OH^- \longrightarrow Hg + HgO + H^+$$

Golgi-Cox method adapted for wax embedding (Pugh & Rossi, 1993)

Fixation:
Integral in method.

Sections:
None: fresh tissue slices.

Preparation of solutions:

Golgi-Cox fixation/ impregnation solution

A.	5 % mercuric chloride ($HgCl_2$)	20 ml
B.	5 % aqueous potassium dichromate	20 ml
C.	5 % aqueous potassium chromate	20 ml
D.	Distilled water	40 ml

Mix A to B. Mix C with D, then add to the mixture of A and B.

Method:
1. Fresh tissue slices, not thicker than 5 mm, are placed on a layer of glass wool and left in the Golgi-Cox fluid in the dark for up to 16 weeks at 20-25°C.
2. Blocks are washed overnight in 1 per cent solution of potassium dichromate ($K_2Cr_2O_7$).
3. Blocks are processed into paraffin wax using the following schedule:

70 % ethanol	2 hours
100 % ethanol	4 x 2 hour changes
Chloroform	3 x 2 hour changes
Wax (56°C)	4 x 2 hour changes

4. Sections are cut between 5 and 200 ums.

Blackening:
1. Dewax sections in xylene and take to water.
2. Drain and invert over a fully saturated solution of NH_3. Allow 10 min. for sections up to 10 um, 15 min. for sections up to 30 ums, and 30 min. for sections above 30 ums.

3. Wash in running water for 5 min.
4. Immerse in 15 per cent Amfix to decolorize the background (approx 10 min.).
5. Wash in running water for 5 min.
6. Dehydrate clear and mount in DPX

Result:

A proportion of neurons and their dendritic processes — black
Occasional astrocytes in subpial layer — black
Occasional astrocytes in white matter — black.

Vital staining methods:

The vital dye may be injected into the living animal (intravital) or removed tissue may be incubated in vital dye solution (supravital).

Methylene blue is a common vital dye for axon. Methylene blue reduced to its colorless leucobase, in which both the indamine and paraquinoid chromophore are reversibly disrupted (Kiernan and Berry, 1975).

$(CH_3)_2N$ — methylene blue — $N(CH_3)_2$ $\xrightarrow{[H]}$ $(CH_3)_2N$ — leucomethylene blue — $N(CH_3)_2$

The unionized leuco-base is the re-oxidized to the colored form by oxygen or air exposure.

Supravital staining of nerve fibers and endings

Preparation of solution:
Methylene blue solution:

Medicinal methylene blue (zincfree) — 50 mg
Distilled water, pyrogen free — 100 ml
Sodium chloride — 0.85 g
Dissolve in the order stated.

Ammonium molybdate (stored at 4—6°C):
Ammonium molybdate — 8 g
Distilled water — 100 ml

Method:
1. Inject methylene blue into the tissue and leave for 5-10 minutes.
2. Excise the tissue and cut longitudinally into strips not thicker than 3 mm.
3. Place tissue on Kleenex tissue soaked in saline in a Petri dish. A suitably sized funnel is inverted over the specimen and oxygen passed at the rate of 1 to 4 litters per minute for 1 hour. The specimen should be turned during this time in order to expose all surfaces.
4. Transfer tissue to cold ammonium molybdate and leave overnight at 4-6°C.
5. Wash in several changes of distilled water for 30 min.
6. Fix tissues in 10 per cent formalin for 24 hours
7. Cut frozen sections at 50-100 um.
8. Sections are dehydrated in absolute alcohol and cleared in xylene.

Results:
Nerve fibers and endings — blue.

Silver impregnation methods:

The silver methods for axon include impregnation and devolvement steps:

Impregnation consists of immersing the section in a solution containing silver ions and during this step, large numbers of silver ions become chemically bound to neurofilament polypeptide of axon neurofibril by the imidazole side-chains of histidine (Peter 1955) or disulfide and sulphydryl groups of cystine (Barnett & Seligmam 1954). This attachment, however, does not allow visualization because small numbers of silver ions are reduced to metallic silver and this site of reaction called nuclei silver or seeded silver or in situ silver.

In the development step, the section is transferred to a solution that contains a reducing agent mixed with a substance that can form soluble complexes with silver to reduce unreduced silver in the first step until their amount and size are sufficient for microscopic detection. A commonly used one contain sodium sulphite and hydroquinone as below.

$$2Ag^+ + \text{(hydroquinone)} + 2OH^- \longrightarrow 2Ag(s) + \text{(p-benzoquinone)} + 2H_2O$$

hydroquinone   p-benzoquinone

The contrast of axons impregnated with silver can be improved by using gold chloride and this process called gold toning.

$$3Ag + (AuCl_4)^- \rightarrow Au + 3AgCl + Cl^-$$

Palmgren's method for nerve fibers in paraffin-embedded material (Palmgren 1948)

Fixation:
Formal saline or Bouin's fixative.
Sections:
Paraffin or double-embedded sections, 6-10 um. Sections should be coated with nitrocellulose.
Preparation of solutions:
Acid formalin

40 % formaldehyde	25 ml
Distilled water	75 ml
1 % nitric acid	0.2 ml

Silver solution

Silver nitrate	15 g
Potassium nitrate	10 g
Distilled water	100 ml
5 per cent acetic acid	1 ml

Reducer

Pyrogallol	10 g
Distilled water	450 ml
Absolute ethanol	550 ml
1 per cent nitric acid	2 ml

Allow to stand for 24 hours before using.
Toning bath

Gold chloride	1 g
Distilled water	200 ml
Glacial acetic acid	0.2 ml

Intensifier

50 % ethyl alcohol	100 ml
Aniline oil	2 drops.

Fixing bath
5 % sodium thiosulfate.
Method:
1. Take sections to distilled water.
2. Wash sections in acid formalin for 5 min or longer.
3. Wash in three changes of distilled water for 5 min.
4. Leave in silver solution for 15 min. at 20-25°C or 4-5 min at 35°C.
5. Without rinsing, drain the slide and add reducer that has been heated to 40-45°C. Rock the slide gently and add fresh reducer. Leave for 1 min. A beaker placed on a hot plate is useful for this stage.
6. Rinse in 50 % alcohol for 5-10 seconds.
7. Wash in three changes of distilled water. Examine microscopically and, if necessary, repeat from step 2, reducing the time in the silver solution and decreasing the temperature of the reducer to 30 C.
8. Tone in gold chloride until yellow brown has faded.
9. Transfer directly into intensifier for 15 seconds or longer. Sections which contain nervous tissues only should be intensified after previously rinsing in 2 % oxalic acid.
10. Wash in tap water.
11. Fix for a few seconds in 5 % sodium thiosulfate.
12. Wash in water.
13. Dehydrate and remove nitrocellulose in absolute alcohol. Clear and mount.
Result:

Nerve fibers	brown or black.

Linder's method for nerves in paraffin sections of soft and mineralized tissue (Linder 1978)

Fixation:
Formal saline, formal calcium or Bouin's fluid.

Sections:
Paraffin, 6-10 um. Mineralized tissues are decalcified with formic acid or EDTA.
Preparation of solutions:
Buffer stock solution
2.4.6- collidine   6.6 ml
Distilled water   450 ml
Adjust pH 7.2 – 7.4 with 10 per cent nitric acid, and make up to 500 ml with distilled water.
Diluted buffer
Buffer stock   8 ml
Distilled water   92 ml
Silver cyanate impregnating solution
Distilled water heated to 60°C   84 ml

1 % silver nitrate   4 ml
0.38 % sodium cyanale   4 ml
Buffer stock solution   8 ml
Physical developer stock solution
Sodium sulfite ($Na_2SO_3,7H_2O$)   20 g

Sodium tetraborate ($Na_2B_4O_7,10H_2O$)   4.75 g
Distilled water   450 ml
Heat the solution to about 50°C, and add gelatine (Belgium Gold label)   10 g.
Physical developer working solution
Physical developer stock solution   95 ml

2 % hydroquinine   5 ml
1 % silver nitrate   2 ml
Add the silver nitrate, stirring constantly.
Method:
1. Remove paraffin, celloidinize sections and bring to distilled water.
2. Place in dilute buffer; soft tissues are left 10-20 minutes at 60°C, decalcified tissues overnight at 40-45°C.
3. Transfer directly to silver impregnating solution; soft tissues are incubated for 10-30 min. at 60°C, decalcified tissues are incubated for 90 min. at 40-45°C.
4. Wash in several changes of distilled water for a total of about 3 min.

5. Transfer sections into the physical developer working solution at about 25°C. The progress of development can be monitored by washing with distilled water and examining under the microscope. When results are judged to be optimal, the sections are washed in distilled water, dehydrated, cleared in xylene and mounted in Canada balsam or DPX.
Results:
Myelinated and non-myelinated nerve fibers
                                                                black
Striated muscle fibers   brown.

Eager's method for degenerating axons (1970)

Fixation:
Formal saline.
Sections:
Frozen, 30 ums.

Preparation of solutions:
Ammoniacal silver solution
1.5 % silver nitrate   40 ml
95 % ethanol   24 ml
0.88 Ammonia   4 ml
2.5 % sodium hydroxide   3.6 ml

Reducer
Absolute alcohol   90 ml
Distilled water   810 ml
1 % citric acid   27 ml
10 % formalin   37 ml

Method:
1. Place frozen sections into 2 per cent formalin.
2. Rinse sections in distilled water.
3. Transfer sections into 2.5 per cent uranyl nitrate for 5 min.
4. Rinse in distilled water and place in ammoniacal silver. Leave until brown, 3-15 min.

5. Transfer directly to reducer and leave until no further color change occurs, 2-5 min.
6. Rinse in distilled water.
7. Fix in 0.5 per cent sodium thiosulfate.
8. Wash, dehydrate, clear and mount.

Results:

Degenerating fibers	brown to black
Normal fibers	pale yellow.

The Myelin sheath

It is a fatty tubular covering around the axon formed by oligodendroglia cells in the CNS and by Schwann cells in the peripheral nervous system. Myelin contains protein, cholesterol, phospholipids and cerebrosides. During injury or disease, the myelin breakdown. Demonstration methods of myelin detect both normal and degenerating myelin.

Staining of normal myelin:

This divided into three groups

Hematoxylin method:

Weigert (1891) was the originator of the hematoxylin methods for myelin using chrome mordanted material. The principle of his methods is the reduction of chrome salts to chromium dioxide by myelin, this acts as a mordant and forms a lake with subsequent hematoxylin stain. Of numerous modifications of the Weigert principle, those of pal (Weigert – Pal) method in which dye lake is mixture of lithium carbonate and hematoxylin to attachment with myelin and differentiation step occurs firstly by oxidizer agent (potassium permanganate) which aids in restricting the dye lake to the myelin and red cells while Pal's bleach (second differentiator) makes further oxidation and completes differentiation process. The kultschitzky's modification of the Weigert-Pal method is based on the formation of chromium dioxide by interaction of chrome salts with the phosphatides and cerebrosides which are constituents of normal myelin, in which chromium dioxide acts as a mordant and forms a lake with hematoxylin.

Other hematoxylin stains for myelin use iron mordant and applied to the section rather than the block are Weil's and Loyez's methods. On Weil's method, staining solution consists of hematoxylin and ferric ammonium sulphate which combines with phospholipids of myelin especially choline moist of sphingomyelin and guanidyl groups of arginine side chains, the differentiation accomplished firstly by ferric ammonium sulphate which removes most of the excess dye and secondly by borax ferric cyanide (oxidizer) which removes any remaining non-specifically bound hematoxylin lake and from colorless product. In the Loyez's method iron alum followed by staining in lithium carbonate Hematoxylin and subsequently differentiation like Weil's method.

Weil's method for myelin sheaths (Weil 1928)

Fixation:
Formal saline or formal calcium.

Sections:
Paraffin, 10-15 um. Frozen, 20-30 um. Nitrocellulose, 20-30 um.
Frozen sections are brought through alcohols up to xylene and back again to water.

Preparation of stain:

4 % aqueous iron alum	50 ml.

50 ml of 1 % hematoxylin made from 10 % alcoholic hematoxylin (5 ml) and distilled water (45 ml).
Mix together immediately before use.

Method:
1. Wash sections in distilled water
2. Place sections in stain for 10-45 min at 50-60°C.
3. Wash well in tap water.
4. Differentiate in 4 per cent iron alum, just long enough to distinguish the gray matter or the degenerated areas.

5. Wash well in several changes of distilled water.
6. Complete the differentiation in Weigert's borax ferricyanide solution.
7. Wash well in several changes of distilled water, followed by tap water.
8. Dehydrate, clear and mount.

Results:

Myelin	black
Background	yellow.

Solochrome cyanine R is used in much the same way as Weil's ferric-hematin but a solution of solochrome cyanine R with added ferric salts can be kept for many years without deterious and differentiation of stain requires only a single step. The blue complex solution is anionic and with composition $[Fe(dye)]^{2-}$. (Kiernan 1984).

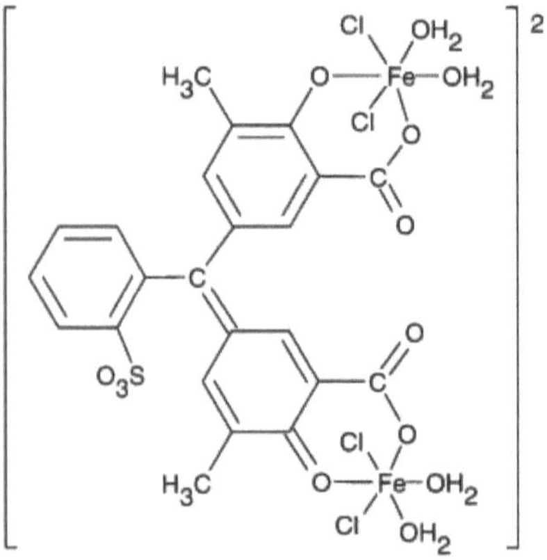

$[Fe_2(dye)]^-$ Blue. $\lambda_{max} = 585$ nM

The solochrome cyanine technique for myelin in paraffin sections (Page 1965)

Fixation

Formal saline or formal calcium.

Sections:

Paraffin, 6-10 um. Cryostat section, 10 ums.

Preparation of solution:

Solochrome cyanine RS	0.2 g
Distilled water	96 ml
10 % iron alum	4 ml
Concentrated Sulphuric acid	0.5 ml

Method:
1. Take sections to water.
2. Stain for 10-20 min at room temperature.
3. Wash in running water.
4. Differentiate in 5 per cent iron alum until all the nuclei are unstained. Wash frequently in distilled water, and examine.
5. Wash in running tap water.
6. Counterstain if desired.
7. Dehydrate, clear and mount.

Result:

Myelin sheaths   blue.

Copper phthalocyanine dyes methods

The copper phthalocyanine dyes luxol fast blue MBS and methasol fast blue 2G in alcoholic solution, have the property of combing with and staining the phospholipids of myelin.

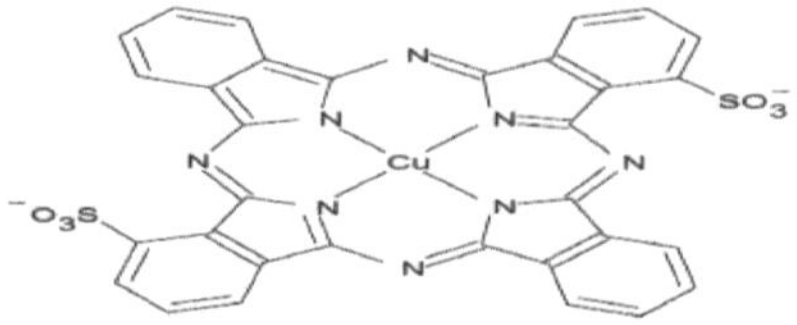

The staining mechanism occurs by one of an acid-base reaction with salt formation, the base of myelin lipoproteins replaces the base of luxol fast blue.

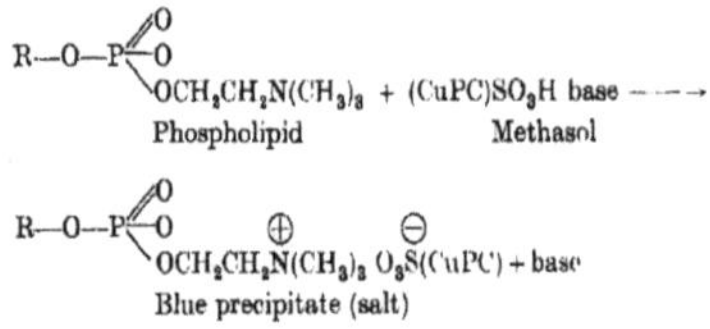

176

Kluver and Barrera (1953) used the first dye and counter stained with cresyl fast violet, and subsequently various modified and simplified version of the technique have been developed.

The combination of luxol fast blue with common technics like periodic Acid-Schiff, oil red O, phosphotungestic acid, hematoxylin and silver nitrate techniques found in use in the majority of laboratories.

Kluver & Barrera Luxol fast blue stain for myelin with NissI counterstain (Kluver & Barrera, 1953)

Fixation: Formalin.
Sections: Paraffin, 10-15 um.
Preparation of solutions:
Luxol fast blue

Luxol fast blue	1 g
Methanol (absolute)	1000 ml
10 per cent acetic acid	5 ml

Mix reagents and filter. This may then be stored for up to 18 months before use.
Cresyl violet solution

| Cresyl violet | 0.5 g |
| Distilled water | 100 ml |

Filter before use.
Cresyl violet differentiator

| Alcohol | 100 ml |
| Glacial acetic acid | 250 ul |

Method:
1. Take sections on slides to 95 per cent alcohol (not water).
2. Stain in luxol fast blue solution, 2 hours at 60°C, or 37°C overnight.
3. Wash in 70 per cent alcohol.
4. Wash in tap water.
5. Differentiate in saturated lithium carbonate solution until gray and white matter are distinguished. This may be more easily controlled by using 0.05 per cent lithium carbonate followed by 95% alcohol instead.
6. Wash in tap water.
7. Check differentiation under the microscope. Repeat step 5 if necessary.
8. Stain in cresyl violet solution, 10-20 min.
9. Wash in tap water.
10. Differentiate in cresyl violet differentiator, 4-8 sec.
11. Check differentiation under microscope (Nissl and nuclei only).
12. Dehydrate, clear in xylene and mount.

Result:

| Myelin | blue/green |
| Cells | violet/pink. |

Lipids staining methods
These methods based on the detection of unsaturated fatty acids or phospholipids and sphingolipids. The lipids of myelin are 17-22 carbon atoms in length and some linkages are unsaturated (- CH= CH -) therefore osmium tetroxides and combines with these unsaturated linkages (Kiernan & Berry 1975).

$$
\begin{array}{c} H-C \\ \| \\ H-C \end{array} + OsO_4 \longrightarrow \begin{array}{c} H-C-O \\ | \quad\quad\; Os \\ H-C-O \end{array}
$$

The sudan dyes (including oil red O) are non-ionic azo dyes with hydrophobic molecules that fit into the hydrophobic domain of myelin lipids, and the simple way of this mechanism is the dye is more soluble in the lipids than its solvent.

Staining of degenerating Myelin:
Marchi and Algeri (1985) was first described method for degenerating myelin. The principle of this method is reduction of osmium tetroxide by myelin lipids, the reduction process prevented in normal myelin by addition of potassium dichromate or potassium chloride (oxidizer) to osmium solution. They are a number of theories as to why degenerating myelin is not affected by this differentiation process, one pos-

tulate that normal myelin lipids are hydrophilic and readily absorb both the osmium and oxidizer therefore the oxidizer preventing the reduction process, in contrast to degenerating myelin lipids which are hydrophobic and absorb osmium only without oxidizer so the reduction process occur.

Marchi's method, Swank-Davenport modification (Swank & Davenport, 1935)

Fixation:
Formal saline.
Sections:
Frozen.
Preparation of impregnating solution

1 % osmium tetroxide	20 ml
1 % potassium chlorate	60 ml
Formaldehyde	12 ml
Glacial acetic acid	1 ml

Method:
1. Cut thin slices of tissues, 3-5 mm thick.
2. Rinse tissues for 5-10 min in 1 per cent potassium chlorate.
3. Transfer tissues to the impregnating solution and leave for 7-12 days at room temperature, in the dark.
4. Wash in running tap water for 1-2 days.
5. Cut frozen sections at 25-90 um. Mount in glycerine-jelly or dehydrate, clear and mount in Canada balsam.
6. Dehydrate and embed in paraffin wax or nitrocellulose.

Results:

Degenerate myelin   black

Depending on the age of the demyelination, the reaction products may vary from being ring-shaped, coarse irregular, extra cellular globules or fine intracellular granules inside macrophages.

Normal myelin   light brown.

There is no connective tissue proper in the central nervous system (CNS) except in the meninges covering the brain and the blood vessels in addition to synaptic contact regions, instead there are the neuroglia (nerve glue). There are four types of glial cells

Astrocytes

They are large stellate cells of two types:
Protoplasmic astrocytes which are ectodermal in origin, present in gray matter of central nervous system, branched with multiple short thick processes, their cytoplasm rich by granules known as gliosomes and secrete opioid substance called enkephalin.

Fibrous astrocytes are other type of astrocyte which are similar to protoplasmic astrocytes, but they are present in white matter of the central nervous system have long, slender, smooth processes that branch in frequently and their cytoplasm rich in straight neuroglia fibers without granular.

Oligodendroglia

They are ectodermal in origin, present in both gray and white matter, have small branches with large deeply stained nuclei and form a myelin sheath.

Microglia

They are spindle shaped cells, mesodermal in origin, present in gray and white matter, have few short processes with flat oval darkly stained nuclei, have an amoeboid movement and change into phagocytic cells during inflammation of neurons, so it called police man of the brain.

Ependymal cells

They are derived from the spongioblast cells, and they are true simple cuboidal ciliated cells which line the central canal of the spinal cord and brain ventricles.

Staining of Neuroglia:
The methods described below are the most reliable of a great variety of techniques and their modifications, and are recommended.

PTAH stain for astrocytes

Principle:
It is a dye-lake complex between hematin and phosphotungestic acid, in which the amount of phosphotungestic acid is far greater than the amount of hematin (20:1) in the staining solution to give blue lake. This blue lake links with fibrillary protein of astrocyte filaments to give blue color, while neurons stained by the phosphotungestic acid to give red-brown color.

Fixation:
Formalin.

Sections:
Paraffin, 5-10 um.

Solutions:
A. PTAH:

Hematoxylin	1g
Phosphotungstic acid	20 g
Distilled water	1000 ml

B. Permanganate:

Potassium permanganate	1g
Distilled water	100 ml

C. Oxalic acid

Oxalic acid	5 g
Distilled water	100 ml

Method:
1. Take section to water.
2. Mordant sections in Zenker's for 60 min at 50° C.
3. Wash in running tap water, 15 min.
4. Place in Lugol's iodine, 15 min.
5. Decolorize in 95% alcohol for 60-90 min.
6. Wash in distilled water, three changes.
7. Oxidize in permanganate solution, 3-5 min.
8. Decolorize in oxalic acid solution, 5 min.
9. Stain in PTAH solution, 12-24 hours at room temperature.
10. Rinse rapidly with 96 per cent alcohol.
11. Dehydrate rapidly in three changes of absolute alcohol.
12. Clear in xylene; mount.

Result:

Astrocyte fibrils	blue
Nuclei	blue
Myelin	blue
Neurons	pink.

Steart's modification of Holzer's method for astrocytic processes and glial fibers

Principle:
The crystal violet links with all glial fibers to give blue color, then decolorization step by the alkaline aniline-chloroform mixture remove the blue color from all glia except astrocyte due to strong combination of crystal violet and astrocyte fibrillary protein.

Fixation:
Formalin, Helly's or Bouin's fixatives.

Sections:
Paraffin, 6-10 um.

Preparation of solutions:
Mordant

1 % phosphomolybdic acid	10 ml
Absolute alcohol	40 ml

Chloroform—alcohol mixture

Chloroform	160 ml
Absolute alcohol	40 ml

Crystal violet stain

Crystal violet	2 g
Absolute alcohol	20 ml
Chloroform	80 ml

Differentiating solution

Aniline oil	80 ml
Chloroform	120 ml
Ammonia, concentrated	10 drops

Method:
1. Bring sections to absolute alcohol.
2. Flood slide with mordant for 5-10 min.
3. Pour off and wash in absolute alcohol.
4. Flood slide with chloroform-alcohol mixture.
5. Drain off and quickly pour on the crystal violet stain, agitating for 30 seconds.
6. Drain slide and rapidly wash off excess stain in running tap water.
7. Pour on 10 per cent potassium bromide solution and continue until no green discoloration remains.
8. Drain slide and blot with dry fluff-free filter paper. Allow to air dry.
9. Differentiate in differentiating solution until the background is nearly colorless. The time for this can be very variable and should be controlled under the microscope. In prolonged cases, tip off differentiator and add fresh.
10. Rinse well in xylene.
11. Mount in synthetic mountant.

Results:

Glial fibrils	blue
Nuclei	pale blue
Background	colorless.

Cajal's gold sublimate method for astrocytes

Principle:
It is gold-impregnation by gold chloride in presence of mercuric chloride. The astrocyte fibrillary proteins are responsible from gold reduction to metallic gold.

Fixation:
Formal saline.

Sections:
Loose paraffin sections, 15-20 um. Frozen, 20 ums.

Solutions:

a) 5% Mercuric chloride.
prepared by dissolving in distilled water with gentle heat.

b) *Gold chloride solution*

1% brown gold chloride	8 ml
Distilled water	40 ml

c) 5% Cupric sulfate hydrated

d) Glacial acetic acid

e) *Formal ammonium bromide*

Ammonium bromide	0.6 g
Formalin	14 ml
Distilled water	100 ml

Gold sublimate impregnating solution

Solution b	10 ml
Solution e	40 ml

Method:
1. Dewax loose paraffin sections in xylene and bring them down to distilled water through graded alcohol.
2. Rinse sections in several changes of distilled water.
3. Place in formal ammonium bromide for three days. Sections should not overlap.
4. Rinse thoroughly with distilled water.
5. Place sections in the gold sublimate impregnating solution and leave at room temperature (20-22°C) in subdued light for 1 hours and 30 min. Sections must lie flat and not overlapping and allow 10 ml of solution per section. To the impregnation bath, for every 10 ml of solution, add 120 ul of glacial acetic acid and 40 ul of solution c. Mix well and make sure that the sections remain flat and not overlapping. After 3 hours of total impregnation, at regular intervals, check sections microscopically. Proceed on if the astrocytes are clearly visible; otherwise return sections to the gold bath for further staining for up to 8 hours.
6. Place sections in 1% acetic acid for 30 min.
7. Rinse in distilled water.
8. Place section in 5% sodium thiosulfate for 10 min.
9. Rinse sections in distilled water, dehydrate, clear and mount.

Results

Fibrous and protoplasmic astrocytes dark purple to black.

Background   purple.

Penfield's combined oligodendroglia and microglia method (Penfield 1928)

Principle:

Both oligodendroglia and microglia reduce silver solution.

Fixation:

Formalin ammonium bromide or formal saline.

Sections:

Frozen sections, 15-20 um.

Preparation of solution:

Silver carbonate solution

10 % silver nitrate   5 ml
5 % sodium carbonate   20 ml
Ammonia is added, sufficient to dissolve the precipitate.
Distilled water up to   75 ml
Filter before use.

Method:

1. Leave sections in 1 % ammonia overnight to remove the formalin.
2. Transfer directly to 5 % hydrobromic acid and leave for 1 hour at 37°C.
3. Wash in three changes of distilled water.
4. Place sections for 1 hour or more in 5 percent sodium carbonate.
5. Impregnate sections in silver carbonate solution for 3-5 min.
6. Transfer directly to 1 per cent formalin in distilled water.
7. Wash in distilled water.
8. Tone in 0.2 per cent gold chloride until gray.
9. Wash in water.
10. Fix in 5 per cent sodium thiosulfate for 2-5 min.
11. Wash, dehydrate, clear and mount in Canada balsam.

Results:

Microglia and oligo-dendroglia   dark grey.

Weil & Davenport's method for microglia and oligodendroglia

Principle:

Similar to penfield method.

Fixation:

Formal ammonium bromide or formal saline.

Sections:

Paraffin sections are cut at 15-20 um and transferred directly into two successive baths of xylene. Place sections in absolute alcohol, then in 50 per cent alcohol. Wash in distilled water. Frozen sections are cut at 20-25um and left in 10 percent ammonia for 2 hours before staining.

Preparation of solution:

To 2 ml of concentrated ammonia, add 5 per cent silver nitrate, until a slight permanent turbidity is formed. The solution should be orange-brawn in color.

Method:

1. Wash sections well in distilled water.
2. Impregnate in silver solution for 3-4 seconds.
3. Transfer to 3 per cent formalin in distilled water, moving them continuously. Leave for 30 seconds.
4. Wash in distilled water.
5. Fix in 5 per cent sodium thiosulfate for 2-5 min.
6. Wash, dehydrate, clear and mount in Canada balsam.

Results

Oligodendroglia, microglia and astrocytes black

Further reading:

Biclschowsky, M. (1902) Die Silber impragnation der Axenzylinder. Zentralblatt fur Neurologic, 21: 579.

Barnett RJ, Seligman AM, Histochemical demonstration of sulfhydryl and disulfide groups of protein. J Nut Cancer Inst 14769-804, 1954.

Eager. R.P. (1970) Selective staining of degenerating axons in the central nervous system by a simplified method spinal cord projections to external cuneate and inferior olivary nuclei in the cat. Brain Research, 22: 137-141.

Kiernan, J.A. (2015) Histological and Histochemical Methods: Theory and Practice. 5th edition, Scion Publishing.

Kiernan, J.A. and Berry, M. (1975). Neuroanatomical methods. In Bradley, P.B. (ed.), *Methods in Brain Research*, pp. 1–77. London: Wiley.

Kluver, H. & Barrera, A. (19 53) A method for the combined staining of cells and fibres of the nervous system. Journal of Neuropathology and Experimental Neurology 12: 400.

Marsland, T.A., Glees, P. & Erikson, L.B (1954) Modification of the Glees, silver impregnation for paraffin sections. Journal of Neuropathology and Experimental Neurology, 15: 587.

Marchi, V. and Algeri, G. (1885). Rivista sperimentale di freniatriae medicina legale delle alienazioni mentali. Sulle degenerazioni discendenti consecutive a lisione della corteccia cerebrale. *Riv. Sper. F reniât.*, Il, 492.

Page, K. (1965) A stain for myelin using solochrome cyanin. Journal of Medical Laboratory Technology. 22:224.

Palmgren, A. (1948) A rapid method lor selective silver staining of nerve fibres and nerve endings in mounted paraffin sections. Acta Zoologiea. 29: 377-392

Penfield, W. (1928) A method of staining oligodendroglia and microglia. American Journal of Pathology. 4: 153.

Peters A: Experiments on the mechanism of silver staining. I. Impregnation. Quart J Microsc Sci 96:84-102, 1955.

Pugh, B.C. & Rossi, M.J. (1993) A paraffin wax technique of Golgi-Cox impregnated CNS that permits the joint application of other histological and immunocytochemical techniques, journal of Neural Transmission (Suppl.) 39: 97-105.

Weil, A. (1928) A rapid method for staining myelin sheaths. Archives of Neurology and Psychiatry 20: 392.

Weigert, C. (1891) Zur marksche idenfiirbung. Dentsches Medizinisches Wochenschrift. 1184.

Swank, R.L. & Davenport, H.A. (19 35) Chlorate-osmic formalin method for degenerating myelin. StainTechnology, 10. 87-90.

Enzyme histochemistry have ability to detect an early metabolic change in biopsy and autopsy tissues before disease manifestation on H&E staining or immunohistochemistry.

Now it has been largely replaced by immuno-histochemistry. But there are some classical methods which are of diagnostic value. The two most common uses of enzyme histochemistry in histopathology laboratories are: Skeletal muscle biopsy and Colonic biopsy in cases of suspected Hirschsprung's Disease.

Definition

Enzymes are biocatalyst proteins synthesized by living cells that increase the chemical reactions in biological systems by temporarily combining with their specific substrates without being changed in the overall process.

Types of enzymes:

Hydrolases

This class of enzymes includes: esterases, phosphatases, peptidases, lipases, glycosidases and pyrophosphatases.

Oxidoreductases

This class of enzymes includes: oxidases, peroxidases and dehydrogenases.

Transferases

These enzymes transfer a functional group from one compound to another as phosphorylase.

Lyases

They catalyse the removal of groups from substrates resulting in formation of double bonds of carbon, like decarboxylase.

Type of enzymatic histochemical reaction:

A- simultaneous capture

It is the most important techniques for demonstrating of enzymes. In which the enzyme catalyses substrate to produces primary reaction product (PRP) then the latter combines with diazonium salt to produce the final reaction product (FER).

B- Post-incubation coupling

It is similar to simultaneous capture, but here the primary reaction product (PRP) has to be sufficiently insoluble and remain at the site of production for the duration of the initial incubation till the final reaction product (FRP) produced in a separate solution media.

C- Self-colored substrate

In this type we use colored soluble substrate which hydrolysed by enzyme into insoluble colored product and soluble grouping which the latter removed by enzyme hydrolysis. This type is not need coupling by diazonium salts.

D- Intramolecular rearrangement

The enzyme hydrolyses soluble colorless substrate in primary product undergoes molecular rearrangement to colored in soluble product.

Fixation:

Cold acetone serves the purpose of enzyme detection. Buffered formal-saline and 95% alcohol are used.

Phosphatases

Phosphatases are hydrolytic enzymes that break the bond between an alcohol and a phosphate group.

$$
\begin{array}{c}
\text{OH} \\
| \\
\text{O}\!=\!\text{P}\!-\!\text{O}\!-\!\text{R} \;+\; H_2O \;\longrightarrow\; ROH + H_3PO_4 \\
| \\
\text{OH}
\end{array}
$$

The released phosphate is made visible by a variety of techniques like gomori-type metal precipitation method or alternatively, the alcoholic residue of the substrate (produced by enzyme hydrolysis of the substrate) reacts with a diazonium salt to produce a highly colored insoluble azo dye.

They are classified on the basis of their optimal pH level into alkaline phosphatases which exhibit maximum activity at around pH 9.0 and acid phosphatases which exhibit maximum activity at around pH 5.0.

Most phosphatases are non-specific i.e. hydrolysis of a wide range of organic phosphate esters while few of them are specific (i.e. hydrolysis specific substrates) like 5-nucleotidase, ATPase and glucose-6-phosphatse.

Demonstration of non-specific phosphatases

This group demonstrated by both precipitation methods and azo dye methods.

1-Metal precipitation method:

This method is a simultaneous coupling reaction, in which the alkaline phosphatase hydrolyses the substrate (sodium B-glycerophosphate) to produce phosphate ions that link with calcium ions to form calcium phosphate.

$$
\begin{array}{c}
\text{CH}_2\text{-OH} \\
| \qquad\quad \text{ONa} \\
\text{CH-O-P} \!\!<\!\! \text{O} \quad \xrightarrow[\;H_2O + Ca^{2+}\;]{\text{Enzyme}} \quad \begin{array}{c}\text{CH}_2\text{-OH}\\ |\\ \text{CH-OH} + Ca_3(PO_4)_2 \downarrow\\ |\\ \text{CH}_2\text{-OH}\end{array}\\
| \qquad\quad \text{ONa} \\
\text{CH}_2\text{-OH}
\end{array}
$$

Sodium salt of 2-glycerophosphate   Glycerin   Calcium phosphate (white)

And this in turn is treated with cobalt nitrate to produce a precipitate of cobalt phosphate.

$$
Ca_3(PO_4)_2 + 3\,Co^{2+} \;\longrightarrow\; Co_3(PO_4)_2 \downarrow
$$

Calcium phosphate   Cobalt cations   Cobaltous phosphate

This reaction product cannot be seen with light microscope and further treatment is needed with dilute ammonium sulfide to produce a visible black precipitate of cobalt sulfide.

$$
Co_3(PO_4)_2 + 3\,S^{2-} \;\longrightarrow\; 3\,CoS \downarrow
$$

Cobaltous phosphate   Sulfide anions   Cobaltous sulfide (black)

The acid phosphatase hydrolyses the substrate (sodium B-glycerophosphate) to produce phosphate ions that link with lead ions to form lead phosphate.

$$
\begin{array}{c}
\text{CH}_2\text{-OH} \\
| \qquad\quad \text{ONa} \\
\text{CH-O-P} \!\!<\!\! \text{O} \quad \xrightarrow[\;H_2O + Pb^{2+}\;]{\text{Enzyme}} \quad \begin{array}{c}\text{CH}_2\text{-OH}\\ |\\ \text{CH-OH} + Pb_3(PO_4)_2 \downarrow\\ |\\ \text{CH}_2\text{-OH}\end{array}\\
| \qquad\quad \text{ONa} \\
\text{CH}_2\text{-OH}
\end{array}
$$

Sodium salt of 2-glycerophosphate   Glycerin   Lead phosphate (white)

And this in turn is treated with ammonium sulfide to produce a precipitate of lead sulfide.

$$
Pb_3(PO_4)_2 \;+\; 3\,S^{2-} \;\longrightarrow\; 3\,PbS \downarrow
$$

Lead phosphate (white)   Sulfide anions   Lead sulfide (brownish black)

Alkaline phosphatase: The Gomori calcium method (1951, modified)

Fixation:
Formal calcium at 4°C.

Sections:
Pre-fixed cryostat preferred.

Preparation of incubating medium:

2 % sodium b-glycerophosphate	2.5 ml
2 % sodium veronal	2.5 ml
2 % calcium nitrate	5.0 ml
1 % magnesium chloride	0.25 ml
Distilled water	1.25 ml

The final pH of the incubating medium should be between 9.0 and 9.4. The sodium veronal acts as the buffer vehicle and the magnesium ions as an enzyme activator.

Method:
1. After suitable fixation, bring sections to water, incubate at 37°C for 25 min to 6 hours.
2. Wash well in distilled water.
3. Repeat wash.
4. Treat sections with 2 per cent cobalt nitrate, 3 min.
5. Wash well in distilled water.
6. Repeat wash.
7. Immerse sections in 1 per cent ammonium sulfide, 2 min.
8. Wash well in distilled water.
9. Counterstain in 2 per cent methyl green (chloroform extracted).
10. Wash well in running tap water.
1 1. Mount in glycerin jelly.

Results:

Alkaline phosphatase activity   brownish-black
Nuclei   green.

Acid phosphatase: The Gomori lead method

Fixation:
Formal calcium at 4°C. Formal vapour.

Sections:
Pre-fixed cryostat preferred.

Preparation of incubating solution:

0.05 M acetate buffer pH 5.0	10 ml
Sodium b-glycerophosphate	32 mg
Lead nitrate	20 mg

The lead nitrate must be dissolved in the buffer before the sodium P-glycerophosphate is added. The pH of the incubating medium should be approximately 5.0.

Method:
1. Place sections in incubating solution at 37°C for 1/2-2 hours.
2. Wash in distilled water.
3. Immerse in 1 per cent ammonium sulphide (fresh), 2 min.

4. Wash well in distilled water.
5. Counterstain in either 2 per cent methyl green, or Mayer's carmalum.
6. Wash in tap water.
7. Mount in glycerin jelly.

Results:

Acid phosphatase activity   black
Nuclei   green or red.

2- Azo dye methods:
These also simultaneous coupling methods, in which involve the use of a diazonium salts to provide a means of visibly locating the reaction product produced by the action of the enzyme on the substrate. According to type of substrate employed, there are two methods:

A- Azo dye coupling method using simple naphthols:
The sections are incubated in a substrate containing simple naphthol (sodium- α naphthol phosphate) and a diazonium salt (fast blue RR). The enzyme liberates α-naphthol which couples with fast blue RR to form an insoluble colored precipitate.

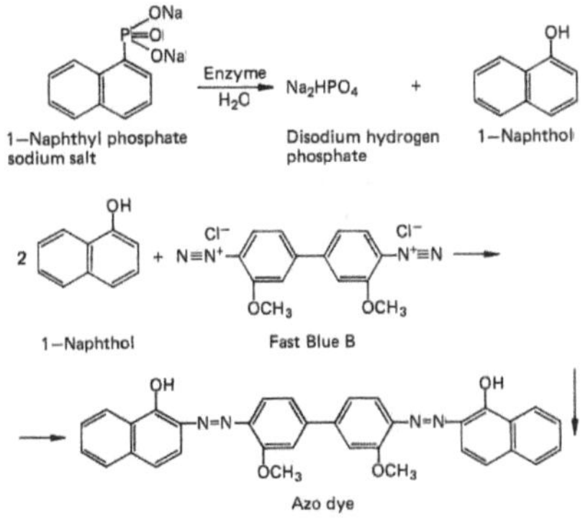

Alkaline phosphatase: azo dye coupling method using α-naphthyl phosphate

Fixation:
Formal-calcium at 4 CC. Formal vapour.

Sections:

Prefixed cryostat preferred.

Preparation of incubating medium:

Sodium α- naphthyl phosphate   10 mg

0.2 M Tris buffer (stock solution A) pH 10.0

     10 ml

Diazonium salt (fast red TR)   10 mg

The final pH of the incubating medium should be between 9.0 and 9.4. The sodium a naphthyl phosphate is dissolved in the buffer, the diazonium salt is added and the solution well mixed. The solution is then filtered and used immediately.

Method:

1. After fixation, bring sections to water, incubate at room temperature for 10-60 min.

2. Wash in distilled water.

3. Counterstain in 2 per cent methyl green (chloroform extracted).

4. Wash in running tap water.

5. Mount in glycerin jelly.

Results:

Alkaline phosphatase activity   reddish-brown

Nuclei   green.

Acid phosphatase: azo dye coupling method

Fixation:

Formal calcium at 4°C. Formal vapour.

Section:

Pre-fixed cryostat preferred.

Preparation of incubating medium:

Sodium - α-naphthyl phosphate   10 mg

0.1 M acetate buffer, pH 5.0   10 ml

Fast garnet GBC   10 mg

The sodium a-naphthyl phosphate is dissolved in the buffer and the diazonium salt added. The solution is then filtered and used immediately.

Method:

1. Incubate at 37°C for 15-60 min.

2. Wash in distilled water.

3. Counterstain in 2 per cent methyl green (chloroform extracted).

4. Wash in running tap water.

5. Mount in glycerin jelly.

Results:

Acid phosphatase activity   red

Nuclei   green.

B- Azo dye coupling method using substituted naphthols:

The sections are incubated in a substrate containing substituted naphthol (Naphthol AS-BI-phosphate) to produce naphthol-AS-BI and orthophosphate by the action of the enzyme, then the hexazotized pararosaniline reacts with naphthol-AS-BI to produce colored azo dye.

Naphthol AS-BI phosphate

Alkaline phosphatase: naphthol AS-BI method (substituted naphthol)

Fixation:

Formal calcium at 4 CC. Formal vapour.

Sections:

Pre-fixed cryostat preferred.

Preparation of solutions:

a. Naphthol AS-BI stock solution

Naphthol AS-BI phosphate   25 mg

N: N-dimethyl formamide   10 ml

Distilled water   10 ml

Molar sodium carbonate   2-6 drops

The reagents are added in the above order sufficient molar sodium carbonate is added until the pH is 8.0, then add:

Distilled water   300 ml

0.2 M Tris buffer, pH 8.3   180 ml

The solution, which is faintly opalescent, is stable for many months.

b. Incubating solution

Stock naphthol AS-BI solution   10 ml
Fast red TR   10 mg
Shake well, filter and use immediately.

Method:
1. After fixation and bringing sections to water, incubate at room temperature for 5-15 min.
2. Wash in water.
3. Counterstain in 2 per cent methyl green (chloroform extracted).
4. Wash well in running tap water.
5. Mount in glycerin jelly.

Results:
Alkaline phosphatase activity   red
Nuclei   green.

Acid phosphatase: the naphthol AS-BI phosphate method (Burnstone 1958, modified by Barka 1960)

Fixation:
Formal calcium at 4°C. Formal vapour.

Sections:
Pre-fixed cryostat preferred.

Preparation of solutions:

a. Substrate solution
Naphthol AS-BI phosphate   10 mg
Dimethyl formamide   1 ml

b. Buffer solution
Sodium acetate (3H$_2$0)   1.94 g
Sodium barbitone   2.94 g
Distilled water   100 ml

c. Sodium nitrite solution
Sodium nitrite   400 mg
Distilled water   10 ml

d. Pararosanilin-HCl stock solution
Pararosanilin hydrochloride   1 g
Distilled water   20 ml

Hydrochloric acid (cone)   5 ml
Heat gently, cool to room temperature and filter.

e. Distilled water

Preparation of incubating solution:
Solution a   0.5 ml
Solution b   2.5 ml
Solution c   0.4 ml
Solution d   0.4 ml
Solution e   6 ml

For the success of this technique it is essential that equal parts of solutions c and d are mixed together and allowed to stand for 2 min before being added to the incubating medium. The final pH should be between 4.7 and 5.0; it is adjusted if necessary with 0.1 M NaOH.

Method:
1. Incubate sections at 37°C for 15-60 min.
2. Wash in distilled water.
3. Counterstain in 2 per cent methyl green (chloroform extracted).
4. Wash in running water.
5. Either mount in glycerin jelly, or dehydrate rapidly through fresh alcohols to xylene and mount in DPX.

Results;
Acid phosphatase activity   red
Nuclei   green.

Demonstration of specific phosphatases

5-nucleotidase:
It demonstrated by a metal precipitation method of Wachtstein and Meisel (1957) in which the enzyme acts on the substrate (Adenosine-5-phosphate) in the presence of magnesium ion as an activator to produce phosphate ions which the latter precipitated by lead ion to produce lead phosphate (invisible). The ammonium sulfide is used to convert the lead phosphate to visible lead sulfide.

5-Nucleotidase: lead method (Wachstein & Meisel 1957)

Fixation:
Unfixed preferred, or formal calcium at 4°C.
Sections:
Cryostat, free-floating.
Preparation of incubating medium:

1.25 % adenosine-5-phosphate	4 ml
0.2 M Tris buffer, pH 7.2	4 ml
2 % lead nitrate	0.6 ml
0.1 M magnesium sulphate	1 ml
Distilled water	0.5 ml

Method:
1. Incubating medium at 37°C for 30 min to1 hour.
2. Fix in formol saline if unfixed sections used.
3. Transfer sections with glass rod to distilled water.
4. Repeat wash in fresh distilled water
5. 1 per cent ammonium sulfide, 3 min.
6. Wash well in distilled water.
7. Repeat wash.
8. Mount on microscope slides and allow to dry partially in the usual way.
9. Mount in glycerin jelly.
Result:

5-nucleotidase	blackish-brown deposits.

Glucose-6-phosphatase:
It also demonstrated by a metal precipitation method of Wachstein and Meisel (1956) in which the enzyme hydrolyses glucose-6-phosphate in the presence of lead nitrate to form lead phosphate, which is then converted to lead sulfide by dilute ammonium sulphide.

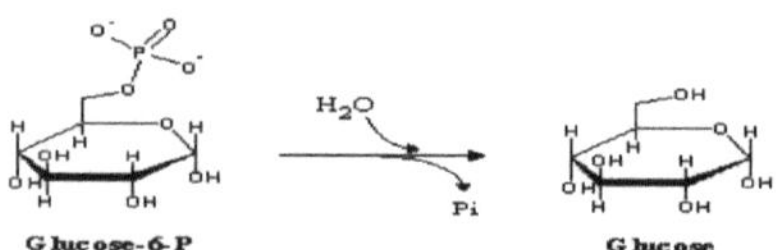

Glucose-6-phosphatase: lead method (Wachstein & Meisel 1956)

Fixation:
None.
Sections:
Cryostat, unfixed.
Preparation of incubating medium:

0.125 per cent glucose-6-phosphate	4 ml
Tris maleate buffer pH 6.7	4 ml
2 per cent lead nitrate	0.6 ml
Distilled water	1.4 ml

Method:
1. Place fresh unfixed cryostat sections into incubating medium at 37°C for 5-20 min.
2. Wash well in distilled water, two changes, 2 min. each.
3. Immerse sections in 1 per cent ammonium sulfide, 2 min.
4. Wash in distilled water.
5. Fix sections in 10 per cent formaldehyde, 15-30 min.
6. Wash in distilled water.
7. Mount in glycerin jelly.
Result:
Glucose-6-phosphatase activity brownish black.

Adenosine triphosphatase (ATPase)

The ATPase reaction is also a metal precipitation method of Wachstein (1960). The enzyme produces phosphate from the substrate (Adenosine triphosphate) which combine with lead ions to produce a precipitate of lead phosphate which finally converted to lead sulphide by treatment with sulphide.

Adenosine triphosphatase (ATPase)

Sections:
Unfixed cryostat.

Solutions:
a. 0.1 M glycine buffer
Glycine   0.75 g
NaCI   0.585 g
Make up to 100 ml with distilled water.
b. 0.1 M glycine buffer with 0.75 M CaCl2
M NaOH until pH 0.1 M glycine buffer (solution a)   50 ml
0.75 M CaCI2(l 1.03 g CaCl2/2H20 in 100 ml distilled water)   10 ml
Mix, then add approx. 22 ml 0.1NaOH until PH 9.4.
c. 0.1 M solution veronal-acetate buffer pH 4.2 and pH 4.6.
d. Incubating solution
ATP   5 mg
Solution b   10 ml
Adjust to pH 9.4 with 0.1 M NaOH or 0.1 M HCI if necessary.
Method:
1. Incubate freshly-cut sections in incubating solution (d) at 37°C.
2. Rinse well in distilled water.
3. Immerse in 2% cobalt chloride for 5 min.
4. Rinse well in tap water, then in three changes of distilled water.

5. Immerse in dilute (1:10) ammonium sulphide solution for 30 seconds (in fume cupboard).
6. Rinse well in running tap water.
7. Stain lightly in Harris's hematoxylin, blue in tap water.
8. Mount in glycerin jelly ar dehydrate, clear and mount in DPX.
Method (at pH 4.2 and 4.6)
1. Pre-incubate freshly cut sections at 4°C inappropriate 0.1 M veronal-acetate buffer (solution c above) for 10 min.
2. Rinse briefly in distilled water.
3. Proceed as from step 1 in the pH 9.4 method above.
Results:
Strong staining pattern (dark or black): ++ or +++.
Weak staining pattern (pinkish): +.
Negative (no staining).

Esterases

Esterases are enzymes capable of breaking the bond between carboxylic acid, alcohol, phenol and a hydroxylated base such as choline (Kiernan 2015).

$$R-O-\underset{O}{\overset{\|}{C}}-R' + H_2O \xrightarrow[(esterase)]{} ROH + HOOC-R'$$

Esterases divided into non-specific estrases like carboxyl esterases, arylesterases and acetyl esterases or specific esterases like lipase, cholinesterases and acetyl cholinesterases. Most esterases are able to hydrolysing a simple ester such as α-naphthol acetate as substrate.

The use of inhibitors is necessary to separate between estrases and more accurate identification of the specific enzymes. The organophosphates like diethyl-p-nitrophenyl phosphate (E600) and di-isopropyl fluorophosphate (DFP) are the most useful inhibitors.

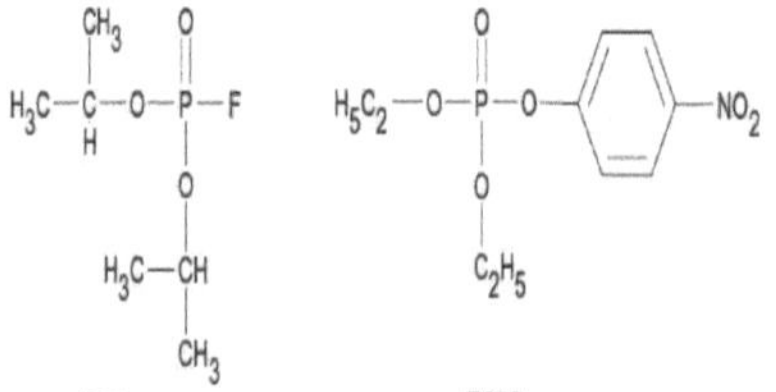

The chemical structures labeled **DFP** and **E600** appear at the top left.

A-Demonstration of non-specific esterases

1- α-naphthyl acetate:

This method depends upon the liberation of α-naphthyl from the α-naphthylacetate. The α-naphthyl then couples with fast blue RR to form an insoluble azo-dye. Davis and ornstein (1959) replaced fast blue RR by hexazotized pararosaniline which the later give better localization of enzyme.

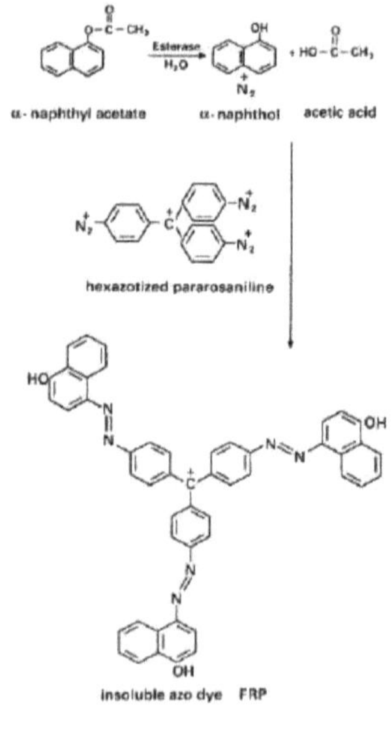

Non-specific esterase: a naphthyl acetate method (Gomori 1950, Davis & Ornstein 1959)

Fixation:
Formal calcium at 4°C. Formal vapour.
Sections:
Prefixed cryostat preferred.

Preparation of solutions:
a. Substrate solution

α-naphthyl acetate	50 mg
Acetone	5 ml

b. Buffer solution

Disodium hydrogen phosphate (Na_2HPO_4)	2.83 g
Distilled water	100 ml

c. Sodium nitrite solution

Sodium nitrite	400 mg
Distilled water	10 ml

d. Pararosanilin-HCl stock solution

Pararosanilin hydrochloride	2 g
2 M hydrochloric acid	50 ml

Heat gently, cool to room temperature and filter.

e. Distilled water

Preparation of incubating medium

Solution a.	0.25 ml
Solution b.	7.25 ml
Solution c.	0.4 ml
Solution d.	0.4 ml
Solution e.	2.5 ml

It is important that equal parts of solutions c and d are mixed together before adding to the incubation medium. Adjust pH to 7.4 if necessary with additional solution b.

Method:
1. After suitable fixation, bring sections to water.
2. Incubate at 37°C for 2-20 min.
3. Wash in running water.

4. Counterstain in 2 per cent methyl green (chloroform extracted).
5. Wash well in tap water.
6. Dehydrate rapidly through fresh alcohol to xylene and mount in DPX.
Results:

Esterase   reddish brown
Nuclei   green.

2- Indoxyl acetate:

It is based upon the liberation of the 5-bromoindoxyl from the hydrolysis of 5-bromoindoxyl acetate.

Which the latter oxidized by the ferri-ferrocyanide to blue product.

Non-specific esterase: indoxyl acetate method (Holt & Withers, 1952;

Fixation:
Formal calcium at 4°C. Formal vapour.

Sections:
Prefixed cryostat preferred.

Preparation of incubating medium:

5 bromo-4-chloro-indoxyl acetate	1 mg
Ethanol	0.1 ml
Tris buffer (0.2 M), pH 7.2	2 ml
Potassium ferricyanide	17 mg
Potassium ferrocyanide	21 mg
Calcium chloride	11 mg
Distilled water	7.9 ml

The 5-bromo-4-chloro-indoxyl acetate is dissolved in the ethanol and the buffer is then added. The remaining chemicals are dissolved in the distilled water and the solution is mixed. It is important that the solution is freshly prepared.

Method:
1. After suitable fixation, bring sections to water.
2. Incubate at 37°C for 15-60 min.
3. Rinse in tap water.
4. Counterstain in Mayer's carmalum for 5 min.
5. Rinse in tap water.
6. Mount in glycerin jelly or
7. Dehydrate through graded alcohols to xylene.
8. Mount in DPX.

Results:

Esterase activity   blue
Nuclei   red.

B- Demonstration of specific esterases

1- lipase
Tween method

The tween compounds are esters of long-chain fatty acids and its numbers indicate the type of fatty acid-20 (lauric), 40 (palmitic), 60 (stearic) and 80 (oleic).

The method is based upon the fact that enzyme hydrolysing the substrate (tween 60) to produce fatty acids which is trapped in situ as an insoluble calcium soaps by calcium ion. These are converted into lead soaps by lead ions and finally backed by ammonium sulphide.

Tween method (Gomori 1952)

Fixation:

Formal calcium at 4°C. Acetone at 4°C.

Sections:

Cryostat. Paraffin.

Preparation of solutions:

Solution a

Tris buffer, pH 7.2

Solution b

Tween 40, 60 or 80	5 g
Tris buffer, pH 7.2	100 ml
Thymol	1 crystal

Solution c

Calcium chloride	200 mg
Distilled water	10 ml

Solution d

Lead nitrate	1 g
Distilled water	50 ml

Preparation of incubating medium:

Solution a	9 ml
Solution b	0.6 ml
Solution c	0.3 ml

Method:

1. After suitable fixation, bring sections to water.

2. Incubate at 37°C for 2-8 hours. If paraffin sections, leave for 24 hours.

3. Rinse sections in three changes of distilled water.

4. Place sections in preheated lead nitrate solution (solution d) at 55°C for 10 min.

5. Rinse sections in distilled water for 2 min.

6. Wash in tap water for 10 min.

7. Place sections in 1 per cent ammonium sulfide for 3 min.

8. Rinse in distilled water.

9. Wash in tap water.

10. Counterstain in Mayer's carmalum for 5 min.

11. Wash in tap water for 1 min.

12. Mount in glycerin jelly.

Results:

Lipase activity	yellow to brown-black
Nuclei	red.

2- Acetyl cholinesterase

The basis for the method is that the acetyl thiocholine cation is hydrolysed by enzyme, and the liberated thiocholine cation (Kiernan 2015)

$$CH_3COS(CH_2)_2\overset{+}{N}(CH_3)_3 + H_2O \longrightarrow CH_3COOH + HS(CH_2)_2\overset{+}{N}(CH_3)_3$$

The latter combines with the copper ions to form the insoluble copper ferrocyanide (Kiernan 2015).

$$\left[Cu-S-\underset{H_2}{C}-\underset{H_2}{C}-\underset{\underset{CH_3}{|}}{\overset{\overset{CH_3}{|}}{N}}-CH_3 \right]^{+} \quad I^{-}$$

Acetyl cholinesterase (from Filipe & Lake 1983)

Preparation of tissue:

Cryostat sections of snap-frozen tissue cut at 10 ums are air-dried and fixed for 30 secs in 4 per cent formaldehyde in 0.1 M calcium acetate (formal calcium). Frozen sections of formal calcium-gum sucrose treated blocks of tissue.

Incubation medium:

Acetyl thiocholine iodide	5 mg
0.1 M acetate buffer pH 6.0	6.5 ml
0.1 M sodium citrate	0.5 ml
30 mmol/l copper sulphate	1 ml
Distilled water	1 ml
4 mmol/l iso-octamethyl pyro-phosphoramide (iso OMPA)	0.2 ml

Add 1.0 ml 5 mmol/l potassium ferricyanide just before use.

Method:

1. Rinse the fixed sections for 10 seconds in tap water.

2. Incubate at 37°C for 1 hour in the above medium.

3. Wash briefly in tap water.

4. Treat with 0.05 per cent p-phenylene diamine dihydrochoride in 0.05 M phosphate buffer pH 6.8 for 45 min at room temperature.

5. Wash in tap water.

6. Treat with 1 per cent osmium tetroxide for 10 min at room temperature.

7. Wash well in tap water, counterstain lightly (10 seconds) in Carrazzi hematoxylin (or Mayer's hemalum), wash, dehydrate, clear and mount in DPX.

Results:

Nerve fibers and cells containing acetyl cholinesterase are stained   dark brown to black.

Oxidases

Oxidases are type of the oxidoreductases that catalyse a reaction between the substrate and oxygen (i.e. they use oxygen as an acceptor thus bypassing all the intermediate components of the electron transport system (Kiernan 2015).

$$2 \begin{bmatrix} reduced \\ substrate \end{bmatrix} + O_2 \underset{(oxidase)}{\rightleftharpoons} 2H_2O + 2\begin{bmatrix} oxidized \\ substrate \end{bmatrix}$$

A number of these enzymes can be demonstrated histochemical like tyrosinase, monoamine oxidase and cytochrome oxidase.

1- Tyrosinase

This enzyme catalyses the oxidation of tyrosine to dihydrophenylalanine (DOPA) and then to melanin. Therefore, the sites of tyrosinase activity were considered to be sites of melanin formation.

Tyrosinase-DOPA reaction for frozen sections (Okun *et al.* 1969, Pearse 1972)

Fixation and sections:

Fresh frozen or formalin-fixed cryostat sections.

Preparation of solutions:

Control incubating solution 'A'

0.1 M phosphate buffer (pH 7.4)	10 ml

Test incubating solution 'B'

L-Tyrosine	2 mg
DL-DOPA	0.2 mg
0.1 M phosphate buffer (pH 7.4)	10 ml

Control incubating solution 'C

DL-DOPA	0.2 mg
0.1 M phosphate buffer (pH 7.4)	10 ml

Control incubating solution 'D'

L-Tyrosine	2 mg
DL-DOPA	0.2 mg

0.1 M phosphate buffer (pH 7.4) 10 ml, and add 1 mg sodium diethyldithiocarbamate.

Method:

1. Label four serial or near serial sections, 'A, B, Cand D'.

2. Place the sections in the appropriate solutions (i.e. slide A in solution A, etc.) for 3 hours at 37°C.

3. Rinse in phosphate buffer, pH 7.4, 2 min.

4. Wash in distilled water, 2 min.

5. Dehydrate through graded alcohols to xylene and mount in DPX.

Results:

Section A Pre-formed pigment only seen.

Section B Black pigments absent from other sections in melanin synthesis.

Section C Little induced pigment.

Section D No new pigment seen.

2- Monoamine oxidase

In this method, the enzyme oxidizes the tryptamine of the incubation solution and the primary reaction product reduces the tetrazolium salt (TNBT) to a black formazan compound.

Monoamine oxidase: tetrazolium method (Glenner *et al.* 1957)

Sections:

Unfixed cryostat.

Incubating solution:

Tryptamine hydrochloride	25 mg
Sodium sulfate	4 mg
Tetra nitro-blue tetrazolium (TNBT)	5 mg
0.1 M phosphate buffer, pH 7.6	5 ml
Distilled water	15 ml

Method:

1. Place sections in incubating medium at 37°C, 45 min.

2. Wash in running tap water, 2 min.

3. Place sections in 10 per cent formal-saline, 30 min.

4. Wash well in tap water, 2 min.

5. Mount in glycerin jelly.

Results:

Monoamine oxidase activity   bluish-black.

3-Cytochrome oxidase:

This method based upon the oxidative polymerization of 3,3'-diaminobenzidine (DAB) to an osmiophilic reaction product.

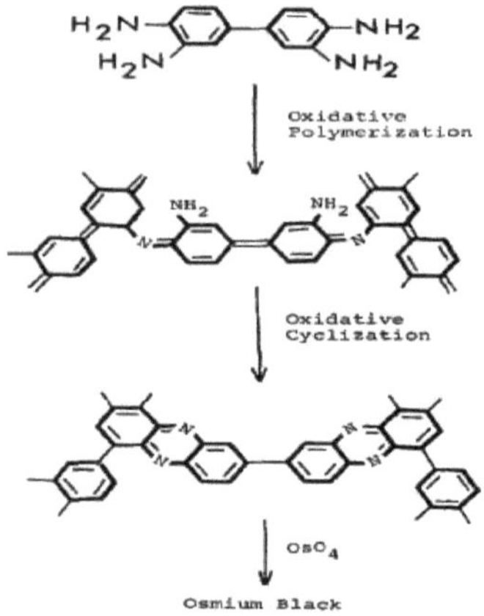

H_2N—   —NH_2

H_2N—   —NH_2

Oxidative Polymerization

NH_2 NH_2

Oxidative Cyclization

OsO_4

Osmium Black

Cytochrome oxidase (Seligman *et al.* 1968)

Tissue:

Cryostat sections (fresh).

Incubating solution:

Catalase (20 ug/ml) (4 mg in 10 ml, remove 2.5 ml and make up to 50 ml in distilled water).

	1 ml
Cytochrome c (type 2)	10 mg
0.1 M phosphate buffer pH 7.4	9 ml
3,3' diaminobenzidine tetrahydrochloride (DAB)	5 mg

Adjust pH to 7.4 before use with 0.1 M NaOH or 0.1 M HCI as required.

Method:

1. Incubate sections at room temperature for 2-3 hours.

2. Rinse in distilled water.

3. Fix in formal-calcium, 15 min.

4. Counterstain in hematoxylin, 15 seconds.

5. Wash and blue.

6. Dehydrate, clear and mount in DPX.

Results:

Brown reaction product at sites of cytochrome oxidase activity.

Dehydrogenases

Dehydrogeneses are a type of the oxidoredctases which remove hydrogen from a substrate and transfer it to a hydrogen receptor (Kiernan 2015).

$$\text{(S)}H_2 + \text{(A)} \rightleftharpoons \text{(S)} + \text{(A)}H_2$$

The released hydrogen is accepted by the coenzymes like nicotinamide adenine dinucleotide (NAD) or nicotinamide the adenine nucleotide phosphate (NADP) and sometimes by the dehydrogenase itself. Finally, the hydrogen accepted by tetrazolium salts like MTT, NBT and TNBT. When these salts receive the hydrogen, it reduced into a colored formazon compound.

Further reading:

Barka, T. (I960) A simple azo dye method for histochemical demonstration of acid phosphatase. Nature. 187:248.

Burstone, M.S. (1958) Histochemical demonstration of acid phosphatases with naphthol AS-phosphales. journal of National Cancer Institute, 21: 523.

Davis, B.J. & Ornstein. L. (1959) High resolution enzyme localisation with a new diazo reagent hexazonium pararosaniline. Journal of Histochemistry and Cytochemistry. 7: 297.

Filipe, M.I. & Lake, B.D. (eds.) (1983) Histochemistry in Pathology. Edinburgh: Churchill Livingstone.

Glenner, G.G., Burtner, H.J. & Brown, G.W. (1957) The histochemical demonstration of monoamine oxidase activity by tetrazolium salts. Journal of Histochemistry and Cytochemistry, 5: 591.

Gomori, G. (1950) An improved histochemical technique for acid phosphatase. Stain Technology, 25: 81.

Gomori, G. (1951) Alkaline phosphatase of cell nuclei. Journal of Laboratory and Clinical Medicine, 37: 526.

Gomori, G. (1952) Histochemistry of esterases. International Review of Cytology, 1: 323.

Holt, S.J. & Withers, R.F.J. (1952) Cytochemical localisation of esterases using indoxyl derivates. Nature, 170:1012.

Kiernan, J.A. (2015) Histological and Histochemical Methods: Theory and Practice. 5th edition, Scion Publishing

Okun, M.R., Edelstein, L.M., Or, N., Hamada, G., Donellan, B. & Lever, W.F. (1970) Histochemical differentiation of peroxidase-mediated from tyrosinase-mediated melanin formation in mammalian tissues. Histochemie, 23: 295.

Pearse, A.G.E. (1972) Histochemistry, Theoretical and Applied,3rd edn. Edinburgh: Churchill Livingstone, vol. 2.

Seligman. A.M. Karnovsky, M.J., Wasserkrug, H.L., Honker, J.S. (1968) Non-droplet ultrastructural demonstration of cytochrome oxidase activity with a polymerising osmiophilic reagent, DAB. Journal of Cell Biology, 38: 1.

Wachstein, M. &Meisel. E. (1956) On the histochemical demonstration of glucose-6-phosphate. Journal of Histochemistry and Cytochemistry, 4: 592.

Wachstein, M. & Meisel, E. (1957) Histochemistry of hepatic phosphatases at a physiological pH. American Journal of Pathology, 27: 13.

Immunohistochemistry (IHC) is a method that combines biochemical, histological and immunological techniques into a simple powerful assay to identify discrete tissue components by the interaction of target antigens with specific antibodies tagged with a visible label. IHC provides valuable information as it visualizes the distribution and localization of specific cellular components within cells and in proper tissue context. IHC detects antigens or haptens in cells of a tissue section by exploiting the principle of antibodies binding specifically to target antigens in biological tissues. The antibody-antigen binding can be visualized in different manners. Enzymes, such as Horseradish Peroxidase (HRP) or Alkaline Phosphatase (AP), are commonly used to catalyze a color-producing reaction. Immunocytochemistry can also be used in detection of organisms in cytological smear preparations such as fluids, sputum samples, and fine needle aspirates. These immunologic techniques make use of antigen antibody interactions, whereby the site of target antigen binding is demonstrated by direct labeling of the specific antibody, or by means of a secondary labeling method. There are numerous IHC methods that can be used to localize antigens. The method selected should include consideration of parameters such as the specimen types and assay sensitivity.

Definitions:

Antigen

A foreign substance presents in the body which stimulates the immune response, and provide a site to where antibodies bind. There are specific set of chemical components that evoke immunogenic response of the antigen which is known as epitope or antigenic determinant site.

Antibody (Immunoglobulin):

Naturally occurring protein in the human body, which acts to identify and remove infection and disease. Each immunoglobulin is composed of a pair of light chains and a pair of heavy chains polypeptides. The light chains of immunoglobulin are of two type, κ (kappa) and λ (lambda). There are five types of heavy chain, α (alpha), γ (gamma), δ (delta), ε (epsilon) and μ (mu), and depending on the nature of heavy chain, immunoglobulins are labelled as IgA, IgD, IgE, IgG, and IgM, respectively. In immunohistochemistry, antibodies are classified as:

Primary antibody:

This is the antibody that is used to detect a specific epitope in tissue.

Secondary antibody:

This is the antibody that is used to detect the primary antibody in tissue. It is typically labeled with a fluorescent probe for fluorescence microscopy or an enzyme that is used to lay down a chromogenic substrate for bright field microscopy.

Antibody Specificity:

The precise detection of specific epitope of the antigen by the antibody.

Antibody-antigen binding:

High degree of antibody-antigen specificity, like the lock and the key.

Avidity:

The overall functional strength of binding capacity of antibody and antigen complex. The avidity of an antibody depends on these factors:

- *Valency:* The more valency of the antibody, the greater is the avidity.
- *Affinity:* The affinity between the individual epitope of the antigen and the corresponding antigen-binding site of the antibody.
- *Structural arrangement:* Three-dimensional structural arrangement of antigen and antibody.

Sensitivity:
The relative amount of antigen that immunohistochemical methods are able to dectect.

Affinity:
The strength of interaction between an epitope and an antibody antigen binding site.

ANTIBODIES:

Monoclonal Antibodies:
Monoclonal antibodies are the product of an individual clone of plasma cells and a myeloma cell line from one animal and continued production of identical antibody by use of hybridoma culture. These antibodies are a homogeneous population and immunochemically identical, directed at a single epitope to which they are raised. Produced in mice or rabbits but for economy reasons, mice are used most frequently for the production of monoclonal antibodies. Monoclonal antibodies are identified by the target name and clone number and have certain advantages like high homogeneity, absence of nonspecific antibodies, ease of characterization and minimal batch-to-batch or lot-to-lot variability.

Polyclonal Antibodies:
Polyclonal antibodies are a heterogeneous mixture of antibodies reacts with many epitopes of the same antigen to which they are raised. It made in different species of large animals like rabbit, donkey, goat, sheep, and chicken so it immunochemically dissimilar. Multiple clones give high levels of labeling for a single antigen because they contain many antibodies to different epitopes on the same protein. There is a chance of batch-to-batch variation in case of polyclonal antibody.

Lectins:
Lectins are plant or animal proteins that can bind to tissue carbohydrates with a high degree of specificity according to the lectin and the carbohydrate group. They can be labeled in similar ways to antibodies, or identified by using lectin-specific antibodies as secondary reagents.

LABELS:

Labels are compounds, usually an enzyme such as peroxidase, attached to the final linking complex, which reacts to allow the visualization of a final reaction product at the site of antigen-antibody reaction. They are four labels of use in immunohistochemisty.

Enzymes:

Enzymes are the most widely used labels in immunohistochemistry, and incubation with a chromogen using a standard histochemical method produces a stable, colored reaction end-product suitable for the light microscope. The most commonly used enzymes in IHC are: horseradish peroxidase and alkaline phosphatase.

Horseradish peroxidase (HRP):
This enzyme (molecular weight 40 kD) is isolated from the root of the horseradish plant (Cochlearia armoracia). Horseradish peroxidase is commonly used as an antibody label for several reasons, includes:

- Its small size does not hinder the binding of antibodies to adjacent sites.
- The enzyme is easily obtainable in a highly purified form and therefore the chance of contamination is minimized.
- It is a stable enzyme and remains unchanged during manufacture, storage, and application.
- Endogenous activity is easily quenched.

It combines with many chromogens like 3,3 α-diaminobenzidene tetrahydrochloride (DAB), 3-amino-9-ethylcarbazole, 4-chloro-1-naphthol, Hanker-Yates reagent and α-naphthol pyronin. Endogenous peroxidase activity is present in a number of sites, particularly neutrophil poly-morphs and other myeloid cells. Blocking pro-cedures may be required, the hydrogen perox-ide-methanol method being the most popular.

Alkaline phosphatase (AP):

Alkaline phosphatase (molecular weight 100 kD) removes (by hydrolysis) and transfers phosphate groups from organic esters by break-ing the P-O bond; an intermediate enzyme-substrate bond is formed briefly. The chief met-al activators for AP are Mg++, Mn++ and Ca++. The enzyme used for IHC labeling is iso-lated from calf intestines. The advantages of using AP is that its substrate-converting reac-tion:

- Linear, which means that incubation with the chromogenic substrate may go longer. This will boost the sensitivity of antigen detection without the risk of over-staining of the tissue sections.
- Nonspecific staining in tissues with high levels of endogenous peroxidase, which limits the application of HRP conju-gates.

There are different AP chromogenic substrates, but those most frequently used are BCIP/NBT (Bromo-chloro-indolyl-phosphate plus Nitro blue tetrazolium), and Fast Red TR (4-chloro-2-methyl-benzenediazonium salt). Endogenous alkaline phosphatase activity is usually blocked by the addition of levamisole to the substrate solution. Levamisole selectively inhibits certain types of alkaline phosphatase, but not intestinal or placental, when used at a concentration of 1 mM. Twenty percent glacial acetic acid is a bet-ter blocker of endogenous alkaline phosphatase activity, as it inhibits all types of alkaline phos-phatase.

Glucose oxidase (GOD) which isolated from the fungus (Aspergillus niger) and Beta-D-galactosidase (Beta-Gal) which isolated from the bacterium (Escherichia coli) are two other enzymes used in IHC in place of HRP if tissues are known to have high endogenous peroxidase levels that may produce nonspecific staining when using HRP substrates.

Colloidal metal labels

Colloidal gold is a suspension (or colloid) of sub-micrometer-sized particles of gold in a flu-id, usually water. It consists of gold particles coated with a selected protein or macromole-cule, such as an antibody, and appears s pink when viewed using the light microscope. Silver may also be used as a conjugate, and it gives a yellow color that is visible directly.

Fluorescent labels

Fluorescence detection methods typically use a small chemical compound (fluorophore) that is excited about a specific invisible wavelength (ultraviolet) and emits light at a longer visible wavelength. The most important properties of fluorophores are: brightness, fading, stock shift and resistance to organic solvents. Currently, there are a lot of different fluorescent com-pounds, or fluorophores sold by numerous ven-dors for IHC applications. There are numerous fluorescent dyes belonging to different families, including but not limited to: Fluorescein (FITC), Rhodamine (TRITC, Rhodamine Red X), Cy® dyes (Cy2, Cy3, Cy5, CY7, etc.), Alexa Fluor® (350, 405, 488, 546, 610, etc.), DyLight® Fluor (DyLight 350, DyLight 488, DyLight 550, etc.) and Oyster® dyes (Oyster-488, Oyster-550, Oyster-645, Oyster-800, etc.). These types of labels are most used in immuno-fuorescene technique.

Radiolabels:

The use of radioisotopes requires autoradio-graphic facilities. And it is no popular as internally labeled antibodies are not widely available.

Fixation:

Fixation has a direct effect upon the preservation of immunoreactivity. The ideal fixative for immunohistochemistry studies should be:

- Give good morphology preservation.
- Not destroy the immunoreactivity of the antigen.
- Prevent extraction, diffusion and displacement of the antigen during the procedural steps following fixation.
- Not interfere with subsequent antigen-antibody reaction employed in the localization of the antigen.

Fixation is always a compromise, and the requirements of a fixative vary according to the different techniques employed in visualizing the structure of the cells or tissues.

Cytological preparations

Acetone-fixed smears or cytospins are often preferred by the immunocytochemist as acetone allows a wide range of primary antibodies to be employed without destroying the epitopes they are attempting to identify. Many cytology laboratories still insist on fixing cytological preparations in alcohol as opposed to acetone and consequently the number of antigens demonstrable is limited, although perhaps the morphology is superior.

Frozen sections

Acetone is preferred by most laboratories. Unfortunately, the preservation engendered by acetone is not complete and often show deleterious morphological changes, including chromatolysis and apparent loss of membranes. This can be partially prevented by ensuring that frozen sections are thoroughly dried both before and after fixation, and by improve acetone fixation to have included the addition of chloroform.

Paraffin sections

It is the most type of sections that are used for immunostaining. Most laboratories use formulae based on formalin such as un-buffered 10 per cent formal-saline or 10 per cent neutral buffered formalin, but some groups prefer picric acid fixation (Bouin's) or mercuric fixation (formal-mercury or B5).

Embedding

Most embedding procedures have little effect on the immunoreactivity of antigens in fixed tissues, and routine schedules for processing fixed specimens into paraffin wax are acceptable. Thin sections from tissues embedded in different types of plastics such as epoxy resin, araldite and methacrylate give excellent morphological details. It is necessary to remove the resin with sodium ethoxide and re-exposed the antigens by antigen retrieval before carry out IHC staining.

Sectioning

Paraffin section generally is cut at 5um or thinner. If lifting and subsequent detachment of the section is a problem, coating the slides with adhesive like Poly-L-lysine, egg albumin, chrome alum gelatin, low viscosity nitrocellulose and rubber solution. Following collection onto slides, the sections are dried overnight in an oven at 37^0 C. Routine dewaxing in xylene and rehydration through a descending alcohol series should be followed by a thorough wash in running water. Frozen sections should be cut at 6 ums, mounted on glass slides coated with one of adhesives outlined above and the air-dried at room temperature.

Section pre-treatment

Prior to immunohistochemical staining, it necessary for tissues to undergo one or more procedures that are aimed at unmasking antigen during fixation, eliminating the identification of endogenous peroxidase and reducing non-specific background staining.

Antigen retrieval

Formalin fixation blocks antigen sites by cross-linking proteins. Antigen retrieval reverses the obstructing effects caused by the cross-linking of formalin (Breaks Methylene bridges caused by hydrogen bonding by the formalin fixation). There are two common methods for antigen retrieval: Enzyme-Induced Antigen Retrieval and Heat-Induced Epitope Retrieval.

Enzyme-Induced Antigen Retrieval:

This group joins Pronase, Protease, Pepsin, Proteinase K and Trypsin. The theory behind the unmasking properties of these proteolytic enzymes is not fully understood. Nevertheless, it is generally accepted that breaking some peptide bonds will make holes in the matrix of cross-linked proteins, allowing the entry of antibody molecules (kiernan2005).

Trypsin

It is a serine protease from the PA clan superfamily, found in the digestive system of many vertebrates, where it hydrolyzes proteins. Trypsin predominantly cleaves proteins at the carboxyl side of the amino acids lysine and arginine, except when either is bound to a C-terminal proline. The process is commonly referred to as trypsin proteolysis or trypsinisation, and proteins that have been digested/treated with trypsin are said to have been trypsinized.

Chymotrypsin

Chymotrypsin is a digestive enzyme component of pancreatic juice acting in the duodenum, where it performs proteolysis, the breakdown of proteins and polypeptides. It synthesized in the pancreas by protein biosynthesis as a precursor called chymotrypsinogen that is enzymatically inactive. The main substrates of chymotrypsin are peptide bonds in which the amino acid N-terminal to the bond is a tryptophan, tyrosine, phenylalanine, or leucine.

Proteases

Proteases are enzymes that catalyze (increase the rate of) proteolysis, the breakdown of proteins into smaller polypeptides or single amino acids. Proteases are involved in digesting long protein chains into shorter fragments by splitting the peptide bonds that link amino acid residues. Some detach the terminal amino acids from the protein chain (exopeptidases, such as aminopeptidases, carboxypeptidase A), others attack internal peptide bonds of a protein (endopeptidases, such as trypsin, chymotrypsin, pepsin, papain, elastase).

The important factors that control enzyme-induced antigen retrieval:

- Concentration- Follow manufacturer's instructions for working concentration.
- Incubation time- Could be 1 to 60 minutes and 10-15 minutes is commonly used.
- Incubation temperature- Is usually at 37 °C.

Heat-Induced Epitope Retrieval:

The use of heat coupled with specific buffered solutions to recover antigens in formalin fixed paraffin embedded tissue has originated since the 1980s for commercial use. Citrate buffer 6.0 pH and EDTA buffer 9.0 pH are commonly used. The rationale behind the heat pretreatment methods is unclear, and four different theories have been suggested. One of these is that heavy metal salts like zinc sulphate, lead thiocyanate and aluminium chloride act as a protein precipitant, forming insoluble complexes with polypeptides, and that protein precipitating fixatives display better preservation of antigens than do cross-link aldehyde fixatives. Second theory is hydrolysis of intermolecular and methylene bridges and weak Schiff bases during formalin fixation by heat-mediated antigen retrieval hot, so the resulting protein conformation is intermediate between fixed and unfixed. A third theory is calcium coordination complexes formed during formalin fixation prevent antibodies from combining with epitopes on tissue-bound antigens. The underlying theory of calcium involvement is that hydroxymethyl groups and other unreacted oxygen-rich groups (e.g. carboxyl or phosphoryl groups) can interact with calcium ions to produce large coordinate complexes which can mask epitopic sites by steric hindrance. The high temperature weakens or breaks some calcium coordinate bonds, but the effect is reversible on cooling, because the calcium complex remains in its original position. A fourth theory is chaotropic effects of water molecules that occur in clusters of 280 molecules and can flip between an expanded and a collapsed structure. Chaotropic ions such as thiocyanate and urea provoke the change from an expanded to a collapsed state, possibly allowing fixed proteins in a tissue section to be made to resemble proteins in solution, with a concomitant increase in epitope visibility. The equipment includes microwave oven, pressure cooker, steamer, autoclave, water bath and the now widely used automated immunocytochemistry platforms with either on-board antigen retrieval technology or external antigen retrieval means. Most HIER devices consist of a primary metal or plastic chamber (into which secondary reagent containers are placed), surrounded by a reliable mechanism for heating the liquid in the secondary containers. The ideal HIER device should be:

a) Incorporates a precision-controlled heat source, capable of maintaining temperatures at or above 100°C.
b) Holds a reasonable volume of retrieval buffer and slides.
c) Minimizes the potential for evaporation and boiling of the HIER solution.

Among the various solutions, citrate buffer at pH 6.0, EDTA at pH 8.0, and Tris-EDTA (pH 9.9 or 10.0) are the most popular. There are three main variables to consider with Heat-Induced Antigen Retrieval:

1. Temperature of retrieval solution: should be around 95-100 °C.
2. Incubation time: varies. Commonly 10-90 minutes and pH value of retrieval solution: depending on which solution is used.

The advantages of heat-mediated antigen retrieval can be summarized as follows:

- Unlike proteolytic enzyme digestion, heating times to demonstrate antigens tend to be uniform, regardless of duration of fixation.
- The intensity of staining and the proportion of cells staining are increased.
- Antigens that are not normally demonstrable in paraffin-embedded tissue can be demonstrated.
- Consistent, reliable, high-quality immunostaining of formalin-sensitive tissue antigens can be produced.

Blocking endogenous enzymes

Endogenous enzymes pose a threat when using enzymatic chromogenic detection protocols: if endogenous enzymes are not blocked they can convert chromogenic substrate solutions into colored precipitates, which is similar to effects produced by exogenously added enzyme conjugates. For practical purposes in immunohistochemistry, both endogenous peroxidase activity and pseudoperoxidase activity can be considered the same. Peroxidase activity results in the decomposition of H_2O_2 and is a common property of all hemoproteins such as hemoglobin (red cells), myoglobin (muscle cells), cytochrome (granulocytes, monocytes) and catalases (liver and kidney).

Various methods have been described for the destruction of peroxidase activity. The most frequently used method is pre-incubation of the sections in absolute methanol containing hydrogen peroxide. Incubation in absolute methanol containing 0.5% hydrogen peroxide for 10 minutes at room temperature has been reported to produce an almost complete abolition of endogenous peroxidase activity, without affecting the immunoreactivity of antigens. There are many types of alkaline phosphatase within the human body like intestine, kidney, osteoblasts, endothelial cell surfaces, neutrophis, stromal reticulum cells, lymphoid tissues, and placenta. And most endogenous alkaline phosphatase activity can be blocked using a 1 mM concentration of levamisole in the final incubating medium. The alkaline phosphatase used in the labeling system is usually intestinal in nature and remains unaffected by levamisole at the recommended concentration.

Blocking background staining

Background staining is probably the most common problem in immunohistochemistry. Specific binding of antibodies to epitopes on tissue antigens occurs via hydrophobic interactions, ionic interactions, and hydrogen bonding. However, the same mechanisms also underlie the nonspecific binding of primary antibodies to irrelevant tissue proteins that result in nonspecific background staining, which is a common problem in IHC experiments. In aqueous media, hydrophobic interactions between macromolecules occur when their surface tensions are lower than that of water. The mutual attractions resulting from this are called van der Waals forces. They can be interatomic as well as intermolecular, and originate through the fluctuating dipolar structure within these macromolecules. Hydrophobic bonding can be minimized by the addition of a blocking protein, by the addition of a detergent such as Triton X, or the addition of a high salt concentration, 2.5% NaCl, to the buffer. Some workers advocate the addition of the blocking serum to the diluted primary antibody. Ionic interactions are produced by non-immunologically attraction of the primary antibody to highly charged groups present on connective tissue elements. Therefore, the subsequent labeling antibodies will be attracted not only to primary antibodies located on the specific antigen but also to the antibody bound to the connective tissue elements. The most effective way of minimizing non-specific staining is to add an innocuous protein solution to the section before applying the primary antibody. The added protein should saturate and neutralize the charged sites, thus enabling the primary antibody to bind to the antigenic site only.

Control

In any IHC staining, it is extremely essential to have proper control because it validates the laboratory test. The control slides indicate the specificity of the test because it is essential to know that the antibody is reacted specifically to the specific epitope of the particular antigen and not with the other antigen. Without their use, interpretation of staining would be hazard and the results of doubtful value. More specifically, controls determine if the staining protocols were followed correctly, whether day-to-day and worker-to-worker variations have occurred, and that reagents remain in good working order. Furthermore, all procedures designed for in vitro diagnostic use must be monitored by reagent and tissue controls.

Negative Control

For negative control, the primary antibody is omitted, or the specific primary antibody replaced by an immunoglobulin which is directed against an unrelated antigen. In the absence of primary antibody, no staining reaction should occur.

Positive Control

The known tissue section with the presence of antigen is used for positive control such as desmin stain wherein one can take uterine myometrial tissue as positive control and normal reactive lymphocytes when staining with an antibody to the leucocyte common antigen to identify a suspected lymphoma.

Immunohistochemical Methods

Many immunohistochemical staining techniques that may be used to localize and demonstrate tissue antigens.

Traditional direct technique

It is the first method for immunohistochemistry in which the labeled primary antibody reacts directly with the tissue antigen. The antibody should be specific for the particular antigen; otherwise non-specific staining may occur. Today, direct immunocytochemistry is not the method of choice

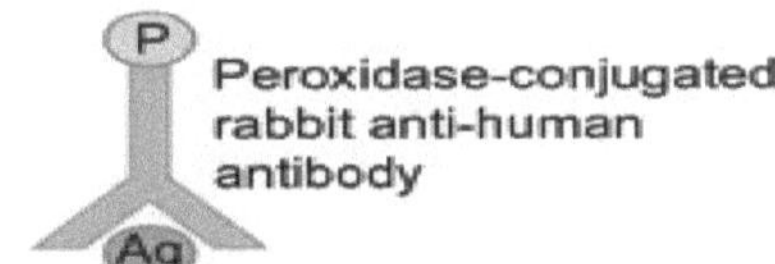

Two-step indirect technique

Firstly, the unlabeled primary antibody acts on antigen, then the labeled secondary antibody is directed against the primary antibody. The secondary antibody is generated by injecting purified IgG from one species of animals as the antigen. It advantages from direct technique by:
1. A single conjugated secondary antibody can be used against different primary antibodies.
2. Higher dilution of primary antibody can be used.
3. Large amount of secondary antibody can be easily produced against the primary antibody.
4. For negative control, the primary antibody can be omitted.

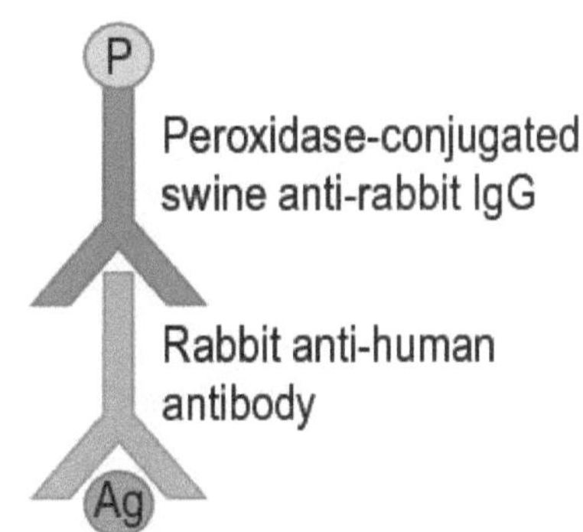

Polymer chain two-step indirect technique

This method uses an unconjugated primary antibody, followed by a secondary antibody conjugated to an enzyme horseradish peroxidase labeled polymer (dextran) chain.

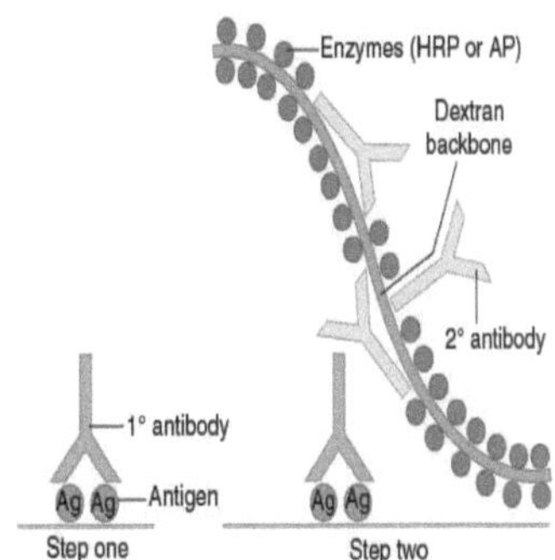

Unlabeled antibody-enzyme complex techniques (PAP and APAAP)

Here, apart from primary antibody and secondary antibody link with complex from peroxidase-anti-peroxidase (PAP) or alkaline phosphatase- anti-alkaline phosphatase (APAAP). It advantages by high degree of sensitivity: peroxidase-antiperoxidase method is 1000 times more sensitive than the indirect conjugated method.

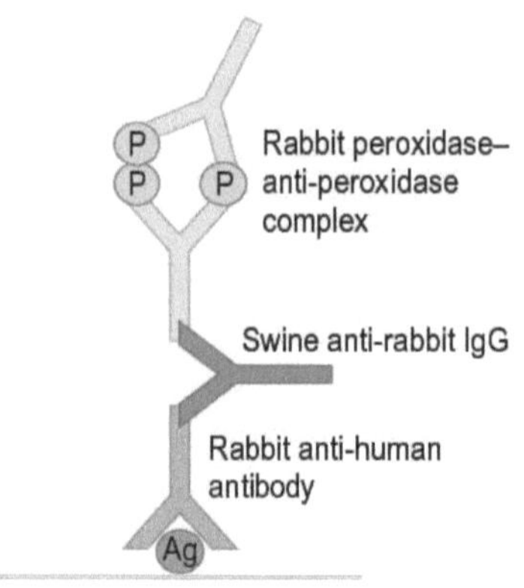

Immunogold silver staining technique (IGSS)

In this method the gold particles are enhanced by the addition of metallic silver layers to produce a metallic silver precipitate which overlays the colloidal gold marker and which can be seen with the light microscope.

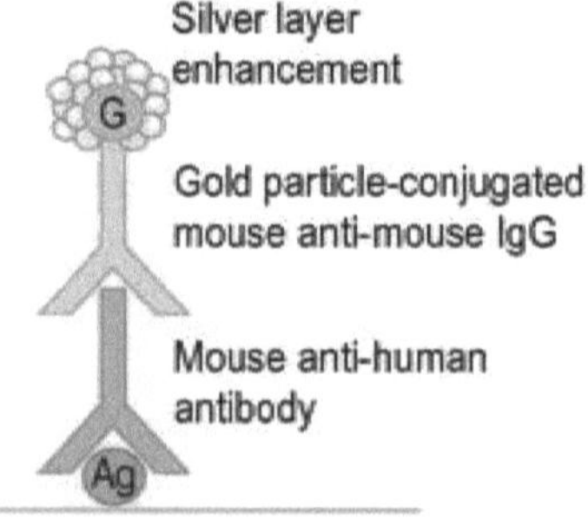

(Strept) avidin-biotin techniques

In this technique, a polymer backbone is used. This may be dextran, polypeptide or dendrimer polymer. The dextran polymer is often used as a polymer backbone. The large number of enzyme molecules (at least 100 peroxidase) and more than 20 secondary antibodies are conjugated within this dextran polymer. This is a three-step method, which has an unconjugated primary antibody as the first layer, followed by a biotinylated secondary antibody. The third layer is either a complex of enzyme-labeled biotin and streptavidin, or enzyme-labeled streptavidin. Biotin is a very small (244 Da) molecule, also known as vitamin B7, that binds avidin with extremely high affinity. Each biotin has just one avidin-binding domain. Streptavidin can be isolated from the bacterium Streptomyces avidini, and like avidin it has four high affinity binding sites for biotin.

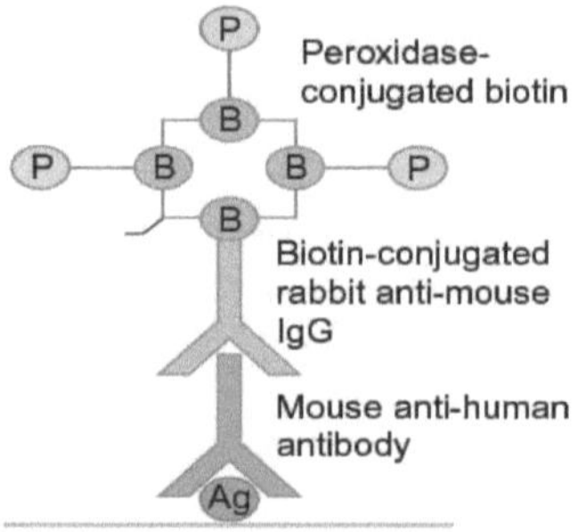

Biotinylated tyramide signal amplification

Tyramide signal amplification (TSA) is a powerful amplification method that allows fluorescent labeling to be significantly amplified. The technique is based around the streptavidin-biotin technique. The primary antibody is followed by subsequent incubations in biotinylated secondary antibody and then either horseradish peroxidase-labeled streptavidin or streptavidin-biotin-horseradish peroxidase complex. Biotinylated tyramine is used in the presence of HRP and hydrogen peroxide. The HRP converts the biotinylated tyramine to reactive biotinylated tyramide. This activated biotinylated tyramide further reacts with tyrosine in the amino acid of the tissue and deposits biotin. This biotin is deposited only in the antigen-antibody reaction site. This biotin is visualized by avidin-biotin technique.

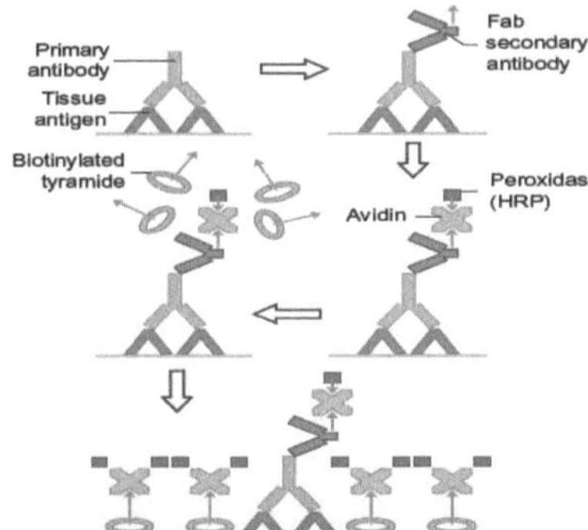

Biotin-free Catalyzed Signal Amplification (CSA II)

Following incubation in the primary antibody, a secondary anti-mouse immunoglobulin conjugated to horseradish peroxidase is bound to the primary antibody. The third layer involves peroxidase-catalyzed deposition of fluorescyl tyramide, which in turn is reacted with peroxidase conjugated anti-fluorescein, producing a greatly enhanced signal.

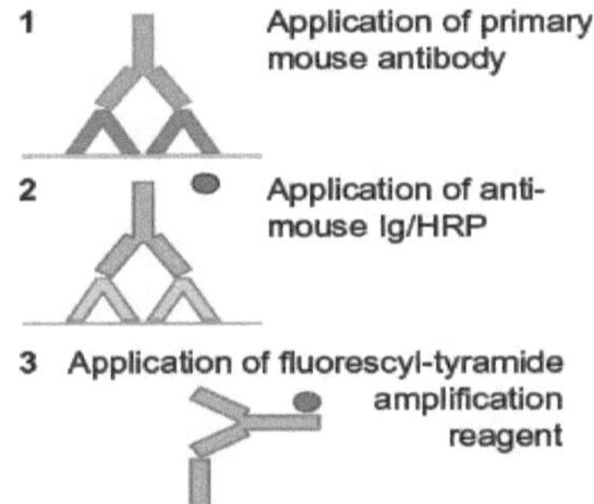

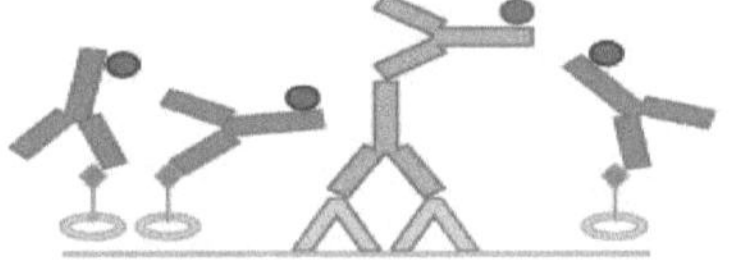

Cytology preparations

Smears, imprints, cytospins, etc., should be air dried for 1–3 hours and then fixed or stored as outlined for frozen sections.

Frozen sections

1. Cut 6 μm frozen sections and place on Superfrost Plus microscope slides or adhesive coated slides.

2. Air dries the sections at room temperature overnight (in urgent cases dry for a minimum of 1–2 hours).

3. Fix sections in absolute acetone at room temperature for 20 minutes. Allow sections to air dry. If required, the sections may be stored at this stage at −20°C or lower. Prior to storage, the slides should be wrapped in foil and then placed in the freezer with a desiccant. When required, the sections should be allowed to return to room temperature before unwrapping.

4. Rehydrate in TBS, apply optimally diluted primary antibody. Antibodies should be diluted in TBS; avoid the use of commercial antibody diluents or the use of detergents such as Triton or Tween. Chromatolysis and loss of nuclear membranes on frozen sections is compounded by the action of detergents.

5. For frozen sections an endogenous peroxidase blocking step is not included, as this can be damaging to the antigens to be demonstrated. The use of a negative control for the identification of endogenous peroxidase activity is preferable. If the endogenous peroxidase activity is excessive, then an alternative enzyme tracer, such as alkaline phosphatase, should be considered.

Paraffin sections

1. Cut 3–4 μm sections and place on clean electrostatically charged glass slides (we recommend Superfrost Plus slides). If using uncharged slides an adhesive should be used. Commercial products such as APES or Vecta-

bond are successful in assisting with section adhesion.

2. Dry the sections overnight in a 37°C incubator. Alternatively, the sections may be placed on a hot plate at 60°C for 15 minutes. Certain antigens, such as estrogen and progesterone receptors, show a reduction in staining when heated on a hot plate and therefore this is not recommended.

3. Where possible, sections should be cut fresh. Sections stored for several weeks prior to immunostaining may show reduced staining intensity. This is the case with estrogen and progesterone receptors.

4. Dewax sections in xylene and bring to absolute alcohol. Xylene substitutes such as Histoclear may be used. To ensure complete removal of wax the xylene/Histoclear may be warmed to 37°C in an incubator.

5. If required, remove fixation pigments.

6. Block endogenous peroxidase activityby incubating in 0.5% hydrogen peroxide in methanol for 10 minutes. This stage may be performed after the primary antibody has been bound onto the antigenic site. It is thought by many users that the methanol/hydrogen peroxide step may slightly alter some of the more labile antigenic epitopes, leading to weak demonstration. We have certainly found this to be the case with the demonstration of CD2 and CD4 in paraffin sections.

7. Rehydrate, wash well in running water.

8. Perform the required/preferred antigen retrieval techniques as detailed below.

Trypsin/chymotrypsin Method

1. Incubate sections in distilled water at 37°C.

2. Prepare 0.1% trypsin in 0.1% calcium chloride in distilled water at 37°C. Adjust pH to 7.8 using 0.1 M sodium hydroxide solution.

3. Incubate the sections in the trypsin solution for 10 minutes at 37°C.

4. Wash sections in cold running tap water to prevent further digestion.

5. Proceed with the immunostaining method of choice.

Protease Method

1. Incubate sections in pre-warmed distilled water at 37°C.

2. Prepare 0.1% protease (Sigma type XXIV, P-8038) in distilled water (at 37°C). Adjust pH to 7.8 using 1 M sodium hydroxide solution.

3. Incubate the sections in the protease solution for 6 minutes at 37°C.

4. Wash sections in cold running tap water to prevent further digestion.

5. Proceed with the immunostaining method of choice.

Pepsin Method

1. Incubate sections in pre-warmed distilled water at 37°C.

2. Prepare 0.4% pepsin solution in 0.01 M hydrochloric acid, pH 2.0, at 37°C.

3. Incubate the sections in the pepsin solution for 15–60 minutes at 37°C.

4. Wash sections in cold running tap water to prevent further digestion.

5. Proceed with the immunostaining method of choice.

Heat-mediated antigen retrieval fluids

Citrate buffer

Citric acid (anhydrous)	21 g
Distilled water	10 liters

Adjust pH to 6.0 using 2 M sodium hydroxide.

Tris-EDTA

Tris	14.4 g
EDTA	1.44 g
1 M hydrochloric acid	1 ml
Tween 20	0.3 ml
Distilled water	600 ml

Add the Tris, EDTA, and acid to the distilled water and adjust pH to 10 with hydrochloric acid, then add the Tween.

Microwave oven heating methodology

1. Using a plastic staining rack, place up to 25 sections in 600 ml of 0.01 M citrate buffer, pH 6.0.

2. Irradiate at a power of 800 W for 22 minutes.

3. Carefully remove the container from the microwave oven and flood with cold water.

4. Proceed with the immunostaining method of choice.

Pressure cooker antigen retrieval methodology

1. Add 1.5 L of appropriate antigen retrieval buffer into the pressure cooker and bring to the boil (without securing the lid).

2. When the antigen retrieval buffer is boiling, carefully place the slide racks into the hot solution and seal the lid.

3. Allow the pressure cooker to reach full pressure 10.3 kPa (15 psi), incubate for 2 minutes (timing starts only when full pressure is reached).

4. Transfer the pressure cooker to a sink and run cold water over the lid until all of the pressure is released.

5. Flood the pressure cooker with cold water. Do not remove the slides until cool.

6. Proceed with the immunostaining method of choice.

Steamer antigen retrieval methodology

1.Place 1 liter of distilled water into the base of the steamer and insert a dry tray into the base.

2.Place steaming tray onto the dry tray.

3.Place the rice bowl into the steaming chamber.

4.Fill the incubation tray with 200 ml of appropriate antigen retrieval buffer and place in the chamber.

5. Place the lid onto the top of the steaming chamber.

6.Set the timer for 1 hour 15 minutes. The equilibration of the bath/rice chamber contents to 95°C is achieved after around 45 minutes.

7.Remove the lid and place the slides in the heated antigen retrieval buffer; replace the lid.

8.Incubate sections for 30 minutes.

9. Remove the antigen retrieval buffer from the chamber and allow the sections to cool for 15 minutes.

10.Wash sections in water.

11.Proceed with the immunostaining method of choice.

Water bath antigen retrieval methodology

1. Place the appropriate antigen retrieval buffer in a plastic Coplin jar.

2. Place the Coplin jar into the water bath and heat to 95–98°C, without boiling.

3. Place slides into the preheated buffer and incubate for 30 minutes.

4. Remove the container from the water bath and allow cooling for 15 minutes at room temperature.

5. Wash sections in water.

6. Proceed with the immunostaining method of choice.

Autoclave antigen retrieval methodology

1. Add 250 ml of appropriate antigen retrieval buffer into the incubation chamber; place in the sections.

2. Place a lid over the incubation chamber to avoid excess evaporation.

3. Place the incubation chamber into the autoclave and close the lid.

4. Set the time for 15 minutes at 120°C.

5. Release the pressure, remove the incubation chamber, and flood with cold water.

6. Proceed with the immunostaining method of choice.

Immunohistochemical staining Techniques

The practical aspects of immunohistochemical staining are simple and straightforward, as the techniques entail only sequential incubations in antibodies and labeling systems separated by washes in buffer.

Washes

Between each step, sections require washing to prevent one reagent contaminating another. 'Gently wash with Tris Buffered Saline (TBS)' indicates several brief washes flooding the slide, followed by draining and wiping around the section to remove excess buffer.

Buffer Solutions

0.5 M Tris-buffered saline

Distilled water	10 liters
Sodium chloride	85 g
Tris (hydroxymethyl) aminomethane	60.5 g

Adjust pH to 7.6 with 50% hydrochloric acid.

Tris-buffered saline containing bovine serum albumin (BSA-TBS)

Tris (hydroxymethyl) aminomethane	12.14 g
Sodium chloride	45 g
Bovine serum albumin	5 g
Sodium azide	6.5 g
Distilled water	5 liters

Adjust final pH to 8.2 with 1 M hydrochloric acid.

Veronal acetate buffer

Sodium acetate trihydrate	0.972 g
Sodium barbitone	1.472 g
Distilled water	250 ml
0.1 M hydrochloric acid	2.5 ml

Incubation

To prevent evaporation of antibodies, incubations must be carried out manual or automated.

Manual

By placing the slides on Perspex strips which run the length of a lidded staining trough, in the bottom of which is a pool of water or a layer of moist tissue paper.

Automated

There are two types of reagent delivery system. Capillary action is used by the Shandon sequenza, Shandon Cadenza and Ventana TechMate (supplied by Dako & Ventana in Europe). And by spraying delivery is used by the Dako Autostainer, LabVision Instrument, Leica HistoStainer, Ventana, Nexes and BioGenex Optimax.

Methods

After the appropriate pre-treatment steps, the following methods can be employed.

Traditional Direct method

1. Bring sections to TBS, drain off, and incubate in non-immune serum.
2. Drain off and wipe around section.
3. Incubate in optimally diluted peroxidase-labeled primary antibody for 1-15 hours in ambient temperature or 4° C.
4. Gently wash in TBS.
5. Incubate in freshly prepared DAB solution.
6. Rinse in TBS and wash in running water.
7. Counterstain in hematoxylin, dehydrate clear and mount.

Indirect technique for monoclonal primary antibodies Method

1. Bring sections to TBS.
2. Drain off slide; wipe off excess moisture around the section.
3. Apply optimally diluted primary monoclonal antibody, 30-60 min.
4. Gently wash slides with TBS.
5. Cover with an optimally diluted peroxidase-conjugated rabbit anti-mouse containing a 1/25 dilution of normal human serum.
6. Gently wash slides with TBS.
7. Incubate in freshly prepared DAB solution for 10 min.
8. Rinse in TBS and transfer to running water.
9. Counterstain in hematoxylin, dehydrate, clear and mount.

Dako EnVision detection technique Method

1. Rinse sections in TBS, then incubate in 10% casein solution for 10 minutes.
2. Drain off excess casein.
3. Apply optimally diluted primary monoclonal antibody for 60 minutes.
4. Wash slides in TBS.
5. Incubate with EnVision polymer reagent for 30 minutes.
6. Wash slides in TBS.
7. Incubate in freshly prepared DAB solution for 10 minutes.
8. Rinse in TBS and transfer to running water.
9. Counterstain in hematoxylin, dehydrate, clear and mount.

Novolink polymer detection technique Method

1. Following antigen retrieval, rinse sections in TBS.
2. Drain off excess TBS and block endogenous peroxidase activity using peroxidase block for 5 minutes.
3. Wash in TBS for 5 minutes.
4. Incubate with protein block for 5 minutes.
5. Wash in TBS.
6. Apply optimally diluted primary antibody for 60 minutes.
7. Wash slides in TBS.
8. Incubate with post primary block for 30 minutes.
9. Wash slides in TBS.
10. Incubate with Novolink polymer for 30 minutes.
11. Wash slides in TBS.
12. Incubate in freshly prepared DAB solution for 10 minutes.
13. Rinse in TBS and transfer to running water.
14. Counterstain in hematoxylin, dehydrate, clear and mount.

Peroxidase-antiperoxidase (PAP) technique Method

1. Bring sections to TBS.
2. Drain off and wipe around section.
3. Incubate in optimally diluted primary antibody for 30-60 min.
4. Gently wash in TBS.
5. Incubate in optimally diluted rabbit anti-mouse antibody for 30 min.
6. Repeat step 4.
7. Incubate in optimally diluted mouse peroxidase anti-peroxidase for 30 min.
8. Repeat step 4.
9. Incubate in freshly prepared DAB solution.
10. Rinse in TBS and wash in running water.
11. Counterstain in hematoxylin, dehydrate clear and mount.

Alkaline phosphatase-anti-alkaline phosphatase (APAAP) for monoclonal antibodies Method

1. Rinse sections in TBS.
2. Drain off excess TBS and incubate in 10% casein for 10 minutes.
3. Incubate in primary antibody at optimal dilution for 30–40 minutes.
4. Wash in TBS.
5. Incubate in optimally diluted unconjugated rabbit anti-mouse bridge antibody for 30 minutes.
6. Wash in TBS.
7. Incubate in APAAP complex at the optimal dilution for 30 minutes.
8. Wash in TBS.
9. Incubate in substrate medium of choice, e.g. fast red solution.
10. Wash in running tap water.
11. Counterstain and mount as desired.

Indirect immunogold technique for monoclonal antibodies Method

1. Take sections to distilled water.
2. Treat sections with Lugol's iodine for 5 minutes, clear with 2.5% sodium thiosulfate, and then wash well in running tap water.
3. Take sections to BSA–TBS (0.1% bovine serum albumin in TBS, pH 8.2), drain and wipe off excess around section.
4. Incubate in 1/20 normal goat serum (NGS) in BSA-TBS for 10 minutes.
5. Drain, wipe off excess serum.
6. Incubate in primary antibody optimally diluted in BSA-TBS for 30–60 minutes.
7. Gently wash in TBS.
8. Incubate in gold-conjugated secondary antibody at optimal dilution in BSA-TBS for 60 minutes.
9. Repeat step 7.
10. Wash in 0.1 M phosphatase buffered saline (PBS), pH 7.6, for three 2-minute changes.
11. Post-fix with 2% glutaraldehyde in PBS for 10–15 minutes.
12. Wash well in several changes of distilled water and enhance staining with silver. (See silver enhancement procedure below.)
13. Counterstain, dehydrate, clear, and mount.

Silver enhancement

The intensity of the gold label may be enhanced by incubation of the sections in a silver solution.

Solutions:

a. Citrate buffer stock solution

Trisodium citrate   23.5 g
Citric acid   25.5 g
Distilled water   100 ml

b. Silver solution

Silver lactate   110 mg
Distilled water   15 ml
Prepare fresh.

c. Hydroquinone solution

Hydroquinone   950 mg
Distilled water   15 ml
Prepare fresh.

d. Gum acacia

50% gum acacia solution   7 ml

e. Silver enhancement solution

Silver lactate solution   15 ml
Hydroquinone solution   15 ml
Molar citrate buffer   10 ml
Distilled water   60 ml
50% gum acacia solution   7 ml

Method:

1. Rinse the sections in 0.2 M citrate buffer for 2 minutes.
2. Incubate the sections in freshly prepared silver enhancement solution at room temperature, protected from the light. Development will take place in approximately 5 minutes.
3. Wash well in distilled water.
4. Wash in 2% sodium thiosulfate, 1 minute.
5. Wash well in running water.
6. Counterstain if desired.
7. Dehydrate, clear, and mount.

Labeled streptavidin-biotin complex technique for monoclonal antibodies Method

1. Rinse sections in TBS, then incubate in 10% casein solution for 10 minutes.
2. Drain off excess casein.
3. Incubate in optimally diluted primary antibody for 60 minutes.
4. Wash slides in TBS.
5. Incubate in optimally diluted biotinylated secondary antibody for 30 minutes.
6. Wash slides in TBS.
7. Incubate in optimally prepared labeled streptavidin or streptavidin-biotin complex for 30 minutes. When using a streptavidin-biotin complex the reagents should be mixed 30 minutes before use in order for the complex to form.
8. Wash slides in TBS.
9. Incubate in DAB substrate solution.

10. Wash in running water, counterstain in hematoxylin, dehydrate, clear and mount.

Tyramide signal amplification of the labeled streptavidin-biotin method

1. Rinse sections in TBS, then incubate in 10% casein solution for 10 minutes.
2. Drain off excess casein.
3. Incubate in optimally diluted primary antibody for 60 minutes.
4. Wash slides in TBS.
5. Incubate in biotinylated secondary antibody for 20 minutes.
6. Wash slides in TBS.
7. Incubate in labeled streptavidin (or streptavidin biotin complex) for 20 minutes.
8. Wash slides in TBS.
9. Incubate slides in biotinylated tyramide reagent for 5 minutes.
10. Wash in TBS.
11. Re-incubate sections in labeled streptavidin (or streptavidin-biotin complex) for 20 minutes.
12. Wash slides in TBS.
13. Incubate in DAB substrate solution.
14. Wash in running water, counterstain in hematoxylin, dehydrate, clear, and mount.

Dako CSAII detection method

1. Rinse sections in TBS, then incubate in 10% casein solution for 10 minutes.
2. Drain off excess casein.
3. Incubate in optimally diluted primary antibody for 15–60 minutes.
4. Wash slides in TBS.
5. Apply anti-mouse immunoglobulins-HRP reagent for 15 minutes.
6. Wash slides in TBS.
7. Incubate in amplification reagent for 15 minutes.
N.B. This incubation should be undertaken in the dark.
8. Wash slides in TBS.

9. Apply anti-fluorescein-HRP for 15 minutes.
10. Wash slides in TBS.
11. Incubate in DAB substrate solution.
12. Wash in running water, counterstain in hematoxylin, dehydrate, clear, and mount.

Visualization substrate solutions

It divides into two groups according to the type of enzyme:

Visualization substrates for peroxidase methods

The peroxidase activity in the presence of an electron donor is first results in the formation of an enzyme-substrate complex, and then in the oxidation of the electron donor. The electron donor provides the "driving" force in the continuing catalysis of H_2O_2, while its absence effectively stops the reaction. The most popular are 3.3'-diaminobenzidine tetrahydrochloride (DAB) and 3-amino-9-ethylcarbazole (AEC).

3,3'-DIAMINOBENZIDINE (DAB)

It produces a brown end product which is highly insoluble in alcohol and other organic solvents. Oxidation of DAB also causes polymerization, resulting in the ability to react with osmium tetroxide, and thus increasing its staining intensity and electron density. Of the several metals and methods used to intensify the optical density of polymerized DAB, gold chloride in combination with silver sulfide appears to be the most successful.

3-AMINO-9-ETHYLCARBAZOLE (AEC)

Upon oxidation, it forms a rose-red end product which is alcohol soluble. Therefore, specimens processed with AEC must not be immersed in alcohol or alcoholic solutions (e.g., Harris' hematoxylin). Instead, an aqueous counterstain and mounting medium should be used. AEC is unfortunately susceptible to further oxidation and, when exposed to excessive light, will fade in intensity. Storage in the dark is therefore recommended.

Dab method

Solutions:
Tris-HCl buffer is recommended for DAB

0.2 M Tris (containing 24.228 g/l)	12 ml
0.1 M HCI	19 ml
Distilled water	19 ml

DAB solution

DAB	5 mg
Tris-HCl buffer (pH 7.6)	10 ml
H_2O_2 (freshly prepared and added just before use)	0.1 ml

This solution should be used immediately after preparation. The sections are incubated at room temperature until a dark brown reaction product is obtained, usually after 5-10 min. The reaction end-product resists alcohol dehydration and clearing in xylene.

3-Amino-9-ethylcarbazole (AEC)

1. Dissolve 10 mg 3-amino-9-ethylcarbazole in 6 ml dimethyl sulfoxide, and then add 50 ml 0.02 M acetate buffer, pH 5.0-5.2.
2. Add 0.4 ml 0.3 per cent hydrogen peroxide and use immediately.
3. Rinse the sections in 0.02 M acetate buffer, pH 5.0, filter the substrate solution onto the sections and incubate for 5-10 min. at room temperature. As the red reaction end-product is soluble in alcohol and xylene, the sections must be mounted in aqueous mounting medium.

Visualization substrates for alkaline phosphatase methods

In the alkaline phosphatase staining method, the enzyme hydrolyzes naphthol phosphate esters (substrate) to phenolic compounds and phosphates. The phenols couple to colorless diazonium salts (chromogen) to produce insoluble, colored azo dyes. Several combinations of substrates and chromogens have been used successfully like fast red TR, hexazotized new fuchsin and nitro blue tetrazolium.

Naphthol AS-MX Phosphate

This can be used in its acid form or as the sodium salt. The chromogens Fast Red TR and Fast Blue BB produce a bright red or blue end product, respectively. Both are soluble in alcoholic and other organic solvents, so aqueous mounting media must be used. Fast Red TR is preferred when staining cell smears.

New Fuchsin

This also gives a red end product. Unlike Fast Red TR and Fast Blue BB, the color produced by New Fuchsin is insoluble in alcohol and other organic solvents, allowing for the specimens to be dehydrated before coverslipping. The staining intensity obtained by use of New Fuchsin is greater than that obtained with Fast Red TR or Fast Blue BB.

Fast red TR solution

Naphthol-AS-MX phosphate, free acid	4.0 mg
N, N-dimethyl formamide	0.2 ml
1 M Tris-HCl buffer, pH 8.2	9.8 ml
Levamisol	2.4 mg
Fast red TR salt	10 mg.

Dissolve the naphthol-AS-MX phosphate in *N, N*-dimethyl formamide in a glass vial and then add the Tris buffer. Add and dissolve the levamisole and fast red TR salt and immediately filter onto the sections. Incubate the sections for 10–20 minutes and, as the bright red reaction product is soluble in alcohol, mount in an aqueous medium. A blue reaction product can be obtained by using 4 mg fast blue BB instead of fast red TR salt in the above recipe. Counterstaining with hematoxylin would not be appropriate with blue salt.

Hexazotized new fuchsin

Naphthol-AS-BI phosphate	5.0 mg
N, N-dimethyl formamide	60 µl

1 M Tris-HCl buffer, pH 8.7	10 ml
1 M levamisole	10 µl
4% sodium nitrite (freshly prepared)	50 µl
5% new fuchsin in 2 M HCl	20 µl

Add the new fuchsin to the sodium nitrite, mix for 30–60 seconds and then add the Tris buffer and levamisole. Immediately before staining, add the naphthol AS-BI phosphate, dissolved in the *N, N-dimethyl* formamide, and filter directly onto the sections. Incubate for 20 minutes. The reaction end-product is bright red, but whilst this is considered to be resistant to dehydration, clearing in xylene, and mounting in resinous mounting media, it is not always consistent. Therefore, it is advisable to water-mount.

Nitro-blue tetrazolium method for alkaline phosphatase Buffer solution

0.2 M Tris-HCl, pH 9.5, containing 10 mM MgCl2

Solution a

5 mg 5-bromo-4-chloro-3-indolyl phosphate (BCIP) is dissolved in 0.1 ml dimethyl formamide (DMF) and then in 1.0 ml of the above buffer.

Solution b

5 mg nitro-blue tetrazolium is dissolved in 0.1 ml DMF.

Solutions a and b are added, with continuous stirring, to 30 ml of the above buffer and filtered. Once filtered, incubate immediately for 20 min-12 hours. The intense blue-black reaction product at the site of alkaline phosphatase activity is soluble in alcohol and xylene, hence aqueous mounting is recommended.

Table 1: Weak or No Staining

Sources	Solutions
Inadequate deparaffinization	Deparaffinize sections longer or change fresh xylene
Inactive primary antibodies	Replace with a new batch of antibodies
Antibodies do not work due to improper storage	Aliquot antibodies into smaller volumes and store in freezer (-20 to -70°C) and avoid repeated freeze and thaw cycles.
Antibody concentration was too low	Increase the concentration of antibodies. Or run a serial dilution test to determine the optimal dilution that gives the best signal to noise ratio.
Inadequate antibody incubation time	Increase antibody incubation time.
Inadequate or improper tissue fixation	Increase duration of postfixation or try different fixatives.
Tissue overfixation	Reduce the duration of postfixation or perform an appropriate antigen retrieval procedure.
Incompatible secondary and primary antibodies	Use secondary antibody that will interact with primary antibody.
Inactive secondary antibody or other reagents	Replace with a new batch of reagents
Inadequate substrate incubation time	Increase the substrate incubation time
Incorrect mounting medium	Choose a correct mounting medium
Reagents applied in wrong order or steps omitted	Check notes or procedure used

Table 2: Over-staining

Sources	Solutions
The concentration of antibodies was too high	Reduce antibody concentration or perform a titration to determine the optimal dilution for primary and secondary antibodies
Incubation time was too long	Reduce incubation time
Incubation temperature was too high	Reduce incubation temperature
Substrate incubation time was too long	Reduce substrate incubation time
Sections dried out	Avoid sections being dried out

Tumour markers (biomarker/indicators) defined as a characteristic that can be measured, evaluated or demonstrated, and can be used as an indicator of normal biological functions, pathogenic processes or pharmacologic responses to a therapeutic intervention (Biomarkers Definitions Working Group.2001). It can be cell surface antigens, nucleic acids, cytoplasmic and nuclear proteins, enzymes or hormones (Kumar et al, 2009). Tumour markers categorized into the following (a single biomarker can belong to two or more categories):

a) Diagnostic markers (for tumors detection such as PSA, PCA3).

b) Predictive markers (predict response to therapy; like HER2, KRAS mutation).

c) Prognostic markers (correlate with disease outcome: invasiveness and metastasis, and can predict patients' survival; for example, TMPRSS2: ETS gene fusion, TP53 mutation, pathological stage, PSA relapse).

d) Pharmacodynamic or therapeutic biomarkers (confirm biological activity; for example, Bcrabl1, EGFR, PARP; and they can be direct targets for drug actions).

e) Surrogate biomarkers (substitute for clinical end points; for example, Bcr-abl1).

f) Risk factor (cancer susceptibility genes that portend risk; for example, genetic variants such as SNPs, copy number variations; they predict risk but may not be causative).

Epithelial tumor markers:

- **Keratin:**

Highly sensitive marker for epithelial cells. It presents in epithelial tumors (carcinoma). Certain non-epithelial tumors (such as mesotheliomas and non-seminomatous germ cell tumors) also stain positive for keratin, and may be distinguished from carcinoma by applying an additional panel of antibodies.

- CK7 (Cytokeratin 7) is frequently found in carcinomas of the lung, breast, uterus and ovaries (serous tumors). These tumors are typically negative for CK20.

- CK20 (Cytokeratin 20) is more common in carcinomas of the colon and stomach. These tumors are usually negative for CK7.

- Transitional cell carcinomas of the bladder and mucinous ovarian tumors are usually positive for both CK7 and CK20.

- Renal cell carcinomas, hepatocellular carcinomas, prostatic adeno-carcinomas, thyroid carcinomas and squamous cell carcinomas (skin, lung and esophagus) are usually negative for either CK7or CK20.

- **EMA (Epithelial membrane antigen):**

High molecular weight protein, helpful in determiningtumor site. It is positive for adenocarcinomas of the breast, lung and kidneys but more often nonreactive to hepatocellular carcinomas, adrenal carcinomas or embryonal carcinomas, and negative for non-epithelial tumors (lymphomas, sarcomas, melanomas).

- **CEA (Carcinoembryonic antigen):**

It is an oncofetal antigen that is present in carcinomas of the gastrointestinal tract, pancreas, lung, breast, ovary, uterus and cervix. It is especially useful for differentiating between adenocarcinoma (CEA-positive) and mesothelioma (CEA-negative). Prostate, thyroid and renal carcinomas are usually non-reactive to CEA.

- **TTF-1 (Thyroid transcription factor-1):**

Is useful in distinguishing lung adenocarcinomas from mesotheliomas. It is positive in thyroid, lung and neuroendocrine tumors (medullary thyroid carcinomas, carcinoid tumors and Small cell tumors of the lung).

- **PSA (Prostate specific antigen):**

Is extremely useful in the diagnosis of prostatic adenocarcinoma. It is also positive in certain pancreatic and salivary gland tumors.

Intermediate Filament Markers:

- *Actin:*

Is a contractile intermediate filament protein present in muscle and some non-muscle tissue. It is a sensitive marker for muscle differentiation and can be used to identify tumors derived from smooth, skeletal and cardiac muscle.

- *Vimentin:*

Is a 57kD intermediate filament that is present in normal mesenchymal cells and their neoplastic counterparts (i.e., sarcoma, melanoma, lymphoma, leukemia, seminoma, and some neural tumors). Melanomas and schwannomas always stain positive for vimentin, so that a negative staining may be used to exclude the diagnosis. It is almost always present in tissue sections because of the background stromal elements, and has limited use as a stand-alone stain, but it can be very helpful when combined with other specific tumor markers.

- *Desmin:*

Is a 53 kD intermediate filament expressed by smooth and striated (skeletal and cardiac) muscle. It is considered to be highly specific for myogenic tumors, including leiomyoma (smooth muscle tumor) and rhabdomyosarcoma (skeletal muscle tumor). It is also used to demonstrate the myogenic component of mixed tumors (i.e., carcinosarcomas or malignant mixed mesodermal tumors).

- *Glial fibrillary acidic protein (GFAP):*

Is a 51 kD intermediate filament protein expressed by central nervous system glial cells, particularly astrocytes. It is most widely used to confirm the diagnosis of astrocytoma (but may also be present in certain cases of ependymomas, oligodendrogliomas and medulloblastomas). Non CNS tumors (meningiomas, metastatic carcinomas and lymphomas) stain negative for GFAP.

- *Neurofilament (NF):*

Expressed in cells of neural origin particularly neurons, neuronal processes, peripheral nerves, sympathetic ganglia, adrenal medulla and neuroendocrine cells. Tumors that show neuronal or neuroendocrine differentiation (e.g., neuroblastomas, ganglioneuromas, neuromas, chemodectomas, and pheochromocytomas) will stain positive for neurofilament.

- *S-100   protein:*

Is a low molecular weight calcium-binding protein that is expressed in CNS glial cells, Schwann cells, melanocytes, histiocytes, chondrocytes, skeletal and cardiac muscle, myoepithelial cells and some epithelial cells of breast, salivary and sweat gland epithelium.

Neuroendocrine markers:

- *Neuron-specific enolase (NSE):*

Is an isoenzyme marker whose presence in tissue provides strong evidence of neural or neuroendocrine differentiation.

- *Chromogranin:*

Is found in the neural secretory granules of endocrine tissues, and is recognized as a marker for neuroendocrine differentiation. Immunoreactivity is typically granular and its distribution is similar to that seen with silver staining methods such as Grimelius stain. A combination of keratin and chromogranin positivity is typical of neuroendocrine carcinoma. Chromogranin positivity with a negative keratin stain is typical of paraganglioma.

- *Synaptophysin   :*

Is a 38 kD transmembrane protein associated with presynaptic vesicles of neurons. It has been identified in normal neurons and neuroendocrine cells.

Germ cell tumor markers

Non-seminomatous germ cell tumors (i.e. embryonal carcinomas, teratomas, choriocarcinomas, and endodermal sinus or yolk sac tumors) generally stain positive for epithelial markers (keratin). For more specific classification, the following germ cell tumor markers are used:

- **HCG** (Human chorionic gonado-tropin): Is synthesized by placental syncytio-trophoblasts, and is a marker for chorio-carcinoma.

- **APP (Alpha-fetoprotein):** Is synthesized by normal liver hepatocytes, and is used as a marker for endodermal sinus tumors showing yolk sac differentiation. Embryonal carcinomas and teratomas containing these elements, as well as hepatocellular carcinomas will also stain positive for APP.

- **PLAP (Placenta-like alkaline phosphatase):** Is produced by the placental syncytio-trophoblasts in late pregnancy, and is used as a marker for germ cell tumors, particularly germinomas. Most embryonal carcinomas, choriocarcinomas and endo-dermal sinus tumors will also stain positive for this antibody. PLAP is positive in majority of seminomas.

Mesenchymal tumor markers

- **Myogenic tumors:** Tumors of skeletal muscle origin are positive for muscle-specific actin and desmin and/or other muscle markers such as myo-D1, myoglobin and myogenin.

- **Fibrohistiocytic tumors:** The use of histiocytic markers like CD 68, or FAM 56, combined with more nonspecific proteolytic enzymes such as alpha-1-antitrypsin and alpha-1antichymotrypsin may be helpful in the diagnosis of malignant fibrohistiocytic sarcomas. An undifferentiated component of sarcoma may react only with vimentin.

- **Vascular tumors:** Endothelial markers for vascular tumors (such as angiosarcomas) include Factor VII relatedantigen, CD31 and Ulex Europaeus1 (UEA).

Melanomas: Melanocytes are derived from neural crest and will be reactive for S100 protein. The intensity of staining for S100 is usually inversely proportional to the melanin content of the tumor. Melanosome (HMB-45) is a widely used, highly sensitive and highly specific marker for the diagnosis of melanoma. Melan-A (MAR T -1) also encodes a melanoma-specific antigen that is present in normal pigmented cells of skin and retina as well as in certain adrenocortical tumors.

- **Lymphomas:** The best screening marker for lymphoma is LCA (leukocyte common antigen), also known as CD45. For immunophenotypic subclassification of lymphoma, the most common markers used include those for T cells (CD3, CD4, CDS), B cells (CD19, CD20, CD23), Reed-Sternberg cells (CD15, CD30), and immunoglobulin light and heavy chains.

Cell Proliferation Markers

- **Ki-67 (MIB-1) and PCNA (proliferating cell nuclear antigen):** Are the most common immunohistochemical markers used to assess proliferation of tumor cells. Increased expression of these antigens is usually associated with greater aggressiveness and higher likelihood of recurrence of metastasis.

Cancer associated genes:

The development and progression of a malignant phenotype of human tumors is related to abnormalities of structure or activity of proto-oncogenes and/or mutation of tumor suppressor genes such as p53. Many cellular oncogenes, including c-erbB-2, c-myc and ras have been found to be activated in cancer, particularly of the breast.

Infectious Agent Markers:

Antigenic markers are now available for a number of infectious agents, including hepatitis A virus, hepatitis B surface and core antigens, hepatitis C virus, human papilloma virus, cytomegalovirus, Epstein-Barr virus, toxoplasma, pneumocystis carinii, helicobacter pylori, cryptosporidium, Cryptococcus neoformans, histoplasma, entamoeba histolytica, and mycobacteria.

For mycobacteria, immunohistochemical techniques are more sensitive, the results are obtained faster than with tissue culture, and they are easier to read than acid-fast stains.

Further reading:

ACCuello (ed.) (1993) Immunohistochemistry II.Wiley, Chichester. ISBN-13:9780471934608.

Bancroft, J.D. and Gamble, M. (eds) (2008). Theory and Practice of Histological Techniques, 6th edn. London: Churchill-Livingstone.

Buchwalow IB, Böcker W (2010) Immunohistochemistry: basics and methods. Springer.

Burry, RW (2010) Immunocytochemistry, a practical guide for biomedical research. Springer.

Hayat MA (2002) Immunohistochemistry microscopy and antigen retrieval methods for light and electron microscopy. Springer, New York.

Johnstone AP, Turner MW (eds.) (1997) Immunochemistry: a practical approach (2-Volume Set). IRL Press, Oxford. ISBN:0199636079.

Kiernan, J.A. (2015) Histological and Histochemical Methods: Theory and Practice. 5th edition, Scion Publishing.

Lin F, Prichard J (eds.) (2015) Handbook of practical immunohistochemistry, frequently asked questions. Springer.

Naish, S.J. (ed.), Immunochemical Staining Methods, Carpinteria, CA: DAKO Corporation.

Oliver C, Jamur MC (eds.) (2010) Immunocytochemical methods and protocols. Humana Press.

Insitu hybridization

In situ hybridization (ISH) is a type of hybridization that uses a labeled complementary DNA, RNA or modified nucleic acids strand (i.e., probe) to localize a specific DNA or RNA sequence in a portion or section of tissue (*in situ*).

Principle

The DNA and RNA strands in fixed tissue denaturing by heating, then specifically annealing with a labeled complementary single strand (probe) when cooled. This is followed by visualization of the hybridized signals with isotopic or colorimetric detection methods.

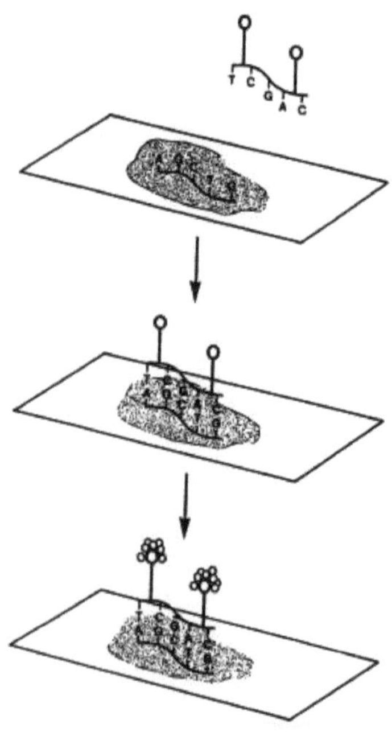

Probes

Four principal types of probes can be used for ISH:

Oligonucleotide Probes

Oligonucleotide probes consisting of 30–50 bases in length. They are produced synthetically by an automated chemical synthesis employing a specific DNA nucleotide sequence. Their short length makes them ideal for accessing targets within FFPE tissue sections, but they are more likely to be dislodged if excessive post-hybridization stringency washes are used. To increase sensitivity, one can use a mixture of oligonucleotides that are complementary to different regions of the target molecule. Labeling oligo-probes for ISH is commonly done with $3'$ end labeling, or "tailing" with relatively few labeled nucleotides incorporated into each probe.

Single-stranded DNA probes

Single-stranded DNA probes, typically (200–500 bp) in length. It can be generated using the polymerase chain reaction (PCR). Using a DNA template and the appropriate primers, probes with high specificity can be produced.

Double-stranded DNA probes

Double-stranded DNA probes are most commonly used to detect DNA targets. It can be prepared by nick-translation, random primer, or PCR in the presence of a labeled nucleotide, and denatured prior to hybridization in order for one strand to hybridize with the mRNA of interest.

Prior to hybridization, a double-stranded DNA probe and its target must be denatured by physical (heat) or chemical (formamide) means to allow annealing.

RNA probes

Often referred to as "riboprobes", these are single-stranded RNA probes that are most commonly used to detect RNA in tissue sections. RNA probes are generated by in vitro transcription from a linearized template using a promoter for RNA polymerase that must be available on the vector DNA containing the template (SP6, T7, or T3).

An alternative method of riboprobe generation is to utilize PCR with appropriate primer sets corporating RNA polymerase promoter sequences at their 5' ends.

Labels

Radioisotope labeling such as ^{3}H, ^{35}S, ^{125}I and ^{32}P is the more traditional way to perform ISH. The ^{35}S-labeled probe is most commonly used, because it gives a reasonable resolution and exposure time (typical exposure about 1 week) compared with other isotopic labeling.

Nonisotope labeling like biotin, digoxigenin, fluorescein, hapten, alkaline phosphatase and bromodeoxyuridine (BrdU) also have been used.

Fixation

The choice of fixative will have an influence on the conservation of nucleic acids and their availability for hybridization; so the ideal fixative for ISH should preserve both RNA/DNA and tissue morphology but still allows penetration of probes. Cross-linking fixatives, such as 4% paraformaldehyde, 4% formaldehyde, or 1% glutaraldehyde are most commonly used. Coagulant fixatives like ethanol and mercuric chloride are not the preferred fixative for use with ISH.

Embedding and sectioning of tissue

However, excellent results can be obtained with cryostat sectioning, Paraffin wax is the most popular embedding medium since sections of

down to 1 um can be cut, and it can be fully dissolved and washed out from the tissue prior to hybridization. Sections are cut at 4–6 μm on an alcohol-cleaned microtome using positively charged or hand-coated slides.

Proteolytic digestion

Proteinase K, pepsin and pronase are commonly enzymes used for digestion to enhance probes penetration, especially after formaldehyde fixation. The concentrations of proteinase K (1–2 g/mL for frozen sections and 20–50 g/mL for paraffin sections) and the length of treatment (5–30 min) depend on tissue type and length of fixation. Prolonged incubation results in overdigestion, resulting in loss of signal and morphologic integrity.

Pre-hybridization

Before hybridization, sections must be prehybridized in a prehybridization solution which contains all the ingredients of the hybridization mixture except the probe to equilibrate the specimen with the hybridization solution prior to the addition of the probe, and to allow anionic macromolecules to block sites of potential nonspecific probe interaction.

Hybridization

Hybridization is carried out under optimal conditions for the annealing of the probe to the target nucleic acid in the tissue. The binding of probe to target occurs due to the interaction of complimentary base pairs; guanine (G) to cytosine (C) and adenine (A) to thymidine (T), or uracil when the target is RNA. Hybridization involves an initial nucleation reaction between a few bases, followed by hydrogen bonding of the remaining sequences. Factors which affect the strength of the bond between the target and the probe include the presence of monovalent cations, organic solvents, the G/C content and heat.

This step involves a series of washes to remove all non-hybridized probes. The sections firstly rinsed with low stringency solutions (high concentrations of salt and low temperature) to remove the unbound probe. Subsequent with high stringency solutions (decreasing salt concentrations and increasing temperature) to reduces mismatching of base pairs.

Detection

Detection will be mainly determined by the probe label used and secondly by the ISH procedure type. Radioisotope labeling is detected with X-ray film and/or emulsion autoradiography while nonisotope labeling is visualized by histochemistry or immunohistochemistry (IHC) detection systems.

Reagents

Diethylpyrocarbonate (DEPC) treated water

Diethylpyrocarbonate	1 ml
Distilled water	1000 ml

Stir while bringing to a boil for 10 minutes (in fume hood). Autoclave to expel DEPC.

2% aminoalkylsilane (positively charged slides)

Aminoalkylsilane (AAS) stored at 4°C	5 ml
Dry acetone	250 ml

Dip clean slides in 2% AAS for 1 minute. Rinse in three changes of deionized water.

Note

These slides may be purchased pre-coated. Make sure they are RNA/DNA free.

Proteinase K

Proteinase K	100 mg
Buffer #1, see below	5 ml

Aliquot and freeze below −20°C.

Hyaluronidase

Hyaluronidase	20 mg
Buffer #1	20 ml

0.1 M triethanolamine (TEA)

Triethanolamine	0.1 ml
DEPC water	100 ml
Acetic anhydride	0.25 ml*

Make fresh.

*Add just prior to use. Stir for 5 minutes, then add an additional 0.25 ml, and stir for another 5 minutes.

1 M Tris (stock)

Trizma base	60.55 g
DEPC water	500 ml
Adjust pH to 8.0 with conc. HCl	20 ml*

*Autoclave.

1 M magnesium chloride (stock)

Magnesium chloride	20.34 g
DEPC water	100 ml*

*Autoclave.

5 M sodium chloride (stock)

Sodium chloride	29.22 g
DEPC water	100 ml*

*Autoclave.

Maleic acid buffer

Maleic acid	100 mM
Sodium chloride	150 mM

Mix 1:10 with water and adjust pH to 7.5 or add Tween 20 (0.3% v/v) for a washing buffer.

Buffer #1: Tris buffered saline, pH 7.5

1 M Tris (stock)	10 ml
5 M sodium chloride (stock)	3.3 ml
1 M magnesium chloride (stock)	0.2 ml
Deionized water	86.7 ml

Adjust pH to 7.5 with HCl.

Buffer #2: Tris buffered saline, pH 9.5

1 M Tris (stock)	10 ml
5 M sodium chloride (stock)	2 ml
1 M magnesium chloride (stock)	5 ml
Deionized water	83 ml

Adjust pH to 9.5 with sodium hydroxide (NaOH).

20x Saline sodium citrate (SSC)

Sodium chloride	348 g
Sodium citrate	167.4 g
DEPC water	1600 ml

Adjust to pH 7.4 with dilute acetic acid, stirring vigorously. Autoclave.

2x SSC

20x SSC	10 ml
DEPC water	100 ml

1x SSC

20x SSC	5 ml
DEPC water	95 ml

Denhart's solution

Ficoll	100 mg*
Polyvinylpyrrolidone	100 mg*
Bovine serum albumin	100 mg
DEPC water	500 ml

*May cause increase in background.

Prehybridization solution

Deionized formamide	5 ml*[1]
20x SSC	2 ml
Denhart's solution	0.10 ml*[2]
50% dextran sulfate	2 ml
Salmon sperm DNA (10mg/ml)	0.30 ml*[3]
Yeast tRNA (10 mg/ml)	25 ml*[4]

*[1] Purified = less non-specific staining
*[2] Reduces non-specific probe binding
*[3] Denature by boiling for 10 minutes
*[4] Blocks non-specific staining

Hybridization solution

Prehybridization solution	1 ml
Labeled probe (500 ng/25 µl)	10 ml

Detection method reagents: choose one

a)	Streptavidin alkaline phosphatase	0.01 ml
	Buffer # 1	5 ml
b)	Anti-digoxigenin	0.01 ml
	Buffer # 1	2.50 ml
c)	Horseradish peroxidase (HRP)	0.01 ml
	Buffer #1	5 ml

Colorimetric detection reagents: choose one

BCIP-NBT

5-bromo-4-chloro-3-indolyl phosphate (BCIP)	0.5 mg/ml
Nitro-blue tetrazolium salt (NBT)	0.3 mg/ml

AEC

3-Amino-9-ethylcarbazole (AEC)	0.08 g
Acetone	10 ml
0.05 M acetate buffer	200 ml
Hydrogen peroxide (30%)	0.10 ml

DAB

Diaminobenzidine (DAB)	22 mg
Tris buffer (stock)	50 ml
Hydrogen peroxide (30%)	0.2 ml

Universal ISH method

Day 1

1. Deparaffinize slides completely. Three changes of xylene and/or substitute for 4–8 minutes each.

2. Dehydrate through two changes 100% (ethanol) EtOH. 1 change 95% EtOH for 3 minutes each. Rinse in DEPC-treated water or use slides already in warmed DEPC-treated water. Rinse in warmed (23–37°C) Tris/saline buffer #1, pH 7.5, and drain.

3. De-proteinize sections in freshly prepared proteinase K solution at 23–37°C, in a moist chamber for 15 minutes.

4. Rinse in Tris/saline buffer #1 at room temperature for 5 minutes. If necessary, digest proteoglycans and/or acetylation before going to next step.

5. Dehydrate slides through one change of 95% EtOH and two changes 100% EtOH for 2 minutes each. Air-dry for 5 minutes. **This step is omitted if prehybridizing (next step).**

6. Apply the prehybridization solution by putting 1–2 drops (60–100 µl) on the sections. Incubate in a moist chamber at room temperature for 1 hour. Blot off all excess prehybridization solution before adding the probe.

7. Apply hybridization fluid (probe) and cover with a heat-resistant film (microwave wrap, coverslips, or chambers). The probe is tailed with either biotin-dUTP or digoxigenin-dUTP.

8. Initiate hybridization by denaturing slides for 5–10 minutes at 92–100°C (try not to exceed 100°C). Use a preheated 'metal' tray to set slides on for optimal denaturization. Cool slides to 37–42°C and incubate in humidity chamber for 18–24 hours. Agitation may enhance reaction. Since this method is not using a commercial kit, the staining continues on day 2.

Day 2

9. Rinse slides twice in 2× SSC and twice in 1× SSC for 5 minutes each at 37°C.

10. Apply a 5% blocking solution at 37°C for 10 minutes.

11. Rinse in buffer #1 for 2 minutes, followed by a 10-minute rinse in buffer #2.

12. Add 1–2 drops of detection reagent to each slide (streptavidin-AP or anti-digoxigenin-AP). Incubate in a humidity chamber for 20–30 minutes at 37°C. During the incubation period, prepare the substrate and warm to 37°C.

13. Rinse slides in three changes of 1× SSC for 5 minutes each.

14. Incubate in substrate for 30–60 minutes at 37°C.

15. Stop reaction by washing in buffer at 37°C for 2 minutes. Rinse in two changes of distilled water (DW) for 2 minutes each.

16. Rinse in two changes of DW for 2 minutes each.

17. Counterstain; this is dependent on the chromogen selected. For BCIP/NBT use nuclear fast red, eosin, or methyl green. For DAB use hematoxylin or methyl green. Go on to step 18 if using BCIP/NBT or DAB. For AEC use methyl green and coverslip out of distilled water using an aqueous mounting medium. Do not go through alcohols or clearing.

18. Dehydrate in increasing concentrations of alcohol.

19. Clear using xylene and coverslip in permanent mounting resin.

Diagnostic applications of tissue ISH

- Detection of abnormal genes
- Identification of viral infection
- Tumor phenotyping.

Fluorescence in situ hybridization (FISH)

Fluorescence in situ hybridization (FISH) or molecular cytogenetics is a molecular cytogenetic technique that uses fluorescent probes that bind to only those parts of a nucleic acid sequence with a high degree of sequence complementarity. The advantages of modern FISH techniques include:

1. Simple, straightforward, standardized techniques.

2. Wide assortment of probes available commercially.

3. Double labeling and use of multiple probes on a single cell.

4. Rapid turnaround times (anywhere from 4 h to a maximum of 48 h).

Principle

FISH procedures involve denaturation of both the probe and the target sequence, then placing the probe and target in contact and allowing them to reanneal. The probe and the target must be visualized, either by direct or indirect fluorescence of the probe.

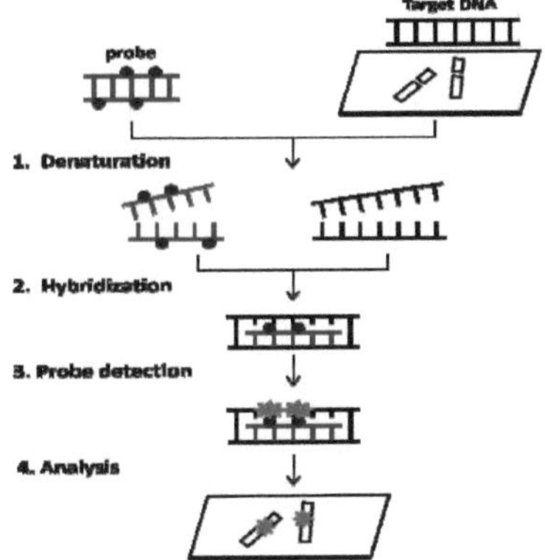

Tissue types

FISH is applicable to most forms of tissue preparation, including single-cell suspensions, frozen sections; formalin-fixed and paraffin-embedded blocks.

Probes

FISH probes used in the clinical laboratory fall into eight categories:

1. **Centromere-specific satellite probes**: which include alpha, beta and classical satellite probes that are complimentary to localized repetitive DNA sequence families at the centromeric and pericentromeric regions of human chromosomes.
2. **Gene probes**: which can be applied to both metaphase and interphase cells, are useful in assessing gene abnormalities.
3. **Telomeric probes**: which are classes of FISH probes containing repeating units of the six base pair sequence TTAGGG.
4. **Whole chromosome painting probes (WCPP)**: which consist of a series of probes complimentary to unique sequences located at specific sites along the length of a single chromosome.
5. **Interspersed repetitive sequences (IRS) probes**: the presence of such sequences in the human genome, Alu or LI repetitive families in particular, can be cloned or PCR-generated to produce Alu or LI FISH probes.
6. **Locus-specific probes**: for the critical regions of human chromosomes are established by creating regional specific libraries from microdissected chromosomal bands.
7. **Total genomic probes**: which are produced by labeling isolated total human DNA.
8. **Riboprobes (RNA probes)**: which are single-stranded antisense or sense RNA probes.

Labeling

FISH probes are usually used as directly conjugated fluorescently labeled, in which the fluorochrome is directly attached to the probe nucleotides like FITC-dUTP (FITC = fluorescein isothiocyonate) and Texas-Red–dUTP (Texas Red = Sulphorhodarnine 101). These directly labeled probes may be labeled in green (such as Spectrum Green or fluorescein), red (Spectrum Orange or Texas Red), blue (Spectrum Aqua), or gold (SpectrumGold).

FISH probes may also be indirectly labeled, via incorporation of a hapten (such as biotin or digoxigenin) into the DNA via nick translation, for example. The probes are then detected using a fluorescently labeled antibody (such as strepavidin and antidigoxigenin).

Counterstain

Propidium iodide dyes the chromosomes red/orange, while DAPI (4,6-diamidino-2-phenylindole) stains chromosomes blue.

Solutions

20× SSC

Sodium chloride   175.32 g
Sodium citrate   88.20 g
Double distilled (dd) H2O   800 ml
pH to 7.0 with 1 M HCl. Bring to 1 liter with ddH2O. Filter through a 0.4 μm filtration unit. Store at room temperature. Expiration: 6 months.

2× SSC

20× SSC   50 ml
ddH2O   450 ml
Store at room temperature. Expiration: 6 months.

Ethanol series

	70%	80%	95%	100%
Ethanol (ml)	350	400	475	500
ddH$_2$O (ml)	150	100	25	0

Store at room temperature.

Denaturation solution (70% formamide/ 2× SSC)

Formamide   35 ml
20× SSC   5 ml
ddH2O   10 ml
Bring pH to 7.0 with 1 M HCl. Store at 4°C. Expiration:1 week.

Post-wash solution (2× SSC/0.1% Nonidet P-40 (NP-40))

20× SSC   100 ml
ddH2O   899 ml
NP-40   1 ml
Bring pH to 7.0 ± 0.2 with 1 M NaOH. Mix well. Store at room temperature. Discard used solution at the end of each day. Expiration: 6 months.

Post-wash solution (0.4× SSC/0.3% NP-40)

20× SSC   20 ml
ddH2O   977 ml
NP-40   3 ml
Bring pH to 7.5 ± 0.2 with 1 M NaOH. Mix well. Store at room temperature. Discard used solution at the end of each day. Expiration: 6 months.

FISH procedure:

Day one

1. Place denaturation solution in water bath at 73°C.

2. Examine slide or coverslip to determine optimal target area.

3. Treat slide (s) in 2× SSC at 37°C for at least 30 minutes.

4. Dehydrate the slide(s) in a cold ethanol series (70%, 85%, and 100%) for 2 minutes each.

5. Allow slides to dry. Store slide(s) in covered slide box until ready to denature.

6. Pre-warm probe to room temperature for about 5 minutes. If probe does not need to be denatured, aliquot 10 μl for each 22 x 22 mm target area; if probe needs to be denatured, aliquot 7 μl hybridization buffer, 2 μl ddH2O, and 1 μl probe into a microcentrifuge tube. Keep probe in darkness as much as possible. Return probe to freezer as soon as possible.

7. Vortex probe briefly and centrifuge for 2–3 seconds.

8. Denature the slide(s) for exactly 2 minutes in the pre-warmed denaturant at 73°C.

Note

A maximum of three slides should be denatured at one time to maintain the correct denaturation temperature.

9. Dehydrate the slide(s) in a cold ethanol series (70%, 80%, and 100%) for 2 minutes each.

10. Wipe the back of the slide(s) and place on a 37°C slide warmer to dry completely. Leave slide(s) on slide warmer until ready to apply probe mixture.

11. Denature aliquoted probe mix for 5 minutes in a 73°C water bath. Vortex probe briefly and centrifuge for 2–3 seconds.

12. Apply 10 μl probe mix to target area and cover with a 22 × 22 mm glass coverslip. Seal with rubber cement.

13. If not denaturing probes and slides separately, probes and slides can be co-denatured on, for example, the ThermoBrite TM Denaturation and Hybridization system from Abbott Molecular Inc. for 2 minutes at 73°C.

14. Following either form of denaturation: incubate slide(s) at 37°C overnight in a humidified chamber (place moist sponge or paper towels in an airtight, opaque container).

Note

Slide(s) may be left in the ThermoBrite TM instrument for hybridization at 37°C for 4–16 hours. A minimum of 4 hours of hybridization is recommended for any probe.

Day two

15. Warm glass Coplin of 0.4× SSC/0.3% NP-40 to 73±1°C. Do not wash more than three slides at a time, to ensure the correct wash temperature is maintained.

16. Remove coverslip and rubber cement from hybridized slide(s). Keep slides covered as much as possible and away from the light.

17. Wash slide(s) in 0.4× SSC/0.3% NP-40 at 72°C for 2 minutes. Agitate slide(s) for 1–3 seconds.

18. Wash slide(s) in 2× SSC/0.1% NP-40 at room temperature for 1 minute. Agitate slide(s) for 1–3 seconds.

19. Allow the slide(s) to dry while protected from the light.

20. Apply 2 μl of DAPI I or DAPI II to slide(s) and cover with appropriately sized glass coverslip.

Main Applications of FISH include:

• Gene mapping

• The identification of numerical and structural chromosome abnormalities

• Interphone cytogenetic

• The identification of the human content of somatic cell hybrids

• The identification of new regions of amplification or deletion

• Positional cloning

• Comparative cytogenetic.

In situ hybridization-polymerase chain reaction

In situ polymerase chain reaction is high sensitive, specific and precise cell localization technique conjugates polymerase chain reaction (PCR) and in situ hybridization (ISH) together. Firstly, the target gene amplified by PCR, and the PCR products remain in cells because of their large molecules or interlacing structures. Then PCR products are detected in situ hybridization with labeled probe. The basic types are direct in situ polymerase chain reaction, indirect direct in situ polymerase chain reaction and in situ reverse transcription polymerase chain reaction (RT-PCR).

Direct PCR amplification protocol

Reagents

1. Pepsin or trypsin at 2 mg/ml (mild digestion) *Note*: Stock solution is 20 mg pepsin + 9.5 ml sterile water + 0.5 ml 2 N HCl.

2. Protease K (harsh)

Dilute 1.0 ml proteinase K at 1 mg/ml in 150 ml of PBS. Use at 55°C.

3. Buffer #1

4. 20×SSC

5. 2×SSC

6. Formamide SSC

Formamide   50 ml

2×SSC   50 ml

7. PCR mixture

00.25 uM primers

10 uM dATP

10 uM dCTP

10 uM GTP

3.5 uM dTTP

Procedure:

1. Fix the tissue with a cross-linking fixative.

2. Cut sections at 5–7 um on an alcohol-cleaned microtome and knife.

3. Place 2–3 sections on positively charged coated slides (spaced evenly apart). Dry overnight flat on a slide warmer, 50–55 C, and then an additional 30 min before deparaffinization.

4. Deparaffinize in three changes of xylene for 3–5 min each. Dehydrate in two changes 100% ethanol for 5 min. Air dry.

5. Digest for 30–90 min. Do not let slides dry out. A humidity chamber is helpful for this step*.

*Quick test for sufficient digestion is: Place slide under a microscope; using a 40x objective look at one cell. When you can count 20 dots in nucleus, digestion is complete.

6. After digestion, rinse slides in double distilled water for 1 min.

7. Dehydrate slides in two changes of 100% ethanol for 2 min each. Air dry for 5 min.

Note

Depending on the type of thermocycler used, the slides are treated differently. For example, some thermocyclers have coverwells that seal and snap tight over the individual tissue section. Other thermocyclers just have a heat block to sit the slides on. To accommodate the individual thermocycler, you may need to circle the tissue with a hydrophobic pen.

8. Cover tissue with PCR mixture and cover with glass coverslip, autoclave wrap or coverwell (use what is recommended by manufacturer of thermocycler).

9. Line the slide girdle of the thermocycler with aluminum foil to prevent leakage from the slides and equipment contamination. For this procedure a Perkin-Elmer thermocycler was used, which was the recommendation of the manufacturer.

10. Place the slides in the aluminum foil trough. Cover each slide with 2 ml of mineral oil.

11. Heat thermal block to 80°C and place on hold for 10 min while setting the thermocycler program. The amplification program used is 15 cycles of 1 min at 96°C, 1 min at 59°C, and 1 min at 72°C.

Note

Amplifi cation program settings will vary.

12. Remove slides from thermocycler and gently remove coverslips, etc. Rinse slides in two changes of xylene for 3 min each to remove mineral oil. Dehydrate and remove xylene with two changes of 100% ethanol for 3 min each. Air dry.

13. Wash slides three times for 5 min each in buffer #1.

14. Place slides in 150 mM NaCl with 0.2% BSA at 50°C for 10 min (this solution should be prewarmed).

15. Drain NaCl from slides and cover with 100 ul alkaline phosphatase-conjugated anti-digoxygenin (1: 50 dilutions in 0.1 M Tris pH 7.5 with 0.1 M NaCl) for 30 min at 37 C in a humidity chamber.

16. Rinse slides in 0.1 M Tris pH 9.5 with 0.1 M NaCl for 1 min.

17. Incubate slides in NBT/BCIP solution (10 ul of NBT/BCIP in 2.0 ml Tris pH 9.5 with 0.1 M NaCl) for 5–15 min. Check the proper end-point under the microscope.

18. Wash slides in distilled water for 2 min. Counterstain with nuclear fast red for 5 min. Rinse in distilled water for 1 min, dehydrate, clear, and mount.

Further reading:

-Bancroft, J.D. and Gamble, M. (eds) (2008). Theory and Practice of Histological Techniques, 6th edn. London: Churchill-Livingstone.

- Bancroft, J. D., Suvarna, S. K., & Layton, C. (2012). Bancroft's Theory and Practice of Histological Techniques (7th ed.). Philadelphia, PA: Churchill Livingstone Elsevier.

- Darby, I.A. (Ed.), 2000. In situ hybridization protocols, second ed. Humana Press, Totowa, NJ.

- Wilkinson, D.G. (Ed.), 1999. In situ hybridization: a practical approach, second ed. Oxford University Press, New York.

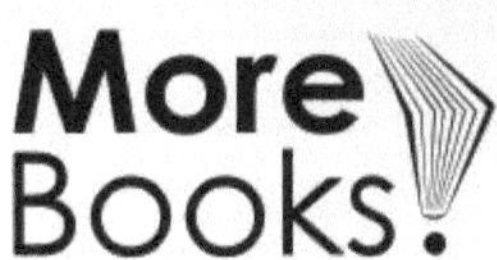

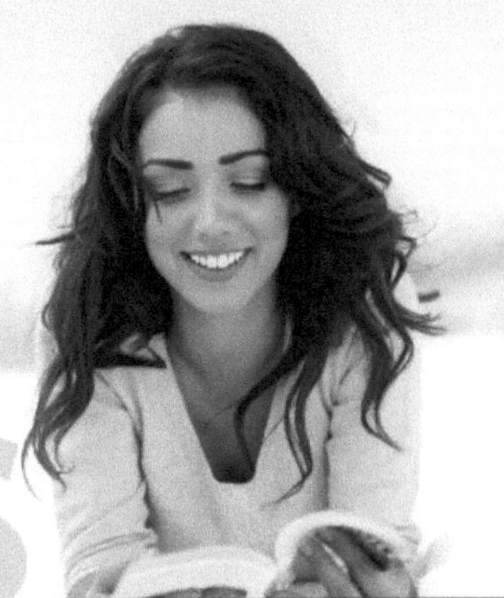

I want morebooks!

Buy your books fast and straightforward online - at one of world's fastest growing online book stores! Environmentally sound due to Print-on-Demand technologies.

Buy your books online at
www.morebooks.shop

Kaufen Sie Ihre Bücher schnell und unkompliziert online – auf einer der am schnellsten wachsenden Buchhandelsplattformen weltweit! Dank Print-On-Demand umwelt- und ressourcenschonend produziert.

Bücher schneller online kaufen
www.morebooks.shop

KS OmniScriptum Publishing
Brivibas gatve 197
LV-1039 Riga, Latvia
Telefax: +371 686 204 55

info@omniscriptum.com
www.omniscriptum.com

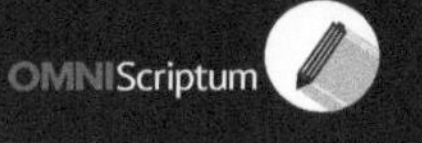

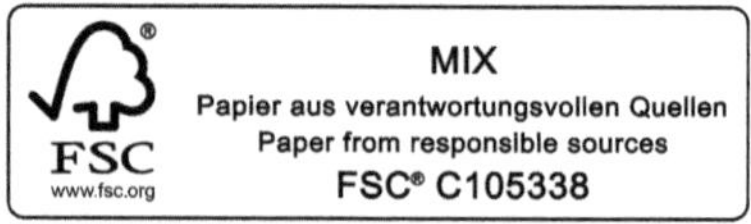

Printed by Books on Demand GmbH, Norderstedt / Germany